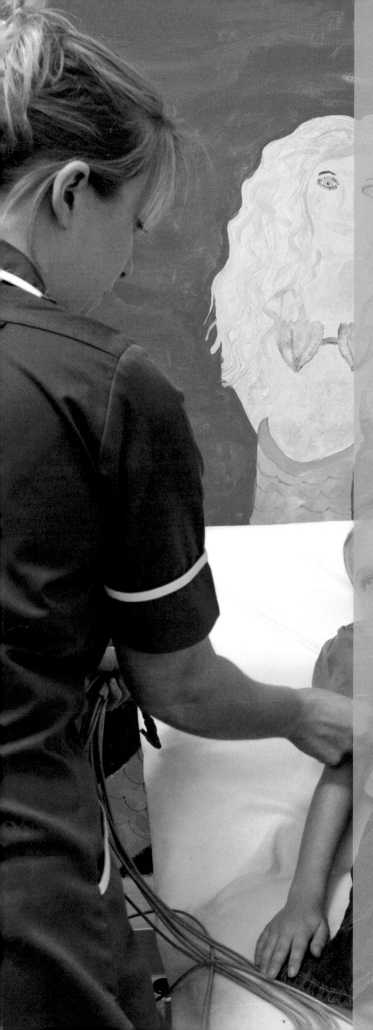

Children and Young People's Nursing
at a Glance

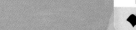

Edited by

Alan Glasper
Professor of Children's and Young People's
Nursing
Faculty of Health Sciences
University of Southampton
Southampton, UK

Jane Coad
Professor in Children and Family Nursing
Faculty of Health and Life Sciences
Coventry University
Coventry, UK

Jim Richardson
Senior Lecturer at the School of Nursing
Faculty of Health, Social Care and Education
Kingston University London and St George's
University of London
London, UK

Series Editor: Ian Peate

WILEY Blackwell

This edition first published 2015 © 2015 by John Wiley & Sons, Ltd.

Registered office: John Wiley & Sons, Ltd, The Atrium, Southern Gate, Chichester, West Sussex, PO19 8SQ, UK

Editorial offices: 9600 Garsington Road, Oxford, OX4 2DQ, UK
The Atrium, Southern Gate, Chichester, West Sussex, PO19 8SQ, UK
350 Main Street, Malden, MA 02148-5020, USA

For details of our global editorial offices, for customer services and for information about how to apply for permission to reuse the copyright material in this book please see our website at www.wiley.com/wiley-blackwell

Library of Congress Cataloging-in-Publication Data

Glasper, Edward Alan, author.
    Children and young people's nursing at a glance / Alan Glasper, Jane Coad, Jim Richardson.
        p. ; cm.
    Includes bibliographical references and index.
    ISBN 978-1-118-51628-7 (pbk.)
    I. Coad, Jane, author.   II. Richardson, Jim, 1957– author.   III. Title.
    [DNLM: 1. Pediatric Nursing–methods–Handbooks.   2. Adolescent.   3. Child.
4. Infant.   5. Nursing Assessment–methods–Handbooks.   WY 49]
    RJ245
    618.92'00231–dc23

                                                    2014005233

A catalogue record for this book is available from the British Library.

Wiley also publishes its books in a variety of electronic formats. Some content that appears in print may not be available in electronic books.

Cover image: Paediatric ECG. LIFE IN VIEW/SCIENCE PHOTO LIBRARY
Cover design by Meaden Creative

Set in 9.5/11.5 pt MinionPro by Toppan Best-set Premedia Limited
Printed and bound in Singapore by Markono Print Media Pte Ltd

1   2015

Contents

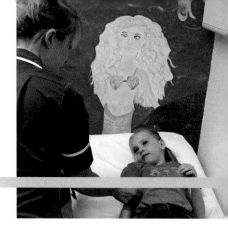

Part 1   Assessment and screening   1

Part 2   Working with families   53

Part 7   Chronic and life-limiting conditions   229

Preface

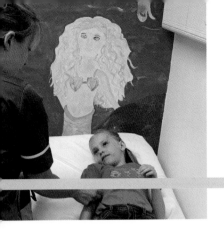

The education of children's and young people's nurses remains a foremost challenge for those wishing to ensure the accuracy and safety of the evidence base for practice. As long ago as 1952, Twistington-Higgins in his book written to commemorate the first 100 years of The Hospital For Sick Children, Great Ormond Street, London, UK, reiterates one of the original aims of the hospital dated 1852, which was: 'To disseminate among all classes of the community but chiefly among the poor a better acquaintance with the management of infants and children during illness by employing it [The Hospital] as a school for the education of women in the special duties of children's nursing'.

That initial aim of one of the early children's hospitals resonates with contemporary children's and young people's nursing and Catherine Jane Wood, one of the early matrons of The Great Ormond Street children's hospital left a tangible legacy of the importance of educating children's and young people's nurses in stating that 'Sick children require special nursing and sick children's nurses require special training' (Wood 1888). In recognition of that laudable aim this new and exciting *at a Glance* book has been written by experienced practitioners and educators in a common quest to capture the complexities delivering nursing practice based on best evidence.

All children's and young people's nurses share a single *espirt de corps* which unites them with their colleagues worldwide and although this book is primarily reflective of children's and young people's nursing in the United Kingdom, others will find it an invaluable guide to the delivery of evidence-based nursing care.

Although the prime focus of the book is to illuminate best clinical practice, my fellow editors and I hope that the format of the *at a Glance* series will provide quick and easy access to important care delivery information packaged in an engaging and informative style. This book will be of interest to undergraduate student nurses and existing registrants wishing to remind themselves of the complexities of children's and young people's nursing which encompasses care delivery across the lifespan of the child from birth through to the emergence of the young person and future adult. In the pages of this book you will find concise information to help you deliver that care to this wide and disparate client group that makes up the landscape of contemporary childhood.

For those students wishing to test their knowledge and understanding of the content there is a comprehensive bank of multiple choice questions on the companion website.

This book could not have been completed without the organizational expertise and help of Brenda Nash. My fellow editors and I are in her debt.

Alan Glasper

References

Twistington-Higgins T. (1952) *Great Ormond Street 1852–1952*. Watford: Odhams Press Ltd.

Wood CJ. (1888) The training of nurses for sick children. *Nursing Record* December 6, 507–510.

Contributors

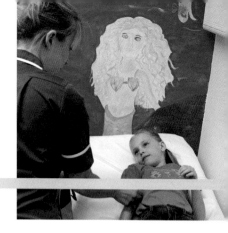

Owen Arthurs
Consultant Paediatric Radiologist
Great Ormond Street Hospital for Children
London, UK

Justine Barksby
Lecturer in Learning Disability Nursing
School of Health Sciences
University of Nottingham
Nottingham, UK

Nicola Barnes
Nurse Practitioner for Complex Epilepsy
Great Ormond Street Hospital
London, UK

Cathryn Battrick
Matron
Southampton Children's Hospital
Southampton, UK

Marie Bodycombe-James
Senior Lecturer
Specialist Community Public Health Nursing
Swansea University
Swansea, UK

Margaret Bourke
Adolescent Mental Health Nurse
St Patrick's Mental Health Services
St Patrick's University Hospital
Dublin, Ireland

Maria Brenner
Lecturer and Programme Co-ordinator
College of Health Sciences
University College Dublin
Dublin, Ireland

Anne Brocklesby
Senior Lecturer in Child Nursing
Canterbury Christ Church University
Kent, UK

Mark Broom
Academic Manager Family Care
Faculty of Life Sciences and Education
University of South Wales
Pontypridd, UK

Pauline Cardwell
Lecturer (Education)
School of Nursing and Midwifery
Queen's University
Belfast, Northern Ireland

Carol Chamley
Carol Chamley
Senior lecturer
Children and Young People's Nursing/Nurse Researcher
Coventry University
Coventry, UK

Collette Clay
Senior Lecturer in Midwifery
Faculty of Health and Life Sciences
Coventry University
Coventry, UK

Jane Coad
Professor in Children and Family Nursing
Faculty of Health and Life Sciences
Coventry University
Coventry, UK

Andrea Cockett
Head of Department
Child and Adolescent Nursing
King's College London
London, UK

Angela Cole
Clinical Nurse Specialist for Children and Young Adults with IBD
Barts Health NHS Trust
London, UK

Sarah Corkhill
Lecturer in Children's nursing
School of Nursing and Midwifery
Keele University
Keele, UK

Doris Corkin
Senior Lecturer (Education)
School of Nursing and Midwifery
Queen's University
Belfast, Northern Ireland

Mick Cullen
Paediatric Gastroenterology Nurse Specialist
Southampton Children's Hospital
Southampton, UK

Jeanette David
Paediatric Clinical Skills Specialist Resuscitation Officer –
Paediatric Lead
Gloucestershire Hospitals NHS Foundation Trust UK
Cheltenham, UK

Maggie Duckett
Midwifery Lecturer
Southampton University Clinical Nurse Specialist
Solent Sexual Health ServicesSouthampton, UK

Kath Evans
Head of Patient Experience
Nursing Directorate
NHS England

Filippo Festini
Professor of Paediatric Nursing
Department of Health Sciences
University of Florence, Italy

Siobhan Fitzgerald
Clinical Nurse Specialist Airway Management
Our Lady's Children's Hospital Crumlin
Dublin, Ireland

Ellie Forbes
Matron for Child Health
South Devon Healthcare NHS Foundation Trust
Torquay, UK

Elizabeth Gillespie
Team Leader
Community Children's Nursing Team
Southbank Child Development Centre
Glasgow, UK

Alan Glasper
Professor of Children's and Young People's Nursing
Faculty of Health Sciences
University of Southampton
Southampton, UK

Elizabeth Gormley-Fleming
Senior Lecturer Children's Nursing
University of Hertfordshire
Hatfield, UK

Karen Grant
Education and Practice Lead
Southampton Children's Hospital
Southampton, UK

Jennifer Grehan
Lecturer and CPD co-ordinator (Diagnostic Imaging)
School of Medicine and Medical Science
University College Dublin
Dublin, Ireland

Karen Griffiths
Senior Lecturern Children's Nursing
Faculty of Health Sciences
Staffordshire University
Stoke-on-Trent, UK

Sheila Hayes
Clinical Nurse Specialist Airway Management
Our Lady's Children's Hospital Crumlin
Dublin, Ireland

Melissa Heywood
Clinical Nurse Consultant
Victorian Paediatric Palliative Care Program
The Royal Children's Hospital
Melbourne, Australia

Dean-David Holyoake
Senior Lecturer in Child and Adolescent Mental Health
University of Wolverhampton
Wolverhampton, UK

Kate Howard
Deputy Director of Nursing
AHP's and QualityNorthamptonshire Healthcare NHS
Foundation Trust
Northampton, UK

Frances Howlin
Lecturer in Children's Nursing
School of Nursing, Midwifery, and Health Systems
University College Dublin
Dublin, Ireland

Elaine Huntingdon
Senior Lecturer in Children's Nursing
Liverpool John Moores University
Liverpool, UK

Emma Inness
Senior Lecturer in Children's Nursing; Advanced Nurse
Practitioner in Paediatric Rheumatology
Oxford Brookes University
Oxford, UK

Lucille Kelsall-Knight
Senior Lecturer in Children's Nursing
University of Wolverhampton
Wolverhampton, UK

Janet Kelsey
Associate Professor Health Studies (Paediatric)
Plymouth University
Plymouth, UK

Olivet Kewley
Senior Lecturer in Child Nursing
Liverpool John Moores University
Liverpool, UK

Kate Khair
Nurse Consultant Haemophilia
Great Ormond Street Hospital
London, UK

Kate Knight
Senior Lecturer Children's Nursing
Liverpool John Moores University
Liverpool, UK

Narinder Kular
Nurse Consultant Paediatrics Complex Care
Shropshire Community Health NHS Trust
Bridgnorth, UK

Karine Latter
Lead Nurse Specialist Cleft Lip and Palate
Nottingham University Hospital
Nottingham Children's Hospital
Nottingham, UK

Helen Laverty
Health Lecturer
Learning Disability Nursing
University of Nottingham
Nottingham, UK

Sandra Lawton
Nurse Consultant Dermatology
Nottingham Children's Hospital
Nottingham University Hospitals NHS Trust
Nottingham, UK

Angela Ledsham
Lecturer/Practitioner PICU
University Hospital Southampton NHS Foundation Trust
Southampton University
Southampton, UK

Gayle Le Moine
Senior Lecturer in Child Nursing
Canterbury Christ Church University
Canterbury, UK

Stella Lovell
Senior Lecturer in Child Nursing
Canterbury Christ Church University
Canterbury, UK

Lindy May
Nurse Consultant Paediatric Neurosurgery
Great Ormond Street Hospital
University College London
London, UK

Orla McAlinden
Lecturer in Children and Young People's Nursing
School of Nursing and Midwifery
Queen's University Belfast
Northern Ireland
BT9 7BL

Isobel McDermott
Senior Lecturer in Midwifery
Faculty of Health and Life Sciences
Coventry University
Coventry, UK

Patricia McNeilly
Lecturer
School of Nursing and Midwifery
Queen's University
Belfast, Northern Ireland

Nick Medforth
Professional Lead: Child Health and Care
Faculty of Health and Applied Social Sciences
Liverpool John Moores University
Liverpool, UK

Victoria Moore
Staff Nurse
Children's Haematology Unit
Royal Belfast Hospital for Sick Children
Belfast, Northern Ireland

Colman Noctor
Advanced Nurse Practitioner
St Patrick's Mental Health Services
St Patrick's University Hospital
Dublin, Ireland

Sharon Nurse
Senior Teaching Fellow, Midwifery
Queen's University
Belfast, Northern Ireland

Patricia O'Hara
Sister, Children's ward
Antrim Hospital
Antrim, Northern Ireland

Theresa Pengelly
Senior Lecturer in Children and Young People's Nursing
Coventry University
Coventry, UK

Vanessa Plares
Practice Educator for Newly Registered Nurses
Nursing and Non-Medical Education Team
Great Ormond Street Hospital NHS Foundation Trust
London, UK

Elisabeth Podsiadly
Senior Lecturer (Neonatal Nursing) Faculty of Health, Social
Care and EducationKingston University and St. George's
University of London
London, UK

Jayne Price
Associate Professor (Children's Nursing)
Faculty of Health, Social Care and Education
Kingston University and St George's, University of London
London, UK

Lavinia Raeside
Advanced Neonatal Nurse PractitionerNICU, RHSC Yorkhill
Glasgow/Southern General Hospital
Southampt Glasgow, UK

Sarah Reed
Lecturer in Children's and Young People's Nursing
University of Southampton
Southampton, UK

Gail Reoch
Senior Lecturer in Children's Nursing
University of Northampton
Northampton, UK

Jim Richardson
Senior Lecturer at the School of Nursing
Faculty of Health, Social Care and Education
Kingston University London and St George's
University of London
London, UK

Sheila Roberts
Senior Lecturer Children's Nursing
University of Hertfordshire
Hatfield, UK

Angela Ryan
Nurse Tutor
Centre of Children's Nurse Education
Dublin, Ireland

Sarah Santo
Clinical Nurse Manager
North West and North Wales Paediatric Transport Service
Warrington, UK

Suzanne Seabra
Senior Lecturer, Children's Nursing
Faculty of Health Sciences
Staffordshire University
Stoke-on-Trent, UK

Sally Shearer
Director of Nursing and Governance for Children
Barts Health NHS Trust
London, UK

Sarah Stead
Senior Lecturer in Child Nursing
Canterbury Christ Church University
Canterbury, UK

Nicola Stevens
Paediatric Diabetes Specialist Nurse
Northampton General Hospital; University of Northampton
Northampton, UK

Kathryn Summers
Senior Lecturer in Child Nursing
Canterbury Christ Church University
Canterbury, UK

Catherine Swailes
Paediatric and Neonatal Clinical Facilitator
Milton Keynes Hospital NHS Foundation Trust
Senior Lecturer in Children's Nursing
University of Bedfordshire
Bedfordshire, UK

John Thain
Senior Lecturer in Children's Nursing
Institute of Health Professions
Faculty of Education, Health and Wellbeing
University of Wolverhampton
Wolverhampton, UK

Angela Thompson
Gastro/IBD Nurse Specialist for Children and Young Adults
Barts Health NHS Trust
The Royal London Hospital
London, UK

Gillian Turner
Senior Lecturer in Specialist Community Public Health
Nursing
Liverpool John Moores University
Liverpool, UK

Alison Twycross
Head of Department for Children's Nursing and
Reader in Children's Pain Management
Editor: Evidence Based Nursing
Department of Children's Nursing
London South Bank University
London, UK

Katy Weaver
Health Play Specialist
Royal Alexandra Children's Hospital
Brighton, UK

Lisa Whiting
Principal Lecturer and Professional Lead
Children's Nursing
University of Hertfordshire
Hatfield, UK

Jane Willock
Senior Lecturer (Child Health) Faculty of Life Sciences and
Education University of South Wales
Pontypridd, UK

Nicola Wilson
Practice Educator
Neurosciences
Great Ormond Street Hospital for Children
London, UK

Mark Woods
Senior Lecturer Clinical Skills
Liverpool John Moores University
Liverpool, UK

Matthew Norridge
Lecturer Practitioner in Paediatric Intensive Care
Kings College London
London, UK

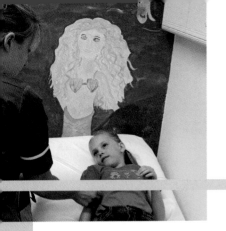

How to use your revision guide

Features contained within your revision guide

Each topic is presented in a double-page spread with clear, easy-to-follow diagrams supported by succinct explanatory text.

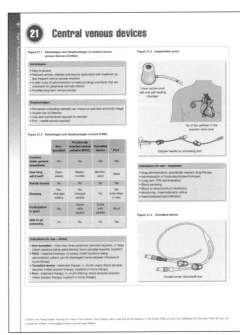

Key point boxes and **red flag boxes** draw your attention to important points.

Key point
• The primary cause of cardiopulmonary arrest in young people is hypoxia. For this reason, if a young person is found unresponsive and not breathing the first action to be taken is for the rescuer to deliver five rescue breaths before seeking further help.

Red flag
• Effective ventilation and oxygenation may prevent a cardiac arrest from occurring in young people.

The website icon indicates that you can find accompanying resources on the book's companion website.

The anytime, anywhere textbook

Wiley E-Text

Your book is also available to purchase as a **Wiley E-Text: Powered by VitalSource** version – a digital, interactive version of this book which you own as soon as you download it.

Your **Wiley E-Text** allows you to:

Search: Save time by finding terms and topics instantly in your book, your notes, even your whole library (once you've downloaded more textbooks)

Note and Highlight: Colour code, highlight and make digital notes right in the text so you can find them quickly and easily

Organize: Keep books, notes and class materials organized in folders inside the application

Share: Exchange notes and highlights with friends, classmates and study groups

Upgrade: Your textbook can be transferred when you need to change or upgrade computers

Link: Link directly from the page of your interactive textbook to all of the material contained on the companion website

The **Wiley E-Text** version will also allow you to copy and paste any photograph or illustration into assignments, presentations and your own notes.

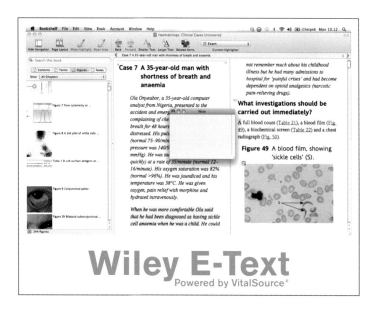

To access your Wiley E-Text:

- Visit **www.vitalsource.com/software/bookshelf/downloads** to download the Book-shelf application to your computer, laptop, tablet or mobile device
- Open the Bookshelf application on your computer and register for an account
- Follow the registration process

CourseSmart

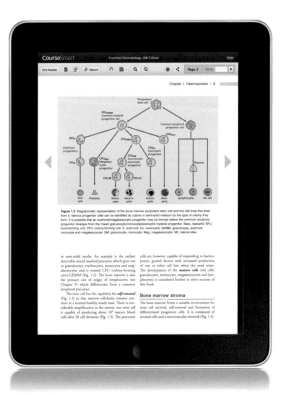

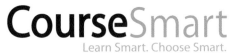

Learn Smart. Choose Smart.

About the companion website

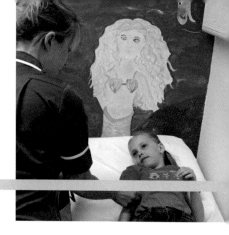

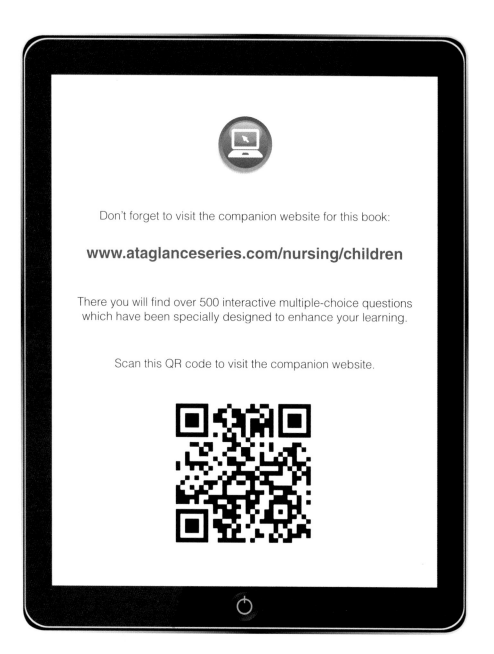

Don't forget to visit the companion website for this book:

www.ataglanceseries.com/nursing/children

There you will find over 500 interactive multiple-choice questions which have been specially designed to enhance your learning.

Scan this QR code to visit the companion website.

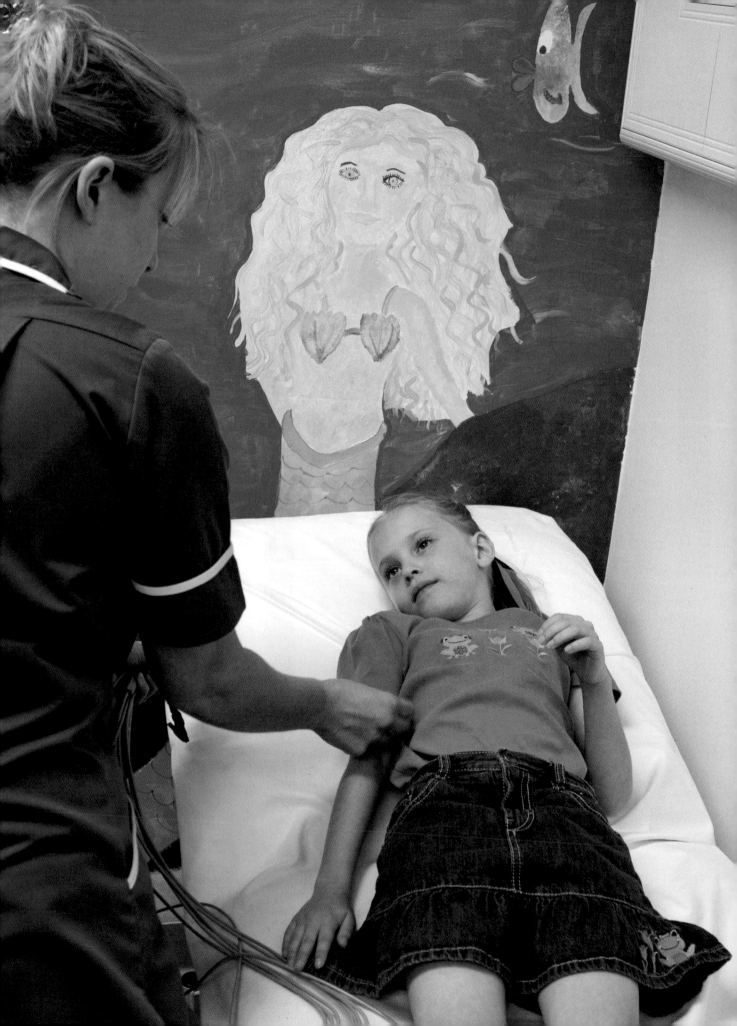

Assessment and screening

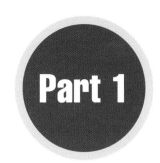
Part 1

Chapters

Don't forget to visit the companion website for this book at **www.ataglanceseries.com/nursing/children** where you will find over 500 interactive multiple-choice questions to supplement your learning.

1

1 Assessment of the child

Figure 1.1 Assessment of the child

Assessment is the gathering of information and formulation of judgements in partnership with the child and family. It is a continuous dynamic process and includes the physiological, physical, psychological, social and the spiritual aspect of the child and the effect that their health problem is having on their development and family life. Accurate assessment of the infant or child is essential to the delivery of safe and effective care. Depending on the child's presenting condition, a focused assessment may be required in the case of the seriously ill child, necessitating prioritization of care until the child's condition is stable.

Assessment leads to the identification of health problems and the development of care plans.

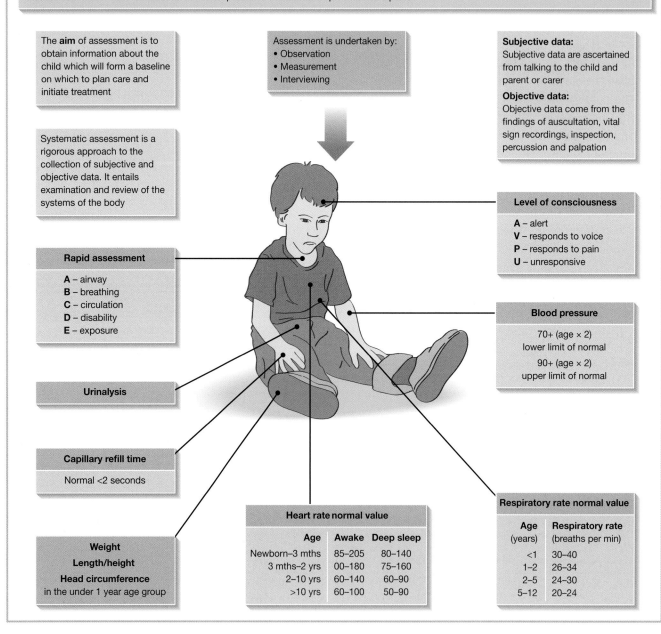

The **aim** of assessment is to obtain information about the child which will form a baseline on which to plan care and initiate treatment

Systematic assessment is a rigorous approach to the collection of subjective and objective data. It entails examination and review of the systems of the body

Rapid assessment

A – airway
B – breathing
C – circulation
D – disability
E – exposure

Urinalysis

Capillary refill time

Normal <2 seconds

Weight
Length/height
Head circumference
in the under 1 year age group

Assessment is undertaken by:
• Observation
• Measurement
• Interviewing

Subjective data:
Subjective data are ascertained from talking to the child and parent or carer

Objective data:
Objective data come from the findings of auscultation, vital sign recordings, inspection, percussion and palpation

Level of consciousness

A – alert
V – responds to voice
P – responds to pain
U – unresponsive

Blood pressure

70+ (age × 2)
lower limit of normal

90+ (age × 2)
upper limit of normal

Heart rate normal value

	Age	Awake	Deep sleep
Newborn–3 mths		85–205	80–140
3 mths–2 yrs		00–180	75–160
2–10 yrs		60–140	60–90
>10 yrs		60–100	50–90

Respiratory rate normal value

Age (years)	Respiratory rate (breaths per min)
<1	30–40
1–2	26–34
2–5	24–30
5–12	20–24

Assessment is the collection of data, both subjective and objective, which aims to achieve a complete picture of the child's health status. Good assessment is a combination of the interpretation of physical data with the information gained from observation of the child and family and from listening to them.

Interviewing – history taking

Gaining the trust of the child and family is an essential element in developing of an effective therapeutic relationship. Introducing yourself to the child and family with explanations of expected outcomes will put the child and family at ease. Age appropriate language should be used. Questions should be directed at both the child and parent. Young people should have an opportunity to talk in private if they wish. When taking a history, a structured approach should be used. This needs to include:
- Presenting complaint
- History of presenting complaint
- Past medical history (birth and neonatal history in infants and young children), immunizations, illnesses and hospitalizations
- Allergies
- Current medication
- Developmental history
- Family history
- Social history – nursery, school.

Observation – subjective data

Subjective data are what the child and parent say along with the visual information gained from the initial encounter with the child and family or while obtaining objective data (physical examination and recording of vital signs). This includes noting:
- The colour of the child: are they pale, mottled, cyanosed, jaundiced, flushed
- Behaviour: alert, crying, agitated, combative, lethargic, drowsy
- Interaction with parents/carers/strangers
- Interaction with environment, wanting to play or sleepy
- Position: normal, floppy or stiff
- The general appearance of the child: e.g. unkempt or clean
- Obvious birthmarks, bruises or rashes
- Dysmorphic features.

Measuring – objective data

All infants and children require a baseline physical assessment. This is a multifaceted process and some aspects are common to all children who require assessment of their health status. The physical assessment is concerned with the analysis and interpretation of data. Privacy and dignity should be maintained during this process. Consent should be obtained prior to undertaking a physical assessment.

Physical assessment includes:
- Basic physical recordings of temperature, pulse rate, respiratory rate, oxygen saturation and blood pressure
- Respiratory assessment, rate of breathing, depth of breathing, noise of breathing, presence of cough, chest movement, nasal flaring, use of other accessory muscles, child's colour, ability to speak/feed, position of the child, peak flow and oxygen saturation level
- Heart rate including pulse volume
- Capillary refill time
- Neurological status using Glasgow coma scale or AVPU
- Level of hydration: obvious signs of dehydration include sunken anterior fontanelle, dull sunken eyes, dry oral mucosa, lethargy, weak cry, decreased urinary output
- Weight
- Height/length
- Head circumference
- Skin assessment using recognized pressure risk assessment tool
- Urinalysis.

All findings need to be documented as they are a legal record of the nursing assessment, the foundation on which care is planned and the basis of communication with multidisciplinary team.

Summary

Assessment is a dynamic continuous process that needs to include the child's and parentor carer's perspectives. Observation is as essential as physical assessment and good communication skills are important.

2 SBAR framework

Figure 2.1 SBAR framework

SBAR is a flexible framework which is widely utilized in health care settings to focus and facilitate communication amongst health care professionals, allowing assessment and management of risk in the care of the acutely ill child or young person (Figure 2.2). This tool enables effective and assertive sharing of information and cultivates a safe approach to patient care. SBAR is an adaptable structure that can be used to shape communication pathways at any stage of a patient's journey, whatever the clinical setting (Institute for Healthcare Improvement).

S – **Situation** – What is currently going on with the patient?

B – **Background** – What are the circumstances leading up to the situation?

A – **Assessment** – What is the problem or concern?

R – **Recommendation** – What do you think should happen next?

Furthermore, in using this tool the health professional is able to identify areas of concern with cognisance of the existing and previous history of the patient's condition. Subsequently, assessing the impact of current issues relating to patient care and making clinical decisions, based on best available evidence, including recommendations of what is required in terms of actions to ensure patient safety and well-being.

Figure 2.2 Simulated scenario using the SBAR tool

Chloe is a 10-month-old baby weighing 9 kg, with a history of gastro-oesophageal reflux (GOR) and faltering growth, which is currently being managed with supplementary enteral feeding via a nasogastric tube (NGT). In addition to this, Chloe has been prescribed oral omeprazole once daily to help manage her GOR. This scenario is explored in greater depth utilizing the SBAR tool to enhance understanding of risk and its effective management.

S – **Situation** – Chloe has dislodged her nasogastric tube (NGT) and is due to commence her oral feed and subsequent enteral 'top-up'. Her named nurse in the children's ward is experienced in passing NGTs and prepares to replace Chloe's NGT. Following insertion, Chloe's nurse notes that the gastric aspirate from the NGT is pH 6 and is concerned about establishing the position of the NGT (NPSA 2005; 2011).

B – **Background** – Chloe remains comfortable throughout the procedure and is soothed by her mother. However, Chloe's nurse recognizes NPSA standards in relation to establishing tube position with a pH ≤ 5.5 and decides to consult medical staff to discuss the issue, including the possible effects of her medication (omeprazole) on the pH result.

A – **Assessment** – Chloe appears well following the procedure, she is due her feed shortly and the nurse is concerned as to how to proceed and wishes to discuss risk management options with the doctor and how best to care for Chloe in this situation, while maintaining her safety.

R – **Recommendations** – Following discussions between the nurse, doctor and Chloe's mother, it is decided to proceed with an oral feed, leaving the NGT in situ and to retest the gastric aspirate pH after her breastfeed, with subsequent reassessment of the situation if the pH remains outside recommended limits.

Summary

The scenario illustrates the utilization of SBAR in the care of Chloe to ensure and maintain her safety, through effective inter-professional communication and patient care. When used appropriately, the SBAR tool is effective in supporting and delivering safe care in a timely manner.

As highlighted by Morrow (2012), this simple framework creates prompts for the user in relation to situational awareness in clinical scenarios and communicating critical information to other health professionals:

Children and Young People's Nursing at a Glance, First Edition. Edited by Alan Glasper, Jane Coad, and Jim Richardson.

Inter-professional working

SBAR is a valuable communication tool when used either uni-professionally or inter-professionally. For example during clinical placement the practice mentor may utilise this SBAR tool to provide feedback on the nursing student's ability to prioritise using this flexible framework, when reporting on a patients' condition and on their theoretical knowledge and problem-solving skills.

Additionally, effective understanding of collaboration and inter-professional working are essential elements within health-care education and practice. During simulated inter-professional learning sessions, nursing and medical students are encouraged to reflect upon this situational briefing tool, which guides them to communicate important information in a predictable structure, when summoning senior nursing or medical help with a deterio-rating child (Morrow 2012).

Communication barriers

The quality of communication between and with patients and healthcare professionals is a critical factor in establishing safe and effective care. Therefore, it is essential that everyone involved within the healthcare team communicates effectively, in order that maximum standards of care can be supported and achieved.

Within the healthcare environment practitioners need to be mindful of language and literacy barriers which may directly or indirectly affect the decision-making process and effectiveness of the communicated message. However, having clear shared goals, role awareness of individual professions and the ability to work independently within a team as well as working together should assist in removing these barriers.

When using SBAR tool the practitioner should aim to:

- Communicate effectively
- Identify priorities
- Utilise decision-making strategies
- Develop problem-solving skills
- Be aware of language and literacy barriers.

3 The nursing process

Figure 3.1 Planning care using the nursing process and nursing models

What is nursing theory?

- Nursing theory is the cognitive knowledge and understanding that is used by practitioners to help them deliver the best possible care based upon best evidence
- Nursing theory is partly drawn from a range of subjects from the arts and science domains that can be applied to the practice of nursing (Colley 2003)

Key point

Nursing theory is knowledge that comes from experiential learning and research and is used by the nurse to guide practice

What are nursing models?

- Nursing models are a combination of theories and concepts that provide a framework to assess, plan, implement and evaluate care
- Many nursing models proposed by theorists (Chalmers 1990)
- Most common are those that include 'activities of daily living'
- Casey's partnership model being based upon the notion of partnership with the family where parents or carers provide care until the child or young person is mature enough to do it themselves

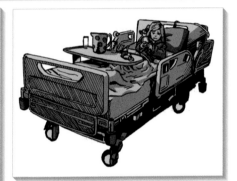

What is the nursing process?

- The nursing process is a framework for organizing individualized nursing care
- Involves four stages: assessment, planning, implementation and evaluation (APIE)
- An essential component is that goals or objectives are measurable to enable care to be evaluated and improved upon: subjective, objective, assessment, planning, implementation, evaluation (SOAPIE)

Key point

The involvement of children and families in planning and implementation of care is recognized by professional bodies as vital in the formation of effective partnership with families and children in the provision of care and health care services

Benefits of care plans

- Improved quality of care
- Improved communication
- Evidence-based practice
- Reduce risk of litigation
- Standardized care
- Continuity of care
- Patient and staff satisfaction

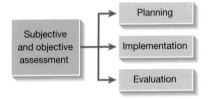

Subjective and objective assessment → Planning

Subjective and objective assessment → Implementation

Subjective and objective assessment → Evaluation

The nursing process is a way of thinking about nursing in a logical and problem-solving manner

- It is a framework for organizing individualized nursing care and promotes continuity of care
- The nursing process has four stages:
  – assessment, planning, implementation and evaluation

Nursing has a theoretical base that has many elements including physiology, psychology, pathology, pharmacology and sociology. To deliver quality care to patients that is focused, safe and organized, it needs to be planned. Documenting the plan of care for a patient and its implementation ensures continuity of care and provides a legal document demonstrating that care has been delivered. Care can be organized using the nursing process and nursing models can help focus care to meet the specific needs of patients.

What is nursing theory?

Nursing theory is the cognitive knowledge and understanding that is used by practitioners to help them deliver the best possible care based on best evidence. Nursing theory is partly drawn from a range of interconnected subjects from the arts and sciences that can be applied to the practice of nursing (Colley 2003). This knowledge comes from experiential learning and research and is part of the rich tradition linked to the development of nursing. The importance of children's and young people's nurses delivering care that is underpinned by evidence-based theory is perhaps reflected in Nightingale's famous pronouncement articulated in her notes for nursing 'Children: they are affected by the same things [as adults] but much more quickly and seriously' (Nightingale 1859: 72).

There are several models that are commonly used in the nursing of sick children and young people (Table 3.1). The most common are 'activities of daily living models' which include Henderson (1978), Roper, Logan and Tierney (1983) and Orem (Aggleton and Chalmers 2000). Additionally, a further model is applied to the care of sick children and can be used in conjunction with other models that were essentially designed for adults. Casey's (2007) model for children's nursing is all about partnership and has become standard practice in UK children's units. The central premise of these activities of daily living models is that normally people maintain their own functions in these areas but in times of illness these may be compromised and require support from health care professionals. In the case of children, some activities of daily living such as keeping the body clean may be compromised simply by developmental age. This is why children's nurses have adopted Casey's theoretical framework based on the notion of partnership and in turn on the philosophy of children's nursing and the notion of the indivisible family unit where parents or carers provide essential care until the child is mature enough to do it themselves. Orem's model is sometimes called the self-care model and is orientated towards restoring an individual to a health status where self-care is possible. It is particularly useful in rehabilitation settings (e.g. after childhood head injury).

Children and Young People's Nursing at a Glance, First Edition. Edited by Alan Glasper, Jane Coad, and Jim Richardson.

Table 3.1 Websites providing further information on a range of nursing models

Virginia Henderson: definitions of nursing	http://www.nursingsociety.org/
Imogene King: general systems framework	http://www.nurses.info/nursing_theory_person_king_imogene.htm
Betty Neuman: systems model	http://www.neumansystemsmodel.com/
Dorothea Orem: self-care framework	http://currentnursing.com/nursing_theory/self_care_deficit_theory.html
Hildegard Peplau: theory of interpersonal relations	http://publish.uwo.ca/%7Ecforchuk/peplau/hpcb.html
Callista Roy: adaptation model	http://www.bc.edu/schools/son/faculty/featured/theorist/Roy_Adaptation_Association.html
Roper, Logan and Tierney: elements of nursing: a model for nursing based on a model of living	http://www.biina.org.uk/news_files/527e5cca89af7.pdf

What is the nursing process?

The nursing process is a framework for organizing individualized nursing care. It involves four stages: assessment, planning, implementation and evaluation (APIE). The intention of the nursing process is to enable continuity of care by thorough documentation of information, to provide continuous observations and ensure effective interventions. However, there has been a much criticism of the nursing process approach to care as it imposes rigid constraints on practice, is cumbersome and outdated (Walsh 1997).

Care plans provide an excellent means through which the rights of children and their families can be respected. They enable children and families to be fully informed and share in decision-making about their care (United Nations 1991; RCN 1992). The involvement of children and families in the planning and implementation of care is recognized by professional bodies as vital in the formation of effective partnerships with families and children in the provision of care and health care services (RCN 1994).

The Nursing and Midwifery Council (NMC) require nurses to respect the patient or client as an individual and recognize and respect the role of patients and clients as partners in the contribution they can make. This includes identifying their preferences regarding care (NMC 2008). The primary rationale for using the nursing process is the creation of a care plan that is used to determine the nursing care given to an individual patient. An essential component is that the goals or objectives of the care plan are measurable to enable care to be evaluated and improved upon.

The nursing process can be perceived as the cognitive vehicle for planning the coordination of care delivered to a patient. Universally, it is the language of nursing and wherever nurses work they will use the same basic steps which constitute the nursing process (i.e. care delivered using four steps: APIE or Soapie). It is important to remember that patient care must be documented and every child should have an individual plan of care that has been determined following a full nursing assessment. In legal terms, **if it was not documented it never happened**.

Planning care

Nursing care has always been planned. However, in recent times the focus of care has changed from the completion of tasks to the provision of holistic care where patients are viewed as individuals with diverse and individual needs (Walsh 2001). Planning care should involve, where possible, the child and family to uphold the overarching family-centred care philosophy of children's and young person's nursing. Planning care involves reviewing all of the identified needs or patient problems and prioritizing them. Glasper (1990) discusses how Maslow's hierarchy of human needs can help nurses objectively plan nursing care. Clearly, if a child has compromised respiratory efforts this must be prioritized before planning dietary intake for example. Care plans are frameworks through which nurses apply the nursing process in addressing the needs of their patients. A nursing care plan is a written statement of the patient's nursing problems and the measures that will be used to effect a solution or mediate these problems (Johnson 1980, cited in Hurst 1993).

Care pathways or critical pathways involve the multidisciplinary team involved in the treatment and management of a patient and provide a programme of care delivery. They provide care that is focused, cost effective and collaborative (Herring 1999). For each clinical problem, the essential steps involved in the care of the patient are set out and planned with regard to that individual's expected progress. They provide a plan of desired patient outcomes, linked to an estimated time frame and the resources available. They can assist in the application of national evidence-based guidelines into local practice. Care pathways have the advantage of improving teamwork, reducing duplication of documentation and provide continuous records of care for a patient (Norris & Briggs 1999). When using care pathways or predetermined core care plans it is important these should still be individualized. Some NHS Trusts have care-planning software that allows nurses to plan an e-care plan for each individual child. When planning care nurses must ensure that the goals of care are achievable.

Summary

The nursing process can be applied in any nursing health care situation and offers a cognitive toolkit to assess, plan, implement and evaluate care. It is easy to use because it is systematic. However, in practice it requires a number of nursing skills: a good understanding of how health problems can impact on an individual child with reference to pathophysiology and social science; excellent interpersonal skills of communication with well-developed listening skills;and technical proficiency in delivering care based on best evidence.

4 Nursing models

Figure 4.1 How to implement nursing models into practice

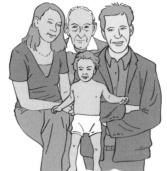

Ways in which personal use of nursing models can be developed

- Used as part of preceptorship or mentorship, clinical supervision to explore nursing actions in more depth
- Development of a personal toolkit using a range of nursing models
- Incorporated into reflective practice

Use of nursing models in practice settings

- As part of the philosophy of care
- As part of multidisciplinary working
- In conjunction with care pathways and guidelines
- As a framework for care planning

Figure 4.2 Suggested activities

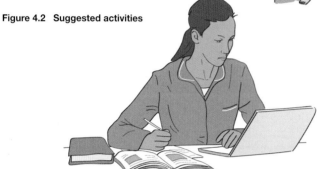

2. Find out a bit more about the three nursing models and compare this to with your reflection. Think of ways in which your newly gained knowledge could enhance your practice.

1. Reflect on a shift, referring to three nursing models outlined in this chapter;
   – i.e. Is there any indication of use of any of these?

3. Find out about two other nursing models not mentioned in this chapter. What are their strengths and how could they be used to develop your practice?

Children and Young People's Nursing at a Glance, First Edition. Edited by Alan Glasper, Jane Coad, and Jim Richardson.

Nursing models are theoretical frameworks, first developed in the 1950s to provide guidance on the delivery of nursing care. There are many different types; however, they all provide direction on how to implement the care for an individual. A nursing model contains concepts, processes and goals that guide care delivery. They are seen by some as being too traditional and not always suited to contemporary care provision; this is because of the continuing drive towards evidence-based practice, which is often based on hard scientific facts.

Models are extremely important in the development of nursing practice, providing direction to children and young people's nurses when planning, implementing and evaluating care. They can be utilized in all settings where children and young people receive care. All nursing models have a focus on meeting the needs of an individual; however, the way that this is defined varies considerably. The models most frequently used are discussed here but there are many others that can also be considered which assist in providing high-quality care that meets the needs of the child and family. A 'pick and mix' approach is helpful, as many nurses find that they draw on more than one nursing model in their practice.

Nursing models used in children and young people's nursing

The partnership model, which was developed in the United Kingdom by Anne Casey in the 1980s, is one that is often most closely identified with children and young people. Unlike many nursing models, it was developed for this specific group, the main focus being the concept of family-centred care. Roper, Logan and Tierney (1985) created the activities of daily living. This is a conceptual model which uses 12 activities of living as the central component with five underpinning factors: biological, psychological, socio-cultural, environmental and politico-economic. Orem's self-care model is based on meeting the self-care needs that the person is unable to meet themselves. Each person has universal self requisites based on human functioning (e.g. a sufficient intake of food), each person has developmental self-care requisites linked to their stage in life, and they also have self-care requisites that arise from their health issue.

How nursing models can be used in practice

All nursing models have a theoretical base. By exploring these concepts, nurses can build on their knowledge base to develop their expertise in becoming caring and compassionate practitioners. Nursing models are often incorporated into care planning. This can be implicit; the philosophy of the partnership model may be used to inform practice but not be directly visible in the care setting. Roper, Logan and Tierney's activities of daily living model (1985) is often easy to detect, for example in admissions documentation. This has led to criticism that it has been reduced to a tick box approach which detracts from a model that has a lot to offer in furthering our understanding of individualized care. It would be unusual to see Orem's self-care model being used directly in practice, but on closer inspection it is often integrated into the care plan, such as encouraging the child and family to take control of their health which is part of the systems approach advocated by Orem.

Summary

Nursing models are theoretical frameworks. Individual practice can be enhanced by applying nursing models in all aspects of care. Evidence-based practice requires an individualized approach and use of nursing models can help to achieve this. Nurses should be encouraged to explore different nursing models and have a flexible approach towards combining them in practice.

The care plan

Figure 5.1 Care plan framework

Identified problem/need

- The need should have been clearly identified during the assessment
- The problem/need should be individualized
- The problem/need covered should be specific, so that if three needs or problems are identified during the assessment, there should ideally be three care plans
- The child and his/her carers need to be involved in the identification of their needs – they are the 'expert' in how the illness makes them feel and the impact it has on the family unit

Short-term goals

- Often used when a period of assessment is needed (e.g. the child is acutely unwell)
- Should be SMART (specific, measureable, achievable, realistic and time-specific)
- Should be mutually agreed by and acceptable to the child and his/her carers
- Should be clear and concise

Long-term goals

- Should be SMART
- Should be mutually agreed by and acceptable to the child and his/her carers
- Should be clear and concise

Interventions

- The child and his/her carers should work in collaboration with the nurse to ensure the interventions are individualized, specific and meet the needs of the child
- The practitioner leading on each of the interventions is skilled and competent to carry them out
- Interventions should be prioritized to meet the needs of the child and his/her carers
- The interventions identified should have a theoretical base
- The practitioner should consider cultural diversity and well as gender, age appropriateness and religious beliefs when planning any intervention
- The core principles of care, compassion, dignity, privacy and quality, should underpin clinical practices

Evaluation

Remember that evaluation should happen continuously
It should include the child and his/her carers
It should provide clear evidence as to whether the interventions are making a difference
It should provide an overview of the child's condition in order to modify care

Review date

Essential in order to measure care outcomes in a timely manner

Figure 5.2 Common care planning problems

- **Incomplete initial assessments** – leading to gaps in care and increased levels of risk
- **Unrealistic care planning** – could give false hope, or increased level of expectation about the child's outcome
- **Lack of clear goals and vague interventions** – leading to difficulties in evaluating care
- **Not individualized** – may lead to inappropriate clinical intervention

Figure 5.3   Example – care plan

Scenario

Jane is 23 and has two children: James who is 4 years and Madelaine who is 18 months. Jane lives by herself with the children and has very little social or family support. Jane calls you and requests a Health Visitor meeting. You arrange to see her at the family home. When you arrive, Jane expresses her concern about James' sleep pattern. She is struggling to get him to bed before 11pm. When he is in bed, James takes a further 30–60 minutes to settle, often disrupting Madelaine. James gets angry at bedtime, he shouts, screams and kicks so that Jane does not follow through any routine. James tells you that he hates bedtime and is old enough to stay up late to watch the television. He denies feeling tired. James is due to start school in September.

Identified problem/need

James lives with his mum and sister in the family home. He is 4 and is due to start school in September. James is not going to bed until 11pm most nights, and when he is in bed does not settle until 11.30pm –12am. Prior to bedtime James shouts, kicks and screams, often disturbing his younger sister. James states he 'hates' bedtime and he is not tired.

Goals

To assess potential bio-psycho-social issues that may prevent James from wanting to go to bed.
For James to have an established sleep routine that ensures flexibility.

Interventions

- For James to be allowed to talk about bedtime – identifying any fears or concerns he may have about this aspect of his daily routine
- To provide James with reassurance in relation to any issues identified, referring on to specialist services as required
- To support Jane in purchasing aids/equipment that may support a new bedtime routine (e.g. new duvet cover of James' favourite cartoon character, night time light, bedtime books)
- To ensure the bedroom environment is supportive of sleep
- Discuss daytime routine with Jane and identify how James could increase his activity levels
- To develop a bedtime routine with Jane – one that is consistent and appropriate for James' age
- To support Jane in the implementation of the routine, providing guidance and positive feedback
- Discuss the implications of the sleep routine on James's initial behaviours (e.g. Jane to expect that initially James will not like these changes to his bedtime routine)
- Discuss with Jane ways in which she can cope with the stresses of providing James with a boundaried approach to bedtime
- Identify how James will be rewarded when small achievements are made

Evaluation

1 July 2013: developed the care plan with James and his mum today, James' opinion was sought. He did not think he should be going to bed any earlier but did add that he would like to go to the park more often. Jane was in agreement. I have left a copy of the care plan with the family so Jane can read it and add any further comments. Jane has requested that we meet again in a week. An appointment has therefore been arranged for 8 July at 2.30pm.

Review

The care plan is to be reviewed after each visit

Children and Young People's Nursing at a Glance, First Edition. Edited by Alan Glasper, Jane Coad, and Jim Richardson.
© 2015 John Wiley & Sons, Ltd. Published 2015 by John Wiley & Sons, Ltd. Companion website: www.ataglanceseries.com/nursing/children

Care plans are arguably the most important part of nursing care (Lloyd 2010). If developed, recorded and used appropriately, they should shape the manner in which the child is cared for, and ensure that each clinical intervention undertaken is suitable, consistent and needs-led.

Care planning is a necessity within the legislative practice; it is the framework that drives the identification of the child's need, highlights professional responsibilities and requires clear evaluation of outcomes. Care planning is also a continuous process, one that requires review and update dependent on the specific requirements of the child and his/her carers.

There are many clearly defined benefits to undertaking the care planning process: ensuring a personalized approach to the child and their carers; providing standardization to the child's care, thus reducing the risk of health inequality; ensuring the child's and his/her carers' voices are heard as part of the planning stage (this approach can increase compliance, and readily supports the maintenance of a therapeutic relationship); and, finally, care planning should be underpinned by choice. Providing suitable options to the child and his/her carers supports the notion of a mutually agreed plan of care.

According to Lloyd (2010), care planning is intrinsically linked to the nursing process.

Assessment

The first stage of the nursing process is the assessment. The aim is to collect and record information pertaining to the health status of the individual child and its effect on the family unit (Corkin et al. 2012: 4). A precise and comprehensive assessment should provide clear insights into the needs of the child, so that issues can be identified and informed interventions can be developed. The problem with the assessment process is that it can sometimes be a hurried exercise (Nazarko 2007) and one that is stifled by closed questioning based on predetermined assessment criteria. Although it can take a brave practitioner to deviate from the approved process, it is a necessity within the setting of children's care to ensure that communication and questioning styles are age appropriate and led by the child's preference.

Where feasible, the child should be included in the assessment process. Where this is not possible, information should be obtained from carers and other physical sources (e.g. referral letters), alongside visual observation and non-verbal communications.

What to assess

Knowing what to assess can sometimes be a challenge. Many organizations use specific assessment documentation or tools, which are often linked to a nursing model. The most common models utilized for this purpose are Roper, Logan and Tierney's – the 12 activities of daily living, family-centered care and Orem's self-care model (Corkin et al. 2012).

In terms of assessment, models are useful; however, it is clearly important to ensure any assessment of the child and his/her carer uses a holistic approach which should encompass elements such as biological health, psychological well-being and social need. It is important to understand the context in which children and their families normally live, their routines and what types of coping mechanisms are utilized. Assessment of the impact the health issue is having on family relationships and the psychological health of carers are important factors that can also impinge on the child's needs.

Using open questions can be helpful in obtaining information. Understanding how communication works and the importance of observation and non-verbal clues are also implicit within the assessment process.

Planning

The care plan should be based on the evidence gained from the assessment; it should be specific and individualized. Goals (either short or long-term, or both) need to be developed that are mutually agreed and acceptable to the child. Planning care should not preclude the need to involve other professional groups, as their impact on the child's well-being may further support the identified need. The manner in which the overarching goals will be achieved should then be developed within the intervention element of the care plan. It is important to stress that any intervention should be aimed at resolving, maintaining or identifying deterioration.

The practitioner needs to ensure that both the goals and interventions are written using an approach consistent with the SMART (specific, measureable, achievable, realistic, time specific) model (Lloyd 2010). Professional responsibility should be highlighted as part of the intervention development process, so identifying who will lead on a specific task in the child's care determines the need for clear communication of the care plan across the team.

Effective communication is an essential part of care planning. It is imperative that children and their carers are given defined opportunities to work with the nurse, making certain they are active partners in the decision-making process. This will ensure that interventions are specific and each child is treated as an individual.

Implementation

This is the third phase of the nursing process, but also an integral part of the care plan. In this phase the identified interventions are implemented. Those practitioners involved should have the skills and knowledge to deliver the care and assess the appropriateness of the planned intervention (Alfaro-LeFevre 2009). It is imperative to continue working closely with the child and his/her carers and to provide clear choices where possible in terms of the planned interventions.

Evaluation

This stage is concerned with the outcome of the care plan. It should be an ongoing process that is led by the needs of the child and his/her response to any intervention. The practitioner should, through the evaluation of the care records, be able to identify changes in the child's well-being and, if needed, redefine the plan of care accordingly. Often, the evaluation process is linked with a reassessment of the child's situation, which in turn could lead to a new care plan being introduced or one being discontinued (if all needs have been met). Again, it is important to ensure that the child and his/her carers are involved, and their opinions are valued and incorporated into future care decisions.

Documentation

Documentation underpins the success of the care plan process. All clinical records should be written in line with local policy and the Nursing and Midwifery Council (NMC) guidelines. Practitioners should be encouraged to write the care plan documentation in a factual and objective manner, avoiding judgemental statements, abbreviations or discriminatory language. Clear and concise documentation reduces the risk of clinical errors, mistakes and complaints. It is also important to ensure the care plan is disseminated across the care team so that all staff are aware of the needs of the child. As a final point, the child and his/her carer should, under normal circumstances, sign the care plan and be provided with a copy if required.

6 Record keeping

Figure 6.1 Record keeping

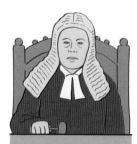

The ELBOW rule

1. No erasures
2. No leaves (pages) pulled out or removed
3. No blank spaces
4. No overwriting
5. No writing in margins

Making amendments to a record

- **Original in black ink only**
- **First amendment in red ink**
- Second amendment in green ink
- **Third amendment in purple ink**

Never obliterate. Any errors to be crossed out with a single line, dated and signed, and followed by correct entry or explanation

There is a link between poor record keeping and health care litigation

All formal record notations should provide an auditable account of the whole of the patient journey

All nurses have a professional and legal duty to keep records that meet the CIA mnemonic:
- Clear
- Intelligible
- Accurate

The NMC record keeping policy defines a record as constituting any carer-related information about the physical or mental health of a named patient or client made on behalf of or by a health care professional:
- Handwritten notes including Post-it trigger notes (especially information given over the telephone)
- Emails
- Electronic monitor printouts
- Tape-recorded telephone conversations (as in 111 calls)
- Text messages

Never write on your skin, your apron or a paper towel!

What constitutes a patient record?

The Nursing and Midwifery Council (NMC) are adamant that good record keeping is an integral component of safe and effective nursing care. In the context of children's and young people's nursing this constitutes any carer-related information about the physical or mental health of a named child or family member made on behalf of or by a health care professional:

- Handwritten notes including Post-it trigger notes (especially information given over the telephone)
- Emails
- Electronic monitor printouts
- Tape-recorded telephone conversations (as in 111 calls)
- Text messages.

The cost to the NHS of health care litigation in England is increasing and poor record-keeping is often cited: 'if it was not recorded it never happened'. Hence, nurses should ensure that their record keeping is meticulous.

CIA mnemonic

The NMC policy is clear in highlighting the importance of nurses keeping records that are accurate and recorded in such a way as to ensure that their meaning is clear. All nurses have a professional and legal duty to keep records that meet the CIA mnemonic:

- Clear
- Intelligible
- Accurate.

Good CIA records are necessary to facilitate synchronous patient care, clinical audit, patient safety and patient decision making, and in promoting continuity of care across inter-

professional and inter-agency boundaries. Importantly, CIA records show how patient decisions were made, and may be used in addressing complaints and subsequent legal processes.

Ensuring good record keeping

There are a number of important principles of good record keeping that nurses can use to help ensure that all their records meet the NMC requirements:

- Importantly, all formal record notations, handwritten or electronic, should provide an auditable account of the whole of the patient journey. Today's nurse is quite likely to use a Post-it note which may be subsequently transcribed into the patient record. There are inherent dangers in temporary trigger note taking and although fully understandable they are best avoided. Any temporary note taking should be formalized within 24 hours in the legal records of care
- Ensure that when giving advice on the telephone, there is a detailed record of what advice was given
- All notes should preferably be made at the time of the incident. In the event that there are no facilities for making notes at the time notes should be made as near to the time of the incident as possible. In addition, the note should state the actual venue of the note taking.

A good way for nurses to get round the problems of temporary trigger note taking is by using small notebooks that meet the following criteria:

- Hardbound, not spiral-bound
- With numbered pages
- With margins.

Children and Young People's Nursing at a Glance, First Edition. Edited by Alan Glasper, Jane Coad, and Jim Richardson.
© 2015 John Wiley & Sons, Ltd. Published 2015 by John Wiley & Sons, Ltd. Companion website: www.ataglanceseries.com/nursing/children

What colour ink should nurses use when making records?

• All entries to notes or records should be made in black ink – never in pencil
• Never alter an entry or disguise an addition to a note or patient record. If you need to amend a note or record, always put a straight line through the original word or sentence as this still allows the original to be read
• All corrected errors must be dated and signed
• Where an amendment is subsequently added, follow the colour code for amendments. Hence, original in **black**, **first amendment in red ink**, second amendment in green ink and any **subsequent amendments in purple ink**
• When making any note, always date and time the entry using the 24-hour clock. This is because dated and timed handwritten notes will be invaluable if a child or family make a personal injury claim which might arise many years later.

All nurses should follow the no ELBOW rule when making notes

1 No **e**rasures (ever)
2 No **l**eaves (pages) pulled out or removed (numbered pages is best practice)
3 No **b**lank spaces (draw a line across any blank space to avoid any unintended additions being made to the original)
4 No **o**verwriting (use the formal method of amendments using the standard ink colours)
5 No **w**riting in margins as this is to be used only for the time and date of the entry (no doodles or text language).

Problems faced by nurses in keeping records

• One of the major problems health care professionals have is inadvertently turning assumptions into fact. For example, a nurse finds a child lying injured by the bed. The entry to the notes made subsequently by the nurse states that the child fell out of bed and injured himself. In reality, the child got out of bed, walked to the toilet and then on the way back slipped on the floor near the bed. Do not make assumptions – especially about illegible medical records – and then make treatment decisions.
• All records should be factual and not include unnecessary abbreviations, jargon, meaningless phrases or irrelevant speculation. Phrases such as 'slept well' should be avoided, especially when they are subsequently amended to read 'the child slept well until he was transferred to PICU at 7.30am'. The dangers of using ambiguous abbreviations such as DNR (do not resuscitate) will not look good in a law court after the child's untimely death when it is revealed by the prosecuting barrister that the term DNR actually meant 'district nurse referral'. Similarly, when the case notes of a child who was claiming compensation for a personal injury sustained after a medication error were examined and the abbreviation FLK noticed, the judge was not pleased to hear it was an inappropriate colloquial abbreviation for 'funny looking kid'!

How long should records for children be kept?

In the case of children, personal injury claims are allowed up to 3 years after their majority (normally 18 years), although in all cases an individual judge may lengthen the period allowed.

Summary

Much potential litigation can be mitigated by clear and accurate record keeping. Importantly, the NMC make it clear that it is a nurse's duty to keep up to date with, and adhere to, all relevant legislation and policies relating to record keeping.

Engagement and participation of children and young people

Figure 7.1 Use of graphic facilitation to capture what children, young people and families want from health services (from visits to primary and secondary schools in the east of England in 2012)

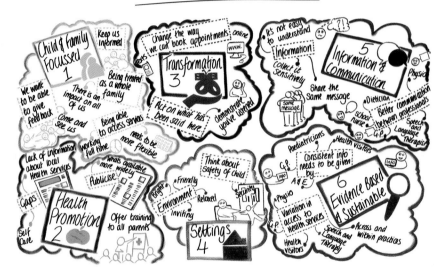

Figure 7.2 Some ideas as to how children and young people can engage and participate in health services

- Provision of direct feedback via a compliment letter, complaint, survey, either in writing, online or via apps
- Engagement in expert patient programmes
- Reviewing current health care services using programmes such as the Department of Health's You're Welcome Standards and the NHS Institute's Fifteen Steps Programme
- Contributing to the design and development of health care environment buildings/services
- Recruitment and selection of staff
- Informing and participating in research programmes
- Participation in the governance of health services
- Involvement in the commissioning of services

Children and Young People's Nursing at a Glance, First Edition. Edited by Alan Glasper, Jane Coad, and Jim Richardson.
© 2015 John Wiley & Sons, Ltd. Published 2015 by John Wiley & Sons, Ltd. Companion website: www.ataglanceseries.com/nursing/children

Children and young people can provide a window into the NHS, sharing powerful insights of what it is like for them to use their local health services. 'I felt really scared' said an 11-year-old describing his experience in an A&E department on a Friday night surrounded by intoxicated adults. Statements such as this reach right to the heart of how much further we still have to go in getting our services right for young people. No country has yet been successful in giving its citizens a truly central role in improving health and health care, preferring to rely on economic and professional levers, yet there is a shift to empowering citizens and one-fifth of our population are children and young people.

The Report of the Children's Outcomes Forum (Department of Health 2012) stated that all health organizations must demonstrate how they have listened to the voices of children and young people. 'We do a great injustice to Children and Young People when as a society, we fail to listen to their views, take on board their perspectives and value their contribution in shaping child health services' (RCPCH 2010). As active citizens, children and young people take actions and make contributions in everyday life that influence their personal circumstances and society. While their age and level of maturity is influential, all, whether a neonate, toddler, non-verbal child with complex needs or an articulate young person, have a right to be listened to and to be active participants in decisions that affect them, the services they utilize and their communities (Unicef 2007).

There are two fundamental levels of participation and involvement: the making of individual health care choices and being confident in interactions with health professionals, and more generic involvement as a service user or as a member of the public to inform the wider development of health services. The NHS Institute for Innovation and Improvement's (2010) work in schools confirms that children and young people express a desire to be involved in decisions surrounding their personal care and also in the development of health services. The National Children's Bureau (2012) highlighted that children and young people want to be listened to, have their recommendations acted on, be informed of what happens as a result of their recommendations and also meet with decision makers so they can explain why their recommendations may not have been taken on board. Children and young people value the opportunity to make a difference and see it as an opportunity to develop skills. High quality productive engagement results in the development of children and young people's self-confidence; it can be enjoyable, sociable and fun.

Children and young people are key stakeholders in health and health care and are not just beneficiaries or passive recipients of services. As health professionals, it is our responsibility to create the mechanisms to facilitate effective engagement of children and young people who are current and future consumers of health care to cultivate true participation and co-production across the NHS.

If health services are to deliver high quality holistic care, the contributions of children and young people needs to be harvested, valued and acted on. Children and young people's engagement and involvement will result in a much richer perspective that will assist in improved outcomes and enhanced services.

What are the practical hints and tips that can assist in achieving effective engagement and participation of children and young people?

- Governance systems and policies need to be in place to ensure that engagement and participation is safe, meaningful, ethical and systematic.
- Consent from the child, young person and their parent or guardian, is essential if names, quotes, drawings or photos are used.
- Records of responses, consultation and engagement should be treated as confidential and should be stored securely.
- Put in place training programmes for staff to address principles of engagement and participation of children and young people in decisions about their individual care and in wider service enhancement programmes.
- Consider collaborating with local authorities as they have statutory youth councils which can be helpful to in progressing engagement activities.
- Consider provision of training for children and young people as it can provide them with transferable skills. Accreditation and recognition can assist in sustained engagement and participation.
- Use a broad range of communication strategies including social media/networking sites to advertise opportunities and to secure engagement and participation.
- Commit to gathering a diverse pool of children and young people. They are not a homogenous group and diverse needs, backgrounds, capabilities and interests should be utilized.
- Aims and objectives of engagement programmes need to stated clearly from the outset.
- Programmes should be frequent, child/youth led and focused.
- Monitor and evaluate the effectiveness of engagement and the wider impact of child and youth participation.
- Put effective feedback mechanisms in place so that children and young people realize the impact of their contributions.
- Children and young people's representation is especially meaningful when young people have a budget and the power to decide its allocation.

What to avoid

- Tokenism: organizations need to be committed to valuing input and acting on suggestions.
- Use of jargon, unnecessarily complex information.
- Exploiting children and young people and not giving credit for their contribution.

Red flag
- Remember: importantly, make it fun and have fun!

8 Observation of the well child

Figure 8.1 Assessment

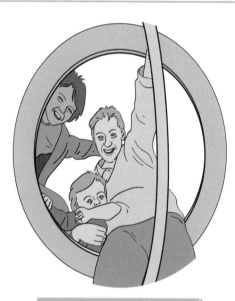

Airway

- Is the child talking or crying?
- Are there any abnormal noises?
- Is the child a normal colour?
- Is there any history of foreign body inhalation?
- Does the child have any history of known airway problems?
- Is the child drooling or unable to swallow his/her secretions?

Circulation

- Is the child a normal colour?
- Does the child have a normal heart rate?
- Is the child warm and well perfused?
- Is the child drinking sufficiently?
- Is the child passing urine sufficiently?
- Is the child vomiting?
- Does the child have diarrhoea?

Breathing

- Does the child have a rate within normal limits?
- Are there any added sounds?
- Is there any increased work of breathing?
- Is the child a normal colour?
- Is the child known to have any underlying breathing problems?
- Can they talk in sentences?
- Does the child appear breathless?

Disability

- Is the child alert?
- Is the child orientated?
- Does the child have normal tone?
- Is the child acting appropriately?

Exposure

- Does the child have a temperature within normal limits?
- Does the child have a rash?
- Is there any sign of trauma: bruising, bleeding, fracture, marks, burns?

If the parent is concerned, and the assessment shows the child is a well child, then reassurance may be all that is required. However, a parent knows their child best; if they are concerned, then ensure you have not missed something important. If you have assessed the child, and they appear to be a well child, but you still have a concern, then ensure they are reassessed by a senior colleague. Remember, a well child can rapidly become an unwell child. An unwell child can rapidly become a well child.

Children and Young People's Nursing at a Glance, First Edition. Edited by Alan Glasper, Jane Coad, and Jim Richardson.
© 2015 John Wiley & Sons, Ltd. Published 2015 by John Wiley & Sons, Ltd. Companion website: www.ataglanceseries.com/nursing/children

Observation of the sick child

Figure 9.1 Observation

Use all your senses to observe what is happening and do not forget to communicate effectively to the child, young person and family throughout. Do not forget that the vital sign normal range varies with the age of the child

Is the **airway** clear?
Can they talk/cry?
Look, listen, feel

Look at their colour: are they cyanosed?
Do they have mottled skin?
Are they flushed?

Count the **breathing** for a minute and record. Observe the pattern, effort, noise, movement

Listen for a stridor which is a 'harsh sound coming from a narrowed upper airway, which can be heard on inspiration and/or expiration' *(Spotting the Sick Child 2012)*. This is a sign of an airway obstruction

Listen for a wheeze which is a 'high pitched sound heard on expiration in, e.g. children with asthma and bronchiolitis. It is caused by a narrowing of the airway, usually due to excess secretions (mucus)' *(Spotting the Sick Child 2012)*

Oxygen saturation should not be measured alone; it needs to be combined with a respiratory assessment. Are they in oxygen?

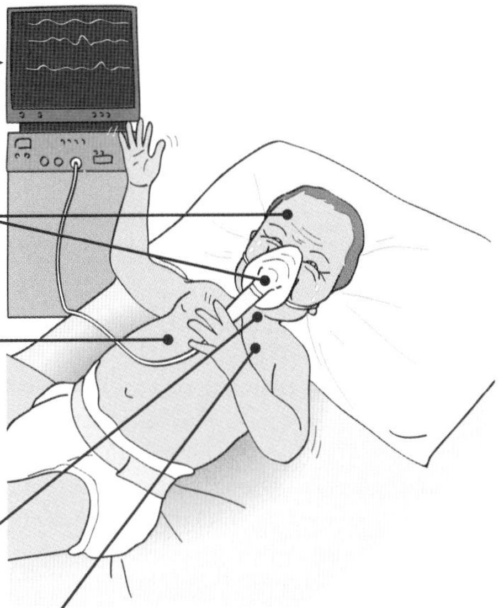

Watch out for signs of respiratory distress:
- Respiratory rate/pattern/effort
- Nasal flaring
- Grunting
- Wheezing
- Stridor
- Dyspnoea
- Recession
- Use of accessory and Intercostal muscles
- Change in chest shape
- Change in movement of chest
- Head bobbing in infants
- Tracheal tug
- Cyanosis
- Oxygen requirement

(McCance and Huether 2010; RCN 2011:6)

To measure capillary refill, press the skin firmly for 5 seconds with your finger, take off and count until the normal skin colouration returns

It may be measured centrally, by pressing on the sternum or the forehead, or peripherally, by pressing on the hands or feet. It may be worth measuring both peripherally and centrally. The peripheral capillary refill time will be affected first, but is also affected by factors such as ambient temperature

Normal children have a capillary refill of less than 2 seconds *(Spotting the Sick Child 2012)*

Observe their urine output
What temperature is their skin?

Check **circulation**. Take the pulse and count beats for a minute. Observe the rate, rhythm and volume

It is important to obtain an accurate temperature.

Listen to parental concerns

Observe the child's behaviour, cry, position, how they interact with others, activity levels.
Check their conscious level (AVPU) (GCS)

Figure 9.2 Things to consider when a child or young person is in distress

Are they in pain? Use a validated age/developmental appropriate tool to assess and document

Have you checked their nappy?

Do they need reassurance from a parent or carer?

Are they hungry/thirsty?

Are they bored? Are they frightened?

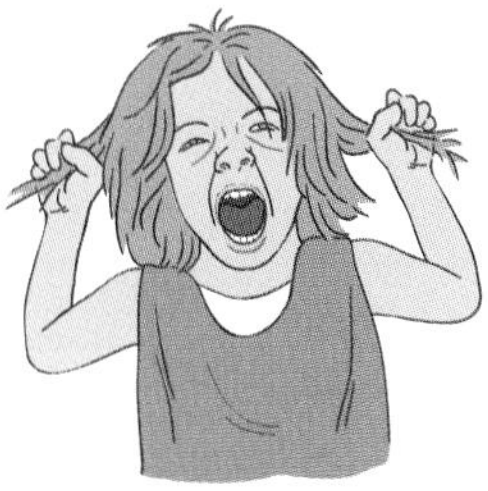

Do they need a soother/comforter?

Are they comfortable?

Do they understand what is happening?

Listen to the child or young person

Listen to the parents and carers

Information gained from the broader assessment of the infant, child or young person should be recorded, e.g. crying, distress, laughing, playing (RCN 2011: 9)
Observations and comments made by the child, young person and parents/carers should be clearly recorded (RCN 2011: 9)

Communicate effectively with the child or young person and family members to gain an understanding of what is happening

Children and Young People's Nursing at a Glance, First Edition. Edited by Alan Glasper, Jane Coad, and Jim Richardson.
© 2015 John Wiley & Sons, Ltd. Published 2015 by John Wiley & Sons, Ltd. Companion website: www.ataglanceseries.com/nursing/children

Introduction

This section will focus on observation of the sick child, in practical steps, and will work in conjunction with a recognized paediatric early warning tool (PEW), effective communication and multi-professional team working.

The importance of observation

Assessment of children and young people is vital, and measurement and monitoring of vital signs are important basic skills for all practitioners (RCN 2011: 2).

This needs to be a systematic process and the views of parents/carers must be included.

A baseline of vital signs including 'temperature, heart/pulse rate, respiratory rate and effort, blood pressure, pain assessment and level of consciousness of all infants, children and young people are initially assessed, measured and recorded on attending hospital and at varying frequencies from then on.' (RCN, 2011: 5). Assessment needs to be a continuous process to be alert for changes.

Respiratory rate

It is vital to measure, record and monitor the respiratory rate, 'as a measure of either respiratory distress, or more systemic problems such as septicaemia.' (Spotting the sick child, 2012).

To measure the respiratory rate accurately, count each breath over a minute (RCN, 2011: 6). Crying or coughing can alter the rate considerably, so try and count when the child is calm.

The normal range varies with the age of the child so check on your PEW chart what the normal range is. As well as counting the breath rate check for respiratory recessions which are the 'indrawing of the respiratory muscles due to an increased effort of breathing' (Spotting the sick child, 2012).

Pulse oximetry

A pulse oximeter machine measures the amount of oxygen saturation in the blood (Spotting the sick child, 2012) using infrared light giving the percentage of the haemoglobin that is oxygenated.

'Normal children should have a saturation of at least 96%. Levels of less than 94% imply significant illness. Levels below 90% are alarming' (Spotting the sick child, 2012). Be cautious with monitoring as movement, skin temperature and probe placement can be factors affecting accuracy. Use your PEW chart to record. Please note that 'children whose normal oxygen saturations fall outside the normal acceptable limits should be documented, for example, a child with a cyanotic heart lesion' (RCN, 2011: 6).

Pulse

'The pulse is measured by lightly compressing the artery against firm tissue and counting the number of beats in a minute' (Dougherty and Lister 2011: 708). The pulse varies with age so check your PEW chart for the normal rate for your child/young person. To measure a peripheral pulse take the radial pulse in an older child, whilst they are most calm if you can, or if a central pulse is needed use the carotid pulse.

In babies under 6 months old, the radial pulses can be difficult to measure, and the brachial pulse may be easier to feel. This is located above the elbow on the inside of the arm (Spotting the sick child, 2012). 'A stethoscope should be used to auscultate the apex heart rate of children less than two years of age. Electronic data should be cross-checked by auscultation or palpation of the heart/pulse rate' (RCN, 2012: 6).

Capillary Refill Time

Capillary Refill Time is 'a measure of tissue perfusion, describing the time it takes for blood to re-enter capillaries after it has been squeezed out' (Spotting the sick child, 2012).

This indicates if a child has a compromized circulation as you are observing to see if their body has constricted the blood vessels to the arms and legs in order to preserve the more important central circulation such as serious bacterial sepsis or dehydration. This is a very useful measure of circulation in children since blood pressure does not drop until the child is extremely ill, and a tachycardia is not a 100% reliable sign (Spotting the sick child, 2012).

Blood pressure

Blood pressure can be difficult to measure in children because they can get upset when the cuff goes tight on their arm. The blood pressure is maintained until very late in the process of shock. This is because children have such good peripheral vasoconstriction to compensate. To measure the blood pressure, it is very important to use the right size of cuff. The cuff should measure two-thirds of the length of the upper arm (Spotting the sick child, 2012).

Sucking, crying and eating can influence blood pressure measurements and these should be noted (RCN 2011: 7).

Temperature

It is important to get an accurate temperature on children. 'A temperature should be recorded on all children who attend with an acute presentation of illness with the device applicable for age' (RCN, 2011: 6).

Key recommendations from the 2007 NICE guideline on fever in children state that 'oral and rectal routes should not be routinely used to measure the body temperature of children aged 0–5 years' (NICE 2007: 15). They recommend that 'in infants under the age of 4 weeks, body temperature should be measured with an electronic thermometer in the axilla' and 'in children aged 4 weeks to 5 years, healthcare professionals should measure body temperature by one of the following methods: electronic thermometer in the axilla, chemical dot thermometer in the axilla and infra-red tympanic thermometer' (NICE 2007: 15). Check your Trust guidelines for which are used. Forehead chemical thermometers are unreliable and should not be used by healthcare professionals (NICE 2007: 15).

Child, young person and family-centred care

It is essential that all observations and assessments are carried out using effective communication appropriate for the age, development and understanding of the child, young person and family.

A full explanation of the procedure, gaining consent, is needed.

10 Septic screening

Figure 10.1 Septic screening

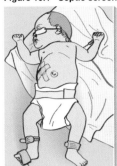

An ABCDE assessment should have been carried out before a septic screen proceeds:

Airway – patent. Apply 15 L oxygen through a non rebreath mask if required

Breathing – effective, check oxygen saturations, respiratory rate and look for signs of respiratory distress

Circulation – is the infant stable enough to wait for IV access or is IO required? Check heart rate, blood pressure, colour and capillary refill time

Disability – AVPU, or amended Glasgow coma score assessment completed, blood sugar sample obtained to rule out hypo-/hyperglycaemia, check pupil size

Exposure – assess for hypo-/hyperthermia. Check for any rashes (in particular petechiae). Look for injuries, bruises, marks or burns

Stabilize the infant before considering septic screen and ensure reassessment is continuous while screening takes place

Septic screen consists of the following:
- Full blood count
- Blood culture
- C-reactive protein
- Urine microscopy sensitivity and culture
- Stool sample
- Chest X-ray
- Cerebrospinal fluid (CSF) if not contraindicated
- Swabs of any wound sites
- Swab of throat, ears, nose or eyes if indicated

What is sepsis?

Sepsis is a whole body inflammatory reaction to infection, usually pathogens in the blood and generally bacteria.

Clinical features include the following:
- Temperature less than 36°C or greater than 38°C
- Low blood pressure (late sign in children)
- Tachycardia
- Tachypnoea
- Limb pain
- Change in behaviour
- Rash
- Cyanosis.

Stabilization of the infant or child

Often, procedures are carried out on sick children and medical professionals lose sight of the basics while they are concentrating on a task, for example taking blood. A shocked, septic, shut-down sick child requires stabilization and continuous assessment of their ABCDE (airway, breathing, circulation, disability and exposure).

It is dangerous to begin any procedure on an unstable child as the procedure may exacerbate a problem and make the infant or child deteriorate further.

Sick infants do not like being handled. They are usually hypoxic, will become increasingly distressed and their tachycardia and tachypnoea may advance. They may deteriorate further and become bradycardic and apnoeic.

Blood tests

Full blood count, C-reactive protein (CRP) blood glucose and cultures can be taken from intravenous (IV) access or intraosseous (IO) access (although usually only enough bone marrow is obtained to carry out a blood sugar assessment). If bone marrow is sent to the laboratory, it is important to indicate that it is not venous blood, as it will look different under the microscope.

If enough blood is obtained, a blood gas assessment is helpful to indicate how acidotic the infant or child is.

The blood test results should be available quite quickly but the cultures take 48 hours to be processed.

Urine

A clean catch urine is recommended and this can cause some challenges, depending on the age and sex of the child. It may sometimes be necessary to obtain a catheter or a suprapubic sample from the infant or child.

Stool sample

This is easier to obtain from an infant's nappy, but if there are frequent abnormal stools, taking a sample is quite simple. Remember personal protection equipment at all times.

Chest X-ray

Ensure the infant or child is stable, has a parent and/or member of staff with them and the X-ray is carried out in a timely manner to help prevent hypothermia and possible deterioration from increased handling.

Results are available fairly quickly and help in the differential diagnosis of sepsis from pneumonia.

Lumbar puncture for CSF sample

This is often contraindicated in a child who is neurologically unstable as it can have catastrophic consequences. It is unlikely that physicians will suggest a lumbar puncture when the patient is unstable, and it should always be questioned if considered.

If a lumbar puncture is required, ensure an ABCDE assessment is carried out before commencing the procedure, ensure it is done in a safe environment with emergency equipment ready including oxygen, bag valve mask, suction and resuscitation trolley in case of further deterioration.

In an infant, observe the airway and breathing continuously, as the position of the infant has the potential to occlude the airway. It may be advisable to ask the parent to step outside the room while the procedure is being undertaken. In an older child, consider analgesia and provide reassurance as it can be a frightening and painful procedure.

Specimens usually take 48 hours to be cultured.

Swabs

Swabs of wound sites, pegs, catheters, discharging ears, noses and throats can be useful in identifying the source of infection and are painfree and quick. The results take 24–48 hours to culture.

Consent

Parental verbal consent should be obtained if at all possible and documented in the notes. A child that is Fraser competent may also consent to a procedure, but also has the right to refuse. The involvement of parents, carers and play specialists may be required.

Remember

1 Stabilize
2 Assess ABCDE
3 Obtain verbal consent if at all possible
4 Consider pain management
5 Document which tests have been carried out and when so results can be expected

11 Advanced physical assessment

Figure 11.1 **Rapid clinical assessment of a seriously ill child will identify any potential respiratory, cardiovascular or neurological failures**
Use the ABCDE approach for a systematic assessment of the child

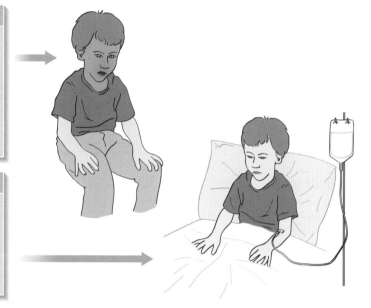

Airway and Breathing

- Is the child awake, talking? Do they sound breathless?
- Can you hear abnormal breath sounds?
- Is the child using accessory muscles to aid breathing?
- Are they breathing fast?
- Do they look pale or cyanosed?
- What position are they sat in?
- What are the O_2 saturations, do they reflect the child's actual condition?

Circulation

- Is the heart rate and BP normal for age range?
- Feel their hands and feet, are they warm or cold?
- Check the capillary refill time
- If they are in nappies, are they wet or dry?
- Are the lips dry and cracked?
- Check the fontanelle

Disability

- Is the child running and playing?
- Are they unsteady on their feet and falling over – do not presume this is normal
- Is the child meeting developmental milestones?
- If the child is crying, is it possible to console them?
- Check the blood sugar level as soon as possible if the child is having a fit or is unduly drowsy or irritable

Exposure

- Check the child's temperature
- Check from head to toe and back to front for the presence of any rashes, scars, bruises or other injuries. Do not presume all injuries are accidental

If in doubt discuss with a senior colleague and report in line with your local safe-guarding policy

---

This chapter follows on from the section on observation of the sick child, further developing these skills in the advanced physical assessment of children. Utilizing the ABCDE approach (ALSG 2005), this section will allow you to identify the deteriorating child and consider appropriate action.

While the majority of children who become unwell will recover with minimal intervention, the rapidity with which a child can deteriorate can lead to anxiety in even experienced practitioners. A rapid clinical assessment of a seriously ill child will identify any potential respiratory, cardiovascular or neurological failures (Lissauer and Clayden 2007). Rapid assessment allows for initiation of appropriate treatment to prevent progression to respiratory or cardiac arrest (Cameron et al. 2006).

The ABCDE approach allows for a systematic assessment of the child to take place:
A – airway
B – breathing
C – circulation
D – disability
E – exposure.

A baseline of vital signs including 'temperature, heart/pulse rate, respiratory rate and effort, blood pressure, pain assessment and level of consciousness' (RCN 2011: 5) should always be carried out as part of this assessment. Look at how the child interacts with the adults and other children around them. Are they playing and interested in their surroundings or are they sitting quietly and apathetically?

Airway

Every cell in the body requires oxygen. A viable airway is the only way for this gas to enter the body. It is vital to establish that the airway is patent on immediate inspection and assessment of the child.

A crying, screaming or talkative child indicates an airway that is patent at that time, whereas a child who appears floppy and quiet may require immediate airway support. If there are any concerns about a child's ability to maintain its airway please follow the Paediatric Life Support Algorithm (see Chapter 23). Look at the child, do they look cyanosed (blue) around the lips and nose? In children with darker skin it may not be immediately apparent, so check the tongue (Jarvis 2011). If the child seems to be drooling excessively ask the parent or carer if this is normal. Difficulty in swallowing can be an indication of an airway problem. What sounds can you hear? A bark, seal-like cough or noisy breathing on inspiration can indicate some narrowing of the upper airway, as in croup for example.

Children and Young People's Nursing at a Glance, First Edition. Edited by Alan Glasper, Jane Coad, and Jim Richardson.
© 2015 John Wiley & Sons, Ltd. Published 2015 by John Wiley & Sons, Ltd. Companion website: www.ataglanceseries.com/nursing/children

Breathing

Once a clear airway is established, breathing can be assessed. Remove the child's top with consent. Remember to maintain privacy, dignity and warmth at all times. Look at the rate of breathing, is it within normal parameter's for the child's age? Is the chest moving equally on inspiration? If it is not, this may indicate a pneumothorax or an injury to the side not moving. Is there any drawing (recession) under the ribs (subcostal), between the ribs (intercostal) or in the sternal notch (tracheal)? While all infants 'tummy' breathe, if this is fast and drawing in excessively it can indicate a breathing problem. Consider the child's general position. Are they in a relaxed position or playing? Children in respiratory distress will often adopt a tripod position. This is where they will sit with their arms stretched out and pushing up against a table or their knees. They will stretch their head back and may possibly be blowing out when breathing in an attempt to improve ventilation. (Lissauer and Clayden 2007). Listen to the child talking. If they are only able to answer in short sentences or not at all then these are signs of respiratory distress. Listen for any noises during breathing. Wheeze is the noise air makes as it is squeezed back out of the lungs. This is not necessarily a sign of respiratory distress in toddlers and infants if the other symptoms discussed are absent, but it can be a source of concern for parents. Oxygen saturation levels, as discussed in other chapters, are a useful measure, but must be considered in the context of the child's overall condition.

Circulation

Assessment of the child's state of hydration and circulation can take place once the respiratory system has been assessed. Checking the pulse is integral to assessing circulation. While palpating the pulse, consider not just the rate of the heart, but the volume and rhythm of the pulse. A thin thready central pulse can indicate shock or severe dehydration. In infants and small children it is often easier to check the brachial pulse than the radial pulse, or consider using a stethoscope placed over the apex of the heart (Jarvis 2011). For infants under 6 months of age, consider checking a femoral pulse when checking the nappy area. Remember, as with all procedures, to explain to the parent or carer what you are doing and why. Look at the child's face and hands. Do they look pale or grey, are the lips dry and cracked? Along with sunken eyes this could indicate a child in shock or dehydrated. In infants with a patent fontanelle ask the parents if it looks sunk in any way compared to its normal appearance. Capillary refill time is an important measure, but bear in mind small infants and toddlers can be very sensitive to environmental changes and will have a sluggish capillary refill time due to a change in room temperature rather than shock. For this reason it is often better to check the capillary refill time on the forehead or chest. Consider urine output and ask the parent or carer how long the current nappy has been on if one is worn. If it is dry after being on for a few hours consider the child's hydration status.

Disability

In the context of advanced assessment, when discussing disability it is not in relation to an existing condition but rather to any acute changes in the child's level of consciousness. The use of the A(lert) V(oice) P(ain) U(nresponsive) system allows for a rapid initial assessment of the child, and goes hand in hand with assessment of the airway (ALSG 2005). Is the child awake and responsive, or floppy and unconscious? The biggest risk to life in an unconscious child is an occluded airway. If the child is awake, ask the attending carers if the child is its usual self, or if anything has changed. Signs of a neurological problem are headaches, vomiting – especially on waking or after a head injury, dizzy spells, altered visual acuity or a change in the appearance of the eyes. In infants, neurological signs can be more discrete, but a bulging fontanelle or inconsolable high-pitched crying is an indication of a problem.

A formal tool for assessing neurological status is the Glasgow coma scale, and an adapted paediatric version is available. This uses a scoring system to assess the level of neurological deficit and can provide an indication as to what treatment may need to be carried out (Glasper et al. 2010). Infants have a poor ability to maintain their blood sugar level when unwell so any signs of an altered level of consciousness in infants and small children should trigger the checking of the blood glucose level.

Exposure

The final part of the advanced physical assessment is an overall review of the child. Infants and small children should be assessed from head to toe for the presence of any rashes, scars, bruises or deformities. Remember to check the axilla, the nappy area, behind the ears and around the nape of the neck. If you suspect there is a non-blanching rash then have a high suspicion for sepsis until proven otherwise. While the majority of rashes seen will be normal innocuous rashes associated with various common childhood conditions, they are often a source of anxiety for carers. If older children present acutely unwell then check for the presence of rashes but allow them the opportunity to undress in privacy before conducting the assessment. If the temperature has not been checked already then this should be done, but remember sepsis can present without fever, particularly in infants. Unusual marks or bruises should not be ignored and in the case of child protection concerns reference should be made to local safeguarding procedures.

12 Developmental assessment

Figure 12.1 Development assessment

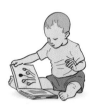

Birth to 2 years (sensorimotor stage)

Physical – rapid growth, key skills developed, gross/fine motor skills, milestones

Cognitive – learn and solve problems, perceptual development, key theorists, reflexes, intelligence, speech and language development: pre-linguistic/linguistic stage, understand and use language

Personality – beginnings of self-concept, trust and mistrust, temperament, gender differences

Social – facial expressions (e.g. smiling), nature versus nurture, attachment/bonding, imitation, developing autonomy

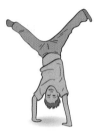

2–7 years (preoperational stage)

Physical – body shape, brain growth, sensory development, nutrition, safety, gross/fine motor skills development: skipping (gross motor skill); using a pencil to draw (fine motor skill)

Cognitive – egocentric, role of education, language development, cultural factors

Personality – self-concept, gender identity

Social – friendships, work of play, consideration of others, family life, moral development, behaviours

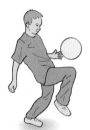

7–12 years (concrete operational stage)

Physical – slow steady growth, motor development, gross motor coordination; fine motor skills, draw detailed pictures

Cognitive – coherent, logical thought processes, appreciate others' perspectives, unable to consider abstract ideas

Personality – developing competence, appreciate own internal traits

Social – sensitive to the importance of friends, level of morality

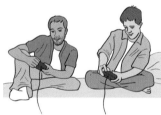
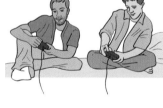

12 years to adulthood (formal operational stage)

Physical – primary and secondary sexual characteristics develop, puberty, growth spurts

Cognitive – abstract and hypothetical thoughts, consider consequences of actions, systematic problem solving, invulnerability

Personality – organized and accurate self-concept, identity formation, developmental self-esteem

Social – personal identity important, peer relationships, conformability, sexual experimentation, autonomy, parental/family conflicts

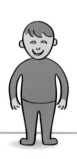
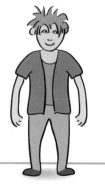

Preterm newborn infants

Term newborn infants (0–28 days)

Infants and toddlers (>28 days to 23 months)

Children (2–11 years)

Adolescents (12–18 years)

Children and Young People's Nursing at a Glance, First Edition. Edited by Alan Glasper, Jane Coad, and Jim Richardson.
© 2015 John Wiley & Sons, Ltd. Published 2015 by John Wiley & Sons, Ltd. Companion website: www.ataglanceseries.com/nursing/children

Assessment

Assessment is a structured comprehensive evaluation of a child's development – including aspects of physical, social, language, intellectual and emotional progress – by a registered health care professional, such as a general practitioner, health visitor or paediatrician. Each child is assessed as an individual, considering their age, expected stage of development and how this information relates to the various identified milestones. Birth and family history, alongside parental and professional observations of the infant's or child's movements, skills, awareness and interactions are important aspects of the assessment process. This process of assessment involves investigations, tests and physical examination and should include the parent in supporting the child.

Genetics and nature versus nurture

Genes are the blueprint of human development and cell function. These may manifest themselves in the inherited characteristics of the infant (e.g. eye and hair colouring). During the prenatal stages of development natural mutations of the genes occur. These genetic factors can impact on the development of the fetus (e.g. Down's syndrome); this is referred to as the 'nature' side of development. The 'nurture' factors that impact on the child's development include the home, family, culture, school, social activities and communities. Risks to any of these factors can impact on the child's overall development (e.g. reading will develop a child's vocabulary; malnourishment may lead to poor brain development and suboptimal IQ). Cultural experiences can impact on the child's social development as beliefs can guide and direct behaviours.

Developmental milestones

A developmental milestone is a skill that a child acquires in a specified period of time. For example, most children learn the skill of walking by the age of 9–15 months. If a child did not walk until they were 22 months this would suggest a delay, which must be closely observed and monitored by the parent and health professional. Children develop along predicted progressive pathways within the main areas of development. These developments are recorded within the child's personal health record – commonly referred to as the 'red book'.

Developmental delay

Development delay is described as a recognized significant delay in the infant's achievement of predicted developmental milestones. This delay may affect only one aspect of development or include all aspects of development – generally referred to as global developmental delay. Natural or environmental factors may be linked to developmental delay and may be indicative of a more permanent setback or disability. Delays in development must be monitored and investigated by the health care professional, in order to give appropriate care and support to the child and family.

Implications for practice

Infants, children and young people are changing every day in terms of their abilities and skills, learning new knowledge and simply growing. Children's nurses need to understand how children grow and develop in order to support children and understand their perspectives of development and how these can be disrupted or affected. Additionally, when children's nurses come in contact with an infant, child or young person they need to be able to plan and provide care that appreciates their stage of development and understanding of what is happening to them and integrate this into care delivery. Children's nurses have a professional and ethical responsibility to preserve and safeguard the public and promote ethical practice in assessment and adherence to professional codes of practice. In performing developmental assessments, obtaining informed consent is considered a fundamental aspect of clinical practice for all health care professionals.

13 Paediatric Early Warning Score

Figure 13.1 Paediatric early warning scores are a systematic tool designed to detect early deterioration in children

Benefits of PEWS

- A full set of vital signs are recorded and repeated as the child's condition dictates
- Aids early recognition of the sick child
- Empowers nursing and medical staff to escalate concerns
- Documents trends in the child's condition – improvement or deterioration
- Reduces risk of cardiorespiratory arrest
- Reduces number of unexpected paediatric intensive care admissions

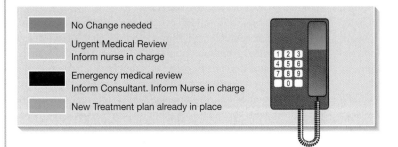

No Change needed

Urgent Medical Review
Inform nurse in charge

Emergency medical review
Inform Consultant. Inform Nurse in charge

New Treatment plan already in place

Once the vital signs have been recorded and scored, the treatment algorithm should be consulted, actioned and documented. The Situation, Background, Assessment and Recommendation tool should be used to communicate findings when escalating concerns

The vital signs that must be recorded are heart rate, respiratory rate and blood pressure. Oxygen saturation should also be recorded.

However, there are many variations of early warning scores in use which may require measurement of other physical signs.

Age appropriate parameters

Age (years)	Respiratory rate	Heart rate (beats/min)	Systolic BP (mmHg)
<1	30–40	110–160	80–90°
1–2	25–35	100–150	85–95°
2–5	25–30	95–140	85–100°
5–12	20–25	80–120	90–110°
>12	15–20	60–100	100–120°

Paediatric Early Warning Score (PEWS) is a systematic clinical tool used to facilitate and detect the signs of clinical deterioration in the patient. Initially, early warning systems were devised as a method of early identification and prediction of which children are likely to deteriorate and necessitate high dependency or intensive care, as it is known that children who die or require intensive care have exhibited signs of deterioration prior to collapse. They are now an integral part of the care of the majority of acutely ill children in hospital. They may have some use as a triage tool in the A&E department. PEWS is a risk management tool and may also be referred to as 'track and trigger'.

Calculating the Paediatric Early Warning Score

The score is calculated by adding the numerical values together that have been assigned to the routine observations that are undertaken on infants and children. Once the score is calculated, the nursing and/or medical staff refer to the algorithm on the chart which will indicate the action required. This multiparameter scoring system includes routine observations: heart rate, respiratory rate, blood pressure, oxygen saturation level, temperature and conscious level. Other observations and treatments may also be considered such as oxygen therapy. Each parameter is allocated a score, which are then added together to give an overall score. The greater the deviation from normal for the physical sign being measured, the higher the score. Generally, if the child's clinical condition is deteriorating the score is high, thus alerting the nursing and medical team that early intervention is required early in anticipation of preventing adverse outcomes. Early intervention may prevent the need for transferring the child to a higher level of care. Early intervention may indicate the need for more frequent observation of the child and a revision of his/her treatment plan.

PEWS provides nursing and medical staff with a framework to escalate their concerns about a child to a more senior team member.

Education on how to use the PEWS tool effectively should be considered.

Limitations

There is currently limited research into the trigger points for scoring and escalating concerns. Inconsistency in the use of PEWS and scoring make is difficult to validate its effectiveness.

There are a variety of scoring systems in existence but with limited methodological assessment to identify their reliability or validity.

Key points
- PEWS has become increasingly used to prevent unexpected intensive care admissions.
- PEWS enables health care professionals to intervene early and prevent deterioration of the child's condition.
- PEWS provides health care professionals with a framework to escalate their concerns.
- There are many scoring systems in use, some of which have limited methodological assessment.

14 Paediatric critical care

Children require intensive care for a variety of reasons; for example, respiratory difficulty due to an airway infection, a mechanical obstruction in the airway, septicaemia (blood poisoning), seizures or a serious traumatic incident.

Most children present to their local hospital and receive immediate care delivered by the emergency department, paediatric and anaesthetic staff. If the child is assessed to be seriously ill he/she will require specialist intensive care advice and treatment in a tertiary children's hospital. A transfer will usually be required. This could involve travelling long distances, especially if the child lives in a rural location.

In 1993 the British Paediatric Association recommended that intensive care for children should be centralized and this led to the requirement for tertiary centres to provide transport for children requiring intensive care.

Results from a number of studies demonstrated decreased morbidity and a lower critical incident rate (e.g. endotracheal tube dislodgement) during transfer by a specialist team.

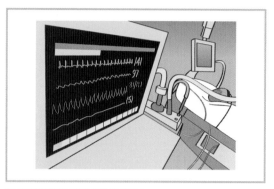

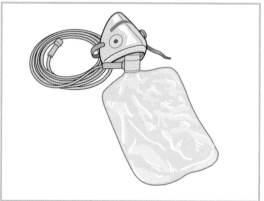

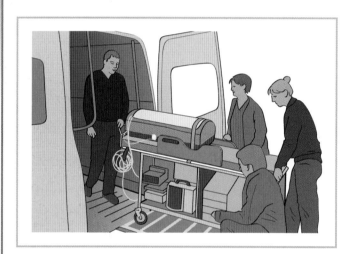

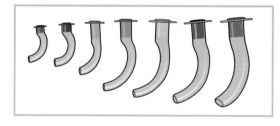

Each geographical region of the United Kingdom has provision to mobilize a specialist paediatric intensive care transport team. This could be a standalone team or a team based in one of the 31 paediatric intensive care units. The Paediatric Intensive Care Society (PICS) has produced standards of practice for the transportation of the critically ill child. This outlined areas such as staffing teams, education, communication and a recommended equipment list. These services also provide advice and support for staff caring for the seriously ill child while the transport team is mobilizing and travelling to the hospital.

Recognition and management of the seriously ill child

The assessment of the vital signs (heart rate, blood pressure, respiratory rate, temperature, capillary refill time) by age is essential to recognize the seriously ill child. Most hospitals now use an early warning score. This is an excellent tool to identify the deteriorating child through changes in their observations. A senior team needs to be alerted to ensure that treatment is administered quickly.

If the child is breathing spontaneously a non-rebreather mask (Hudson type) is recommended. Oxygen administration is essential and should be available via a flow meter that can deliver 15 L per minute.

There are two commonly used airway adjuncts that can be utilized until a definitive airway is achieved. Oropharyngeal airways (Guedel) are available in a variety of sizes and are used to provide a clear passage along the tongue and posterior pharyngeal wall. A nasopharyngeal airway tube is inserted via the nasal passage and is often better tolerated as it is less likely to cause laryngospasm. Insertion of these airway adjuncts should only be undertaken by a trained member of staff.

If the child's breathing requires support this can be achieved by using a self-inflating bag (Ambu bag) or an Ayres T-piece or Mapleson T-piece.

Definitive airway support is achieved when a tube is passed via the mouth or nose into the trachea (windpipe). This requires the expertise of a senior anaesthetist. In order to place the tube, anaesthetic induction agents will be required via intravenous drugs or the inhaled route. Endotracheal tubes range from 2 mm to 8 mm (internal diameter) and require tape to secure to the child's cheeks.

To ensure that the tube is inserted to the correct length a chest X-ray should be requested when tracheal intubation has been

Children and Young People's Nursing at a Glance, First Edition. Edited by Alan Glasper, Jane Coad, and Jim Richardson.
© 2015 John Wiley & Sons, Ltd. Published 2015 by John Wiley & Sons, Ltd. Companion website: www.ataglanceseries.com/nursing/children

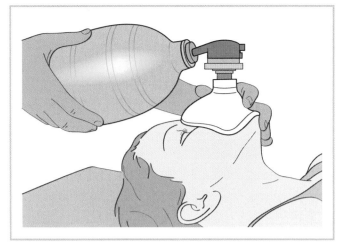

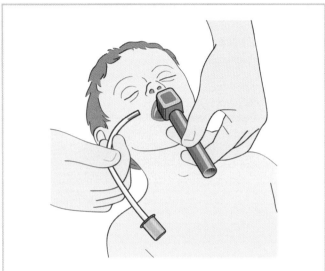

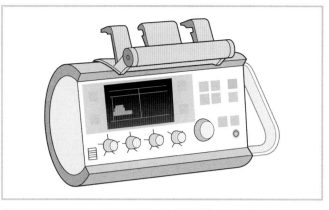

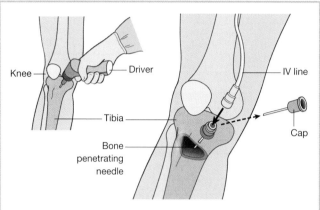

Knee — Driver — IV line

Tibia

Bone penetrating needle

Cap

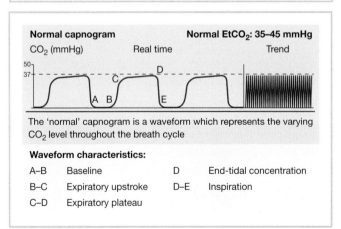

Normal capnogram   **Normal EtCO$_2$: 35–45 mmHg**

CO$_2$ (mmHg)   Real time   Trend

50
37

D
C
A B   E

The 'normal' capnogram is a waveform which represents the varying CO$_2$ level throughout the breath cycle

Waveform characteristics:

A–B	Baseline	D	End-tidal concentration
B–C	Expiratory upstroke	D–E	Inspiration
C–D	Expiratory plateau		

established. Accidental extubation is always a potential risk. Exhaled gases from the lungs contain carbon dioxide. Sampling the exhaled gas can be carried out to alert the team if the tube is dislodged from the trachea. Ventilation can be maintained after intubation by a mechanical ventilator that is suitable for a child.

The child will require a gastric tube to ensure that the stomach can be emptied. Air can be forced into the stomach during bag valve mask ventilation. This air, if not removed, can splint the diaphragm and cause difficulties in establishing mechanical ventilation.

Intravenous access is essential to facilitate drug administration. Peripheral cannulation can be difficult to achieve in the seriously ill child. The insertion of an intra-osseous needle allows rapid delivery of drugs and fluids.

Intravenous drugs are required to ensure the child remains asleep and able to tolerate the endotracheal tube. An infusion of an opiate such as morphine, combined with a sedative (e.g. midazolam) is frequently used. A paralysing agent is also administered to control the child's breathing rate.

Accurate measurement of the child's urine output can be very useful to determine renal efficiency and intravascular fluid volume. A Foley catheter may be required to record urine output hourly.

Blood sampling and analysis is an important diagnostic tool. The results are relied upon to interpret the efficacy of the treatment provided. Blood glucose levels should be frequently checked as all children, especially infants, can become hypoglycaemic when seriously ill.

Neurological assessment using the AVPU scale (alert, voice, pain, unresponsive) is a system by which a health care professional can measure and record the child's responsiveness. Pupil reaction to light should be recorded regularly as changes in the response of the pupil could indicate serious brain disorder or injury.

Communication with the child and parents or carers should never be ignored. Explanation and information will allay fears in most situations so it is important to explain things as clearly and simply as possible.

Key points
- Early recognition of the seriously ill or deteriorating child is crucial
- Alert and request senior medical personnel to the child's bedside
- Prompt treatment and resuscitation as appropriate (children can deteriorate quickly)
- Utilize telephone advice provided by the paediatric intensive care services
- Structured approach to managing a seriously ill child can focus the care delivered
- Effective communication with the child and family is essential

15 Understanding investigations

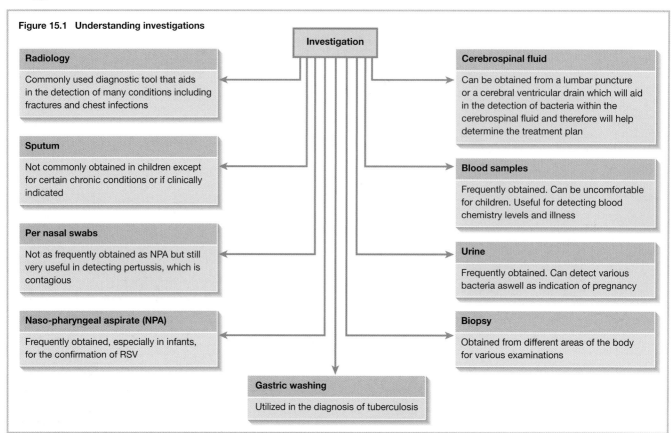

Figure 15.1 Understanding investigations

Investigation

Radiology

Commonly used diagnostic tool that aids in the detection of many conditions including fractures and chest infections

Sputum

Not commonly obtained in children except for certain chronic conditions or if clinically indicated

Per nasal swabs

Not as frequently obtained as NPA but still very useful in detecting pertussis, which is contagious

Naso-pharyngeal aspirate (NPA)

Frequently obtained, especially in infants, for the confirmation of RSV

Cerebrospinal fluid

Can be obtained from a lumbar puncture or a cerebral ventricular drain which will aid in the detection of bacteria within the cerebrospinal fluid and therefore will help determine the treatment plan

Blood samples

Frequently obtained. Can be uncomfortable for children. Useful for detecting blood chemistry levels and illness

Urine

Frequently obtained. Can detect various bacteria aswell as indication of pregnancy

Biopsy

Obtained from different areas of the body for various examinations

Gastric washing

Utilized in the diagnosis of tuberculosis

Children and Young People's Nursing at a Glance, First Edition. Edited by Alan Glasper, Jane Coad, and Jim Richardson.
© 2015 John Wiley & Sons, Ltd. Published 2015 by John Wiley & Sons, Ltd. Companion website: www.ataglanceseries.com/nursing/children

Investigations are carried out to determine the cause of illness and require consent from the child and family. A large number of investigations come under the umbrella of radiology.

Radiology

Radiology includes **plain static X-rays** which can be used to look at bone or soft tissue in any area of the body, chest infections or the position of an endotracheal tube in an intensive care unit patient. It is the most common imaging investigation in hospital. Plain X-rays can be obtained in the radiology department or, if the child is too unwell to be transferred, they can be obtained via a portable machine. **Fluoroscopy** uses pulsed X-rays which create a real time image and is used for procedures such as a barium swallow to examine the gastrointestinal tract, micturating cystourethrogram to examine the bladder and urethra, and intravenous urography to examine the urinary tract. **Ultrasound** uses sound waves and is very useful in examining areas of soft tissue within the body or structures that contain fluid. It is not as useful at examining structures that contain gas because the ultrasound waves pass straight through the gas so there is poor image quality. **Computer tomography (CT)** is a very useful addition to diagnostic medicine. It uses multiple X-ray images and, with the assistance of a computer, creates a cross-sectional image of various parts of the body. It is not only used to distinguish between normal and abnormal structure within the body, but can also be used to assist in procedures whereby instruments need to be placed with accuracy. In **nuclear medicine** a radioisotope is injected into the child or young person via a cannula or butterfly needle. The radioisotope emits gamma rays which are then recorded by a gamma camera. It is a very useful tool in diagnostic medicine. **Magnetic resonance imaging (MRI)** is a way of looking inside the body and producing two- and three-dimensional images without using X-rays. The images are gained by using radiowaves, a magnet and a computer. Metal objects cannot enter into the same room as the magnet. Occasionally, a small amount of contrast is injected into the child or young person so that a clearer picture can be obtained.

Sampling of cerebrospinal fluid

A sample of cerebrospinal fluid (CSF) may be obtained from a lumbar puncture examination (the insertion of a needle into the back) to determine the diagnosis of conditions such as meningitis or encephalitis.

Blood samples

Blood samples are used to determine the different haematological, biochemical, immunological and microbiological components of blood to aid in the diagnosis of illness. They can also be used to determine certain antibiotic and drug levels, which dictate the dose required for the child. Blood cultures can also be obtained if a child's clinical condition is deteriorating as they can detect bacteria in the bloodstream.

Blood samples are obtained frequently as they can be used to determine levels of blood chemistry as well as detect illness. Children generally do not like blood being taken as it can be uncomfortable or painful unless managed well using local anaesthetics and distraction.

Sputum samples

Sputum samples are obtained for the microbiological diagnosis of respiratory tract infections. They are routinely obtained in children with cystic fibrosis.

Gastric washings

Gastric washings can be obtained when children do not produce enough sputum to detect the presence of *Mycobacterium tuberculosis*.

Nasopharyngeal aspirate

A nasopharyngeal aspirate (NPA) sample is mainly obtained for the diagnosis of viral infections such as respiratory syncytial virus (RSV), influenza and parainfluenza.

Per nasal swabs

These are used to help diagnose pertussis. Pertussis, commonly known as whooping cough, is a highly contagious bacterial infection that causes episodes of violent coughing and respiratory obstruction.

Urine samples

Urine samples can be collected in various ways but the most reliable way is via a midstream specimen or a clean catch. This is difficult to obtain in a very young child so it is important to ensure that the nappy area and genitalia are as clean as possible prior to obtaining a urine specimen. Urine samples can be used to detect various bacteria within the urine if sent to the microbiology laboratory for analysis. However, bedside urine tests can detect the presence of blood, protein and other constituents in the urine, which in turn will dictate whether further laboratory tests on the urine need to be considered.

Biopsy

Biopsies can be obtained from different areas of the body to determine the diagnosis of specific conditions. Specimens are sent to a relevant laboratory so that a histopathological and microbiological examination can occur.

There are too many investigations to cover them all in this chapter; however, above is some useful information about the most common ones. It is important to consider the needs of the child and family and to explain why such procedures are being undertaken and, importantly, when the results will be obtained.

16 Understanding blood gas analysis

Figure 16.1 Blood gas analysis

A disturbance in acid–base balance occurs as a result of either respiratory or metabolic disorders. Alteration in the acid–alkali balance in the body is a common problem in sick children that requires urgent intervention. Measurement of these substrates through blood gas analysis is an important part of the assessment of the sick child.

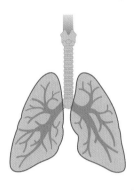
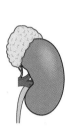

Common causes of acidosis or alkalosis

Metabolic acidosis pH 7.35	• Severe gastroenteritis • Diabetic ketoacidosis (DKA) • Shock: hypovolemic, cardiogenic • Birth asphyxia
Metabolic alkalosis pH >7.45	• Pyloric stenosis • Diuretics • Excessive nasogastric tube losses
Respiratory acidosis	• Respiratory failure due to illness or any other cause, e.g. asthma, inadequate mechanical ventilation, CNS depression
Respiratory alkalosis	• Hyperventilation • Excessive mechanical ventilation

Normal range for acid base and blood gas measurements

Arterial pH	7.36–7.42
Arterial PaCO$_2$	4.7–5.5 kPa
Arterial PaO$_2$	1–14 kPa (8–10 kPa in neonates)
Arterial or venous bicarbonate	17–27 mmol/L
Base excess	>0–2 mmol/L

Analysis of arterial blood gas (ABG)

In order to interpret the ABG of a child correctly, the clinical history, treatment given, findings from examination and previous laboratory investigations need to be considered

A systematic approach such as the 5-step method may be utilized

• How is the child?
• What is the pH?
• What is the PaCO$_2$?
What is the base excess?

Measured (37.0°C)

pH	7.21
pCO$_2$	11.1 kPa
pO$_2$	6.3 kPa
Na$^+$	133 mmol/L
K$^+$	5.6 mmol/L
Ca^{++}	1.37 mmol/L
Glu	5.2 mmol/L
Lac	2.3 mmol/L
Hct	30 %

Derived Parameters

HCO$_3^-$	33.2 mmol/L
HCO$_3$std	27.3 mmol/L
TCO$_2$	35.7 mmol/L
BE(B)	3.6 mmol/L

Changes in the blood gas and acid–base values depending on type of acidosis or alkalosis

*Compensated state	Metabolic acidosis	Metabolic alkalosis	Respiratory acidosis	Respiratory alkalosis
pH	Low	High	Low	High
PO$_2$	Normal	Normal	Normal or low	Normal or high
PCO$_2$	Normal or low*	Normal or high*	High	Low
Bicarbonate	Low	High	Normal or high*	Normal or low*

Indication for measuring blood gas

• Respiratory distress
• Management of mechanical ventilation
• Altered level of consciousness
• Shocked child: sepsis, cardiogenic
• Trauma
• Ingestion of poison
• Metabolic disorders inborn and DKA
• Ongoing evaluation of resuscitation treatments

pH

pH is the term used to describe the acidity or alkalinity of a solution. The pH scale is based on the number of hydrogen ions and is expressed in mmol/L. If a solution has a pH of 7 then it is considered to be a neutral solution such as water where the hydrogen + ions are present in equal concentration with the hydroxyl ions OH+.

A pH below 7 is an acid solution. This dissociates into H+ ions and OH+ ions, with more H+ ions than OH+ ions.

A pH greater than 7 is an alkaline solution. This dissociates into OH+ ions and H+ ions, with more OH+ ions than H+ ions. In the human body there needs to be a balance between intake and removal of H+ if normal body function is to be maintained.

Three systems regulate the acid–base balance:
• Buffers – metabolic
• Lungs – respiratory
• Kidney – metabolic.

In the event of abnormalities, these three systems function together in an attempt to compensate.

Buffers

The function of the buffers is to counteract changes to the pH by either increased absorption or release of H+. The carbonic acid–bicarbonate is the most important buffer system. Carbonic acid (H_2CO_3) is the weaker acid and sodium bicarbonate ($NaHCO_3$) is the weak base. In solution, dissociation occurs:

$$H_2CO_3 \leftrightarrow H+ \quad + \quad HCO_3$$
$$NaHCO_3 \leftrightarrow Na+ \quad + \quad HCO_3$$

When the blood becomes acidic, the sodium bicarbonate disassociates to buffer the acid; this increases the concentration of carbonic acid and decreases the sodium bicarbonate, resulting in an increase in the pH as the carbonic acid is weak.

If the blood is alkaline (strong base), then the concentration of sodium bicarbonate increases and carbonic acid will be utilized as the buffer.

The protein buffer system is activated in the body cells and plasma. The haemoglobin–oxyhaemoglobin buffer system buffers carbonic acid in the blood. The phosphate buffer system works in red blood cells and renal tubular fluids.

Respiration

The level of carbon dioxide CO_2 is regulated by respiration. The respiratory system balances the pH by offsetting the production of H+ ions by clearing the CO_2 through ventilation. This CO_2 dissolves in water, forming carbonic acid which is weak and unstable. If there is an elevation in H+, the respiratory system will increase the rate and depth of the child's breathing in an attempt to remove more CO_2 which inhibits the formation of carbonic acid. This is called respiratory acidosis; the PCO_2 is high and this occurs rapidly. The reverse of this process is called respiratory alkalosis and the PCO_2 will be low.

Base deficit

This indicates the level of base in the blood. Base deficit is the amount of base that needs to be added to return the pH to normal. The base excess is the amount of base that needs to be removed to return the pH to normal. Thus, a high base excess above +3 suggests metabolic alkalosis and if it is less than −3 then metabolic acidosis may be present.

Renal tubular secretion

Renal tubular secretion assists with the control of the pH level of the blood by continuous filtration of bicarbonate ions. If the pH is acidic then the secretion of H+ is increased, sodium Na+ is displaced, which combines with bicarbonate to form sodium bicarbonate which is absorbed into the bloodstream. H+ is lost from the body and the pH becomes less acidic.

Anion gap

The anion gap is calculated to identify the cause of the metabolic acidosis if it is not known. The anion gap is the sum of the:

(plasma sodium + plasma potassium) – (bicarbonate + chloride).

The normal value is 5–12 mmol/L.

Sampling

Blood is taken from the following:
• Artery – usually the radial or femoral
• Arterial cannula
• Capillary prick of heel or ear lobe – this is less accurate as venous and arterial blood is mixed.

This is a painful procedure in the non-ventilated child so careful consideration is given prior to drawing a sample. The Allen test needs to be undertaken prior to arterial puncture from the radial artery. Direct pressure must be applied to the puncture site for 3–5 minutes after sampling has occurred. Capillary refill time should be monitored post procedure.

A pre-heparinized syringe or a capillary tube is required. Avoid dead space and bubbles in the tube blood as this will alter the results.

Minimize metabolism in the sample by placing the specimen on ice if there is likely to be any delay in analysis (i.e. >15 minutes).

The blood is then analysed immediately and a printed result is generated. Fraction of inspired oxygen (FiO) and temperature need to noted when analysing the sample.

17 Understanding blood chemistry

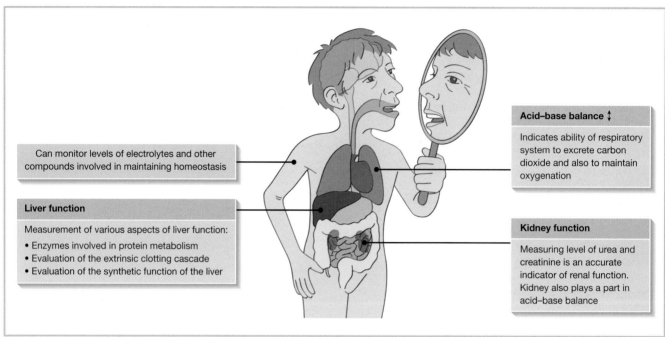

Can monitor levels of electrolytes and other compounds involved in maintaining homeostasis

Acid–base balance ↕

Indicates ability of respiratory system to excrete carbon dioxide and also to maintain oxygenation

Liver function

Measurement of various aspects of liver function:

- Enzymes involved in protein metabolism
- Evaluation of the extrinsic clotting cascade
- Evaluation of the synthetic function of the liver

Kidney function

Measuring level of urea and creatinine is an accurate indicator of renal function. Kidney also plays a part in acid–base balance

Children and Young People's Nursing at a Glance, First Edition. Edited by Alan Glasper, Jane Coad, and Jim Richardson.
© 2015 John Wiley & Sons, Ltd. Published 2015 by John Wiley & Sons, Ltd. Companion website: www.ataglanceseries.com/nursing/children

Electrolytes

Potassium: normal range 3.5–5.0 mmol/L. Important in neuromuscular function. Low level, usually below 3.0 (hypokaleamia) can lead to cardiac arrhythmias. High level, usually above 5.5 (hyperkalaemia) slows heart rate and can cause cardiac arrest.

Calcium: total calcium 2.23–2.57 mmol/L, ionized calcium 1.15–1.27 mmol/L. Allows cardiac muscle to work without becoming tired. Ionized calcium (available for body to use). Low level can lead to decreased muscle contractility.

Sodium: normal range 135–145 mmol/L. Most of body's sodium is in the extracellular fluid. Controls water distribution as well as extracellular volume. Hyponatraemia (usually below 135 mmol/L) = water into cells. Hypernatraemia (usually above 150 mmol/L) = water out of cells.

Phosphate: normal range 0.81–1.45 mmol/L. Intracellular. Critical component of adenosine triphosphate which the body uses as fuel. Also important in muscle function, red blood cells and nervous system. Hypophosphataemia: muscle weakness and reduced cardiac contractility. Hyperphosphataemia: reduced calcium levels, tingling of fingers. Precipitation of calcium phosphate in the kidney.

Magnesium: normal range 0.65–1.05 mmol/L. Intracellular: involved in enzyme reactions. Extracellular: neuromuscular transmission, neuronal control, cardiovascular tone. Low levels (usually below 0.6 mmol/L): muscle weakness, cardiac arrhythmias. High levels (usually above 1.1 mmol/L): bradycardia, reduced skeletal muscle function.

Glucose: normal range 3.58–6.05 mmol/L. Energy source for the body. Hypoglycaemia (usually below 3 mmol/L): confusion, anxiety, weakness, hunger, dizziness, shaking, coma. Hyperglycaemia: increased urine output, excessive thirst, damage to major organs, reduced resistance to opportunistic infections.

Lactate: normal range 0.6–1.7 mmol/L. Produced as an end result of energy production. Level rises in anaerobic respiration and contributes to acidosis.

Chloride: normal range 97–110 mmol/L. Needed to maintain normal cellular and organ function. Also fluid levels. Diarrhoea, nausea and vomiting and increased sweating can decrease chloride levels.

Kidney function

Urea: normal range 2.9–8.9 mmol/L. Waste product produced from protein metabolism.

Creatinine: normal range 53–133 μmol/L. Breakdown product of creatine phosphate in muscle.

Liver function

Ammonia: newborn 42–155 μmol/L; child 9–33 μmol/L. Deamination of amino acids during protein metabolism. Increased levels = reduced synthetic liver function. Can cross the blood–brain barrier and lead to hepatic encephalopathy.

Albumin: 0–5 days 26–36 g/L; 6 days–3 yr 34–42 g/L; 4–6 yr 35–52 g/L; 7 yr+ 37–65 g/L. Plasma protein responsible for maintaining plasma oncotic pressure.

Prothrombin time: 10–14 seconds. International normalized ratio (INR) 0.8–1.2. Clinical evaluation of extrinsic clotting cascade. If longer than normal then could have clotting problems. INR altered if on anticoagulant therapy such as warfarin or heparin.

Alanine aminotransferase (ALT): 0–3 yr 50 units/L; 4–10 yr 40 units/L. Catalyst for protein metabolism.

Aspartate aminotransferase (AST): 1–5 days 35–140 units/L; 6 days–3 yr 20–60 units/L; 4–15 yr 15–40 units/L. Involved in protein metabolism.

If levels of ALT or AST altered then the ability to breakdown protein will be affected.

Alkaline phosphatase (ALP): 0–1 yr 110–320 units/L; 1–9 yr 145–420 units/L; 10–15 yr male 130–525 units/L, female 70–230 units/L. Phosphate metabolism.

Acid–base balance

pH: 7.35–7.45. Measurement of the concentration of hydrogen ions in body fluids. Important in maintaining homeostasis.

(Hydrogen ions: 35–45 mmol/L.)

PCO_2: 4.7–6.0 kPa. Measurement of amount of CO_2 present in blood. If respiratory rate low then level will be raised and if respiratory rate high then level will be low.

Standard bicarbonate: 21–26 mmol/L. Measurement of level of sodium bicarbonate in the blood. Important in maintaining homeostasis.

Base excess: −2 to +2. Measurement of how many extra basic chemicals are present in blood or amount of acid that would have to be added to blood to bring pH back to normal.

PO_2: 9–13 kPa. Measurement of amount of oxygen in arterial blood.

18 Understanding pathology specimen collection

Figure 18.1 Principles of pathology specimen collection

Urine sample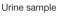

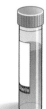

Stool sample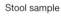

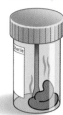

Some additives to blood bottles
- Gel
- EDTA
- Sodium
- Trisodium citrate
- Lithium heparin
- Sodium heparin

Safe transportation

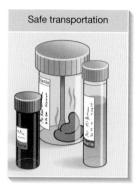

Children and Young People's Nursing at a Glance, First Edition. Edited by Alan Glasper, Jane Coad, and Jim Richardson.
© 2015 John Wiley & Sons, Ltd. Published 2015 by John Wiley & Sons, Ltd. Companion website: www.ataglanceseries.com/nursing/children

Important principles when collecting specimens

It is crucial that the following are adhered to when collecting specimens:
• Required investigations are confirmed with reference to medical records
• Checks are made to ensure it is the correct child and that name, date of birth and hospital number match
• Any labels used must match the child's details
• The correct tubes or bottles are selected prior to sampling
• Correct laboratory request forms are used and labelled
• Expiry dates on the tubes or bottles must be checked
• Tubes and bottles must be intact and not damaged
• Any materials should be prepared before the procedure
• It is the responsibility of the person undertaking the intervention to ensure it is the correct child, tests, tubes and labels
• Any specimens must be stored correctly and transported following local policy and procedures.

Obtaining blood samples

Blood samples can be obtained through a variety of methods:
1 *Heel prick.* Mainly used on neonates where small samples of blood are preferred so as not to reduce their blood volume.
2 *Finger prick.* Often used for measuring blood glucose levels in children with diabetes or in those who have drunk alcohol.
3 *Peripheral venepuncture.* This method involves the insertion of a butterfly cannula or a standard needle to obtain samples for a variety of investigations. This is the most common method utilized.
4 *Large vessel venepuncture.* In some cases it is not possible to obtain blood samples from smaller veins and so larger vessels are utilized.
5 *Arterial blood sampling.* Mainly used for ascertaining blood gas levels and involves taking a sample directly from an artery (often the radial or femoral arteries) or from an arterial line. The former is a distressing procedure and so preparation and analgesia are crucial.

Staff required to obtain blood samples must be trained in the intervention, deemed competent and maintain this. In addition, all staff must prepare the child (where possible), ensure local anaesthetic is applied and monitor their response to the intervention. If unable to perform the technique (e.g. difficult venepuncture), the staff member must seek help from a more experienced colleague. Repeated attempts from inexperienced staff should not occur but in circumstances where it does the nurse must advocate on behalf of the child thus ensuring their safety and wellbeing.

The recommended order to obtain blood samples is:
1 Blood cultures
2 Coagulation tubes
3 Tubes with other additives.

Blood samples are collected either by venepuncture with a standard needle and syringe and then transferred to a tube or a vacutainer system is used. The vacutainer is a tube already attached to a needle or is attached on venepuncture and then the vacuum draws out the blood sample and so a syringe is not necessary.

Once the blood sample has been obtained it is important to ensure that each of the tubes are inverted which allows for the mixing of the blood with the chemical inside the bottle. If the blood is not mixed then it may lead to inaccurate results. The total amount of times that the tube should be inverted is detailed on the side of the blood bottle or tube.

There are various departments that blood samples can be sent to depending on the investigation required:
• Biochemistry
• Haemotology
• Microbiology.

The blood bottles have various additives which aid in the accuracy of the test. It is important to ensure the correct bottle is used as there are different suppliers and so bottles may vary.

Urine collection

Depending on the investigation required, different urine collection methods are utilized including clean catch, catheter, early morning, midstream urine or 24-hour collection.

Early morning sampling is normally collected immediately on the child waking. It is important to collect as much as possible of morning's first urine into the supplied container.

The collection of midstream urine is particularly useful when testing for a bacterial culture. The child or young person must void the first portion of urine into the toilet. Next they must pass the mid-portion of urine into appropriate container to fill it to the mark on the container while not contaminating the inside of the container with the hand. This can be especially difficult for young children as it requires control of the bladder. To ensure a clean specimen of urine that has not been contaminated some departments perform an in–out catheterization procedure; this depends on the age and compliance of the child and the parent's wishes.

Stool specimens

Stool samples are useful in diagnosing bacteria in the gastrointestinal tract. Many children do not like to provide stool samples as they feel embarrassedso it is important to maintain their privacy and dignity. When obtaining a stool sample it is vital to inform the child that they must ensure that the sample avoids contact with urine. It is therefore easier if they pass the stool directly into a bedpan. Once the child has provided the sample the nurse then transfers the specimen into the stool bottle using the spoon that is attached to the lid. The bottle should be sealed and labelled with the child's details, date and time of collection.

Transporting specimens

All specimens must be handled according to local procedures and policies. The primary container for all specimens must be leak-proof and must be labelled with the patient's name and hospital number. Ensure that lids of containers are secure. Each specimen must be placed inside a secondary container for transport. The secondary container is a securely sealed plastic bag labelled with the patient's information and a biohazard symbol if necessary.

All specimen bottles must be individually labelled. Using patient labels is acceptable practice except in the case of transportation of a blood sample for cross-matching purposes. Due to the potential catastrophic effect of a patient being incorrectly cross-matched, the blood bottle that has the cross-match sample in must have the patient's details handwritten on it. Failure to adhere to this requirement will render the sample as void and a new sample will need to be obtained from the patient.

This chapter provides a brief overview of pathology specimen collection and transportation. Practitioners involved in the collection and transportation of specimens must refer to local guidelines and procedures to ensure safe and effective practice.

19 Understanding X-rays

Figure 19.1   How an X-ray is performed

To take a good X-ray you need:
- A radiation source – to provide the X-rays
- Image receptor – like photographic film for a camera
- Cooperation – from both the child and the parent
- Help – from the parent to keep the child still
- A radiographer – to take the X-ray
- A radiologist – to interpret the images
- Protection – for everyone present not being X-rayed
- Communication – to work well together as a team

Image receptor
- This is a square hard box that goes next to the body part of interest
- It houses the technology that holds the image of the patient after the X-ray is taken until it has been processed and converted into an X-ray image (like a photograph before it is processed)
- As X-ray plates can be hard or uncomfortable for distressed patients who may have to lie on them the radiographer knows that speed and comfort are key!

X-ray images
- The X-rays pass through some body structures easier than others, which is why an X-ray image has different shades of grey and white areas
- X-rays pass through air most easily, and so these parts appear black
- X-rays cannot pass through dense bones, and so these parts appear white
- Body tissues between these two extremes appear grey, such as fat, muscle and blood vessels

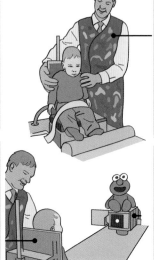

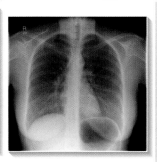

Radiation protection
- General radiation protection when taking X-rays is achieved by wearing a protective lead rubber apron
- Any person holding a patient or by standing behind a protective screen in the room, must be suitable protected
- On the ward a safe standing distance if not wearing a lead rubber apron is no less than 2 metres away from the patient
- It is important that the lead-rubber apron fits correctly, X-ray departments usually have a range of sizes available

Radiation source
- This is what generates radiation (X-rays)
- X-rays are then channelled as an 'X-ray beam' at the body part being imaged
- Light rays are used to indicate exactly where the X-rays are being channelled, like a torch
- An 'X-ray' is used to refer both to the radiation beam that passes through the patient, and the image that is generated from an X-ray machine

Advantages of X-ray
- Imaging which can be performed quickly
- As they are so quick and flexible (think about how an X-ray is taken) they account for the vast majority of imaging undertaken
- They offer a detailed image of each body part at a time

Disadvantages of X-ray
- Uses radiation to take images
- Children do not like having to lie still
- Several body parts being imaged may need a larger dose of radiation or lots of separate X-ray images
- X-rays cannot always be used during pregnancy

Figure 19.2   Types of X-ray

X-rays can be used to image several body parts, examples of which are given below. All of these techniques use X-rays in different ways. X-rays can be used in conjunction with dense contrast material to make tubes and lines appear dark on an X-ray image, such as in studies of vessels or the gut

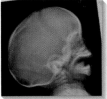

A skull X-ray in a child

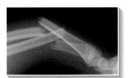

A fractured bone in a child's arm

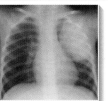

White parts of an X-ray can show abnormalities, such as infection

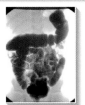

Adding a dense material such as barium helps to show the inside of the bowel, or dense contrast to show blood vessels of the hand

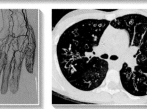

Applying several X-rays at the same time can help create a 3D image of the body (here showing the lungs) using CT

Table 19.1   Procedures and X-ray doses

	Effective dose (mSv)	Equilvalence to how many CXRs?	Equivalence to NBR (2.6mSv/yr)		Effective dose (mSv)	Equilvalence to how many CXRs?	Equivalence to NBR (2.6mSv/yr)
Chest X-ray	0.04	1	6 days	**CT Head**	2.0	50	9 months
Abdominal X-ray	0.4	10	2 months	**CT Chest**	2.5	62.5	11.3 months
Ultrasound exam	0	0	0	**CT Abdomen/pelvis**	5.0	125	22.6 months
Bladder fluoroscopy test	1.5	37.5	6.8 months	**MRI exam**	0	0	0
Swallow fluoroscopy test	1.0	25	6.8 months	**Nuclear medicine test**, e.g. kidneys	0.7	17.5	3.4 months

CXR, chest X-ray; NBR, normal background radiation dose

Children and Young People's Nursing at a Glance, First Edition. Edited by Alan Glasper, Jane Coad, and Jim Richardson.
© 2015 John Wiley & Sons, Ltd. Published 2015 by John Wiley & Sons, Ltd. Companion website: www.ataglanceseries.com/nursing/children

How do X-rays work?

Patients and their families often have questions about the risks and benefits of having an X-ray taken. Understanding X-rays is key to answering these questions.

The X-ray tube points directly at the body region of interest, which lies in contact with the image receptor, either an X-ray cassette or a digital detector. X-rays then travel from the tube through the patient and on to the image receptor. Some structures block the X-rays due to their density and appear white (bone), while air-filled structures allow the radiation to pass through and appear black (lungs). The various shades of grey in between will vary depending on the density of the structures in the image. These X-rays are extremely useful in high patient throughput areas (chest X-ray imaging) or when a speedy answer is needed to an urgent clinical question (e.g. fracture?).

What is radiation?

X-rays use ionizing radiation, which, although fairly safe in small doses, is associated with a very small increased risk of certain cancers later in life. Having a single higher dose, or repeated X-rays over time, can increase this risk. Different procedures use a different dose of X-rays, so it is important to understand the relative differences between these (Table 19.1). Radiographers need to be able to 'justify' any X-ray request as a legal requirement, to ensure that it is the best way to address the medical needs of the patient.

The importance of staying still

X-rays are taken like photographs, a snapshot in time. So a moving patient appears as a blur on an X-ray image, just like a photo. For this reason the radiographer will try to keep the patient as still when they are taking the image as possible, with the help of parents or guardians.

Children often need additional help to stay still. This can include foam pads held by a parent to keep a wriggling child's head still, a chest chair (as in Figure 19.1) can be used to hold both the cassette and the patient in a upright position when they would struggle to keep themselves upright by themselves. Other immobilisation devices may also be used in addition to the help of a holder.

Other types of imaging

Depending on what the doctor's concern is about the patient they might request different types of imaging technique.

Ultrasound uses high frequency sound waves to build an image of an organ or tissue, rather than radiation. A probe is placed over the body part of interest and the sound waves that bounce back from body structures produce an image. This is particularly useful for fluid-filled structures, such as the bladder or imaging an unborn baby during pregnancy, but cannot take pictures of air-filled structures like the lungs, or dense structures like bone.

Fluoroscopy is a method of using a steady stream of X-rays to produce a real-time video image on a monitor screen of what is going on inside a patient. Usually, an extra substance is given to the patient to make certain structures appear dense on the X-ray, such as barium or iodine. This is most useful when moving structures need to be imaged, such as in the gut, where contrast can be given by the mouth (barium swallow), or during imaging of blood vessels (angiography). Fluoroscopy can also be useful to take pictures rapidly elsewhere in the hospital, such as in theatres where a broken limb is being repaired. Using these techniques means that doctors can see the effects of their surgery immediately, or treat problems using catheters in blood vessels.

Computed tomography (CT) is a way of using several X-rays simultaneously to produce a detailed 3D image of a body part using computer software. A CT machine resembles a ring doughnut with the patient table lying in the centre. Within the CT machine are two main parts: an X-ray source and a series of detectors to capture the image. By spinning both of these around the patient, lots of images are taken which resemble cross-sections of anatomy and so are sometimes referred to as 'slices'. The advantage of CT is that it is fast and gives very detailed high quality images. The downside is the high radiation dose to the patient. For this reason, CT should never be undertaken unless clinically justified and a close eye should be kept on the number and frequency of CTs requested on any patient. Often, injections of contrast agents are used to highlight and differentiate structures on a CT scan.

Magnetic resonance imaging (MRI) machines resemble a long tube with a bed inside which a patient must pass into in order for their imaging to be undertaken. It uses no X-rays at all to produce an image, but instead strong magnetic fields are used to image tiny changes in the body's water molecules, and reconstruct these into images by computer. MRI is excellent for detecting very subtle anatomical changes, especially in soft tissues such as the brain. While ionizing radiation is not used, MRI scans can take a long time in a noisy cramped space, and this can be frightening for children. For this reason many children will be medicated to make them sleepy, or given an anesthestic.

Nuclear medicine tests use tiny amounts of radioactive material to look at how certain parts of the body work, like blood flow and activity within certain organs. This requires an injection and then the radioactivity is collected using a gamma camera, which can take a long time. For this reason, it is used only for particular tests in children, such as how the kidney functions, among others.

Pulse oximetry

Figure 20.1 Pulse oximetry

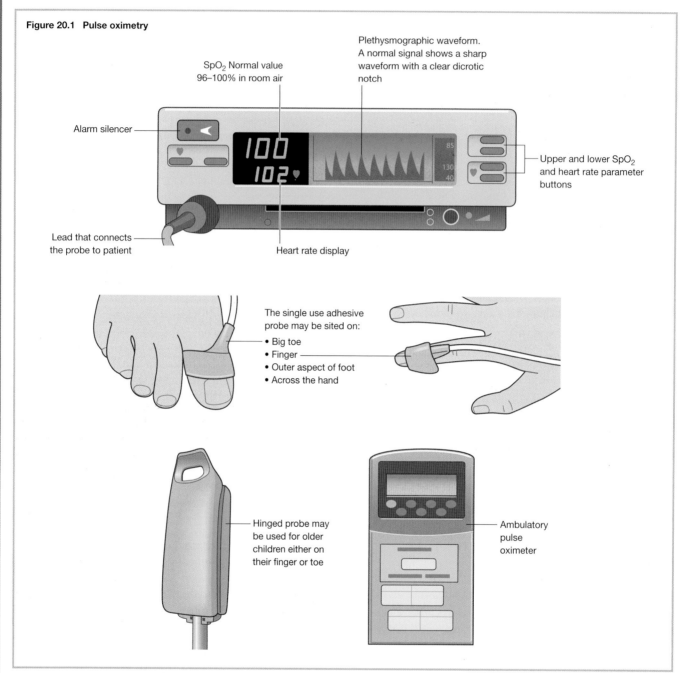

SpO₂ Normal value 96–100% in room air

Plethysmographic waveform. A normal signal shows a sharp waveform with a clear dicrotic notch

Alarm silencer

Upper and lower SpO₂ and heart rate parameter buttons

Lead that connects the probe to patient

Heart rate display

The single use adhesive probe may be sited on:
• Big toe
• Finger
• Outer aspect of foot
• Across the hand

Hinged probe may be used for older children either on their finger or toe

Ambulatory pulse oximeter

Children and Young People's Nursing at a Glance, First Edition. Edited by Alan Glasper, Jane Coad, and Jim Richardson.
© 2015 John Wiley & Sons, Ltd. Published 2015 by John Wiley & Sons, Ltd. Companion website: www.ataglanceseries.com/nursing/children

Pulse oximetry is used in both the acute care environment and the community. It is routinely used as part of the assessment of the respiratory status of infants and children by measuring the oxygen saturation of the arterial blood flow through their extremities. The oxygen saturation level is expressed in SpO_2. Advantages of using pulse oximetry are that it is non-invasive, can be used for continuous monitoring, intermittent monitoring and is accurate if the SaO_2 is >70%.

The pulse oximeter

Pulse oximetry consists of a pulse oximeter monitor which is connected to the patient by a probe. The pulse oximeter display shows the oxygen saturation of the patient, a plethysmographic waveform that indicates the pulsatile nature of the blood flow through the patient's extremities and the heart rate. The heart rate displayed is an average recorded over 5–20 seconds. There is also an audible signal that varies in pitch depending on the saturation level and heart rate level. The pulse oximeter displays a motion indicator that indicates the signal quality, thus identifying the accuracy of the saturation level and heart rate.

As pulse oximetry is based on two physical principles. First, the presence of a pulsatile signal generated by arterial blood which is reasonably independent of non-pulsatile arterial blood and, secondly, oxygenated and deoxygenated blood have different absorption spectra. The two light-emitting diodes emit red and infrared wavelengths through the tissues to a photo detector which work together. The detector measures the colour difference between the oxygenated and deoxygenated haemoglobin during each cardiac cycle so the probe requires a constant supply of arterial blood. The absorption of light by the haemoglobin is dependent on the level of oxygenation. This information is then analysed in the calibration algorithm of the microprocessor of the pulse oximeter and the estimated arterial saturation level is displayed. This is displayed as a percentage and a plethysmographic waveform. A normal signal shows a sharp waveform with a clear dicrotic notch. Movement artefact and decreased perfusion will distort the waveform.

The pulse oximeter probe

The probe is available in two types: hinged clip-on type for the older child or adhesive single use only for the neonate, infant and young child. Some probes are weight specific.

The probe consists of two parts: light-emitting diodes and a photo detector. This needs to be place where a pulse can be detected. In the infant, this will be on the big toe or the lateral aspect of the foot. For the child, the adhesive probe may be sited on the finger or big toe over the nail-bed area or across the hand. With the older child, a finger clip probe may be used on the thumb or big toe. The orientation of the nail-bed is identified on the probe by the manufacturer. The probe position should be changed on a regular basis and only secured as indicated by the manufacturer's instructions.

Indications for use and clinical application

Pulse oximetry is used for monitoring and as a screening tool in infants and children when the following are present:
- Potential for respiratory failure
- Respiratory illness
- Oxygen therapy is being received
- Haemodynamic instability
- Sedation or anaesthesia is required
- Complex surgical procedures have been undertaken
- In infants who are post surgery
- During the administration of continuous respiratory depressant medication (e.g. patient-controlled analgesia)
- During transportation of infants and children between departments or hospitals, who are at risk of respiratory compromise or who are already receiving oxygen therapy.

Limitations of pulse oximetry

Pulse oximetry has a number of limitations that the user needs to be aware of as these may lead to inaccurate readings:
- Inadequate positioning of the probe: excessive light entering straight through the photo detector may give a false high reading
- When the child has low cardiac output, hypothermia or vasoconstriction, peripheral perfusion may be impaired and as oximetry relies on detecting a pulse, it may be difficult for the sensor to detect a true signal
- When the SpO_2 is <70%. The presence of carboxyhaemoglobin which the two wavelengths of light cannot distinguish make pulse oximetery unreliable
- Elevated methehaemoglobin caused by either structural changes of iron in the haemoglobin or drug-induced as with local anaesthesia may lead to tissue hypoxia as oxygen binding to haemoglobin is inhibited
- Smoke inhalation and carbon monoxide poisoning. The pulse oximeter cannot distinguish between haemoglobin saturated with oxygen and that saturated with carbon monoxide
- Motion artefact accounts for a significant number of errors and false alarms, thus shivering can cause problems with detecting saturation level and give a false high pulse
- Use of intravenous dyes such as methylene blue can give false low readings so nurses need to know which dye has been used and its half-life.
- Presence of oedema will lead to inaccurate measurement of saturation level
- High bilirubin levels will affect the accuracy of readings
- Inaccurate readings will also occur in the presence of nail varnish and acrylic nails
- Dried blood and dirt on the skin can also effect accuracy of readings and need to be removed
- Bright overhead lighting and external light may cause overestimation of saturation level.

Key points
- Pulse oximetery is a useful non-invasive monitoring device.
- The correct sized probe needs to be used and it needs to be sited correctly.
- It may be used continuously or intermittently.
- Users need to be aware of the limitations of saturation monitoring.

Central venous devices

21

Figure 21.1 Advantages and disadvantages of central venous access devices (CVADs)

Advantages

- Easy to access
- Reduced anxiety, distress and trauma associated with treatment as less frequent venous access required
- A safer route of administration for vesicant drugs and fluids that are unsuitable for peripheral cannula infusion
- Provides long-term venous access

Disadvantages

- Permanent indwelling catheter can impact on activities and body image
- Greater risk of infection
- Care and maintenance required to maintain
- Port – needle access required

Figure 21.2 Advantages and disadvantages of each CVAD

	Non-tunnelled	Peripherally inserted central catheter (PICC)	Tunnelled device	Port
Insertion under general anaesthetic	No	No	Yes	Yes
How long will it last?	Days–weeks	Weeks–months	Months–years	Years
Needle access	No	No	No	Yes
Dressing	Yes, changed weekly	Yes, changed weekly	No	No (only when in use)
Participation in sport	No	Some with caution	Some with caution	Most
Able to go swimming	No	No	No	Yes

Indications for use – choice

- **Non-tunnelled** – more than three peripheral cannulae required; <7 days irritant solutions being administered, blood samples required, inpatient
- **PICC** – treatment therapy >3 weeks; irritant solutions being administered; patient can be discharged home between infusions or home therapy
- **Tunnelled device** – treatment therapy >1 month–years; blood samples required, irritant solution therapy, inpatient or home therapy
- **Port** – treatment therapy >1 month–lifelong; blood samples required, irritant solution therapy, inpatient or home therapy

Figure 21.3 Implantable ports

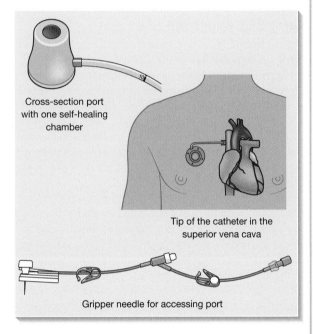

Cross-section port with one self-healing chamber

Tip of the catheter in the superior vena cava

Gripper needle for accessing port

Indications for use – treatment

- Drug administration, specifically vesicant drug therapy
- Administration of fluids/electrolytes/inotropes
- Long-term TPN administration
- Blood sampling
- Blood or blood product transfusion
- Monitoring – haemodynamic status
- Haemodialysis/haemoflitration

Figure 21.4 Tunnelled device

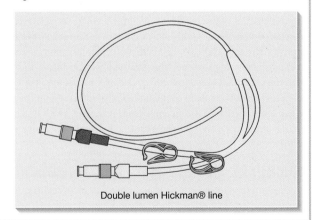

Double lumen Hickman® line

A central venous access device (CVAD) is an intravenous device that is inserted into the central circulation (Green 2008), reducing the need for frequent venepuncture or intravenous cannulation. CVADs are most commonly used for fluid or drug administration and blood sampling. The placement of an indwelling catheter (CVAD) has a crucial role in the administration of treatment to many children and young people with acute and chronic conditions, within various care settings and the home environment.

The type of device selected for use will vary according to:
- Age of the child or young person
- Type of treatment required
- Frequency of use
- Length of time treatment is required:
  - *Short term* – <7 days/weeks
  - *Intermediate* – weeks/months
  - *Long term* – a month or longer/years/indefinite.

Types of CVAD

There are four main types of CVAD:
1 Non-tunnelled devices
2 Peripherally inserted central catheters (PICCs)
3 Tunnelled devices
4 Implantable ports (Scales 2010a).

All CVADs have advantages and disadvantages, which may influence the child or young person's, the parent's or the clinican's choice of device (if appropriate) (GOSH 2013).

Non-tunnelled devices

A short-term venous access device most commonly used within high dependency and intensive care settings within the hospital environment. There are three main insertion sites:
- Internal jugular vein
- Subclavian vein
- Femoral vein (Scales 2010a).

Catheters vary in size – length and gauge – and number of lumens. The line is usually secured in place with skin sutures at the entry point, covered with a sterile semipermeable transparent dressing.

Peripherally inserted central catheters

For intermediate use, the catheter length is measured prior to insertion, and then inserted peripherally. The catheter is advanced through the vein to the required length, until the catheter tip position is located in the superior vena cava (SVC); position is confirmed with imaging. The line is secured in place usually with wound closure strips and then covered with a sterile semipermeable transparent dressing.

Tunnelled devices

For long-term use a skin tunnelled catheter, known as a Hickman® or Broviac® line, is inserted under general anaesthetic. The catheter is tunnelled under the skin for 10–15 cm before the catheter enters the vein, the skin entry site and the vein entry point therefore being a distance apart (Scales 2010b); the catheter tip position is in the SVC. Fibrosis initiated by a Dacron cuff within the device anchors the line in the subcutaneous skin tissues (Scales 2010b). Lines are most commonly single or double lumen, depending on clinical requirements of the patient, with an external clamp.

Regular dressings are not required once the catheter is secured in place.

Implantable ports

For long-term use, skin tunnelled as above, also known as Port-a-Cath® is a form of tunnelled catheter attached to a reservoir (Scales 2010b). The entire device is surgically implanted under general anaesthetic under the patient's skin. The port (chamber) is secured to the underlying tissues with sutures. Ports vary in size and are single or double chamber, depending on the physical size of the patient and clinical requirement of use. Ports are accessed with a non-coring needle – Gripper or Huber needle – which pushes through the skin and silicone septum of the port into the chamber (Johnson 2009). No regular dressing is required once the wound site has healed after insertion. A semipermeable transparent dressing is applied when the needle is *in situ*.

Accessing CVADs

All personnel who use CVADs must have knowledge, be trained and undergo competency assessment in the use and care of these devices (GOSH 2013). The child or young person and family members or carers can be taught and competency assessed as appropriate in accessing CVADs and managing treatment allowing independence for long-term treatment delivery. Before accessing any line, it is important to observe the skin–line entry site, checking for any signs of damage to the line or any attachments and, during access and administration, to observe for signs of leakage of blood or fluids, documenting findings within nursing notes as standard practice. CVADs have a needleless valved access device on the end of the lumen.

Care of CVADs

Guidelines to be followed in all aspects of CVAD care and use, before, during and after procedure(s) are to be adhered to.

General principles

- *Prevention of infection.* Thorough hand washing, decontamination of the hub or needleless device prior to accessing CVAD, maintain principles of asepsis with all equipment, and throughout procedure.
- *Maintenance of a patent catheter.* Adequate flushing, pulsating flushing, heparin flush to fill lumen between use, routine flushing, ensure line is clamped under pressure.
- *Preventing damage of catheter.* 10-mL syringes or larger will need to be used when first accessing any CVAD (GOSH 2013). Smaller syringes produce greater pressure and can result in fracture if the line is blocked.

Nurses have a key role in care of these lines. In addition to performing the practical procedures, they are responsible for the education of the child or young person and family on their CVAD.

Complications

The major risk factor associated with CVADs is of infection either to the exit site or to the line itself, with the potential for septicaemia. Infection is indicated by fever, rigors, redness and/or exudates at the exit site, and in some instances pain and/or swelling.

22 Tracheostomy care

Figure 22.1 Principles of tracheostomy care

Indications

- Upper airway obstruction including:
  – Pierre Robin sequence
  – sub-glottic stenosis
  – bilateral vocal cord palsy
  – tumours, cystic hygroma
- Ventilation insufficiency including:
  – prolonged ventilation
  – tracheomalacia/bronchomalacia
  – neurological disease
  – pulmonary disease
- Protection of the tracheobronchial tree
  – aspiration risk

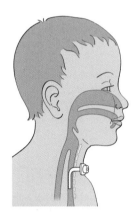

Tracheostomy tubes

An ideal sized tracheostomy tube should be two-thirds the width of the trachea with the tip at least 1 cm from the carina

There are several types of tracheostomy tubes available

Single lumen tubes are most commonly used in paediatrics

The type and size are often determined by the otolaryngologist, some options are listed below:

- Polyvinyl chloride (PVC) or silicone
- Neonatal or paediatric tubes
- Single or double lumen
- Cuffed or uncuffed
- Fenestrated or unfenestrated
- Flextend or customized

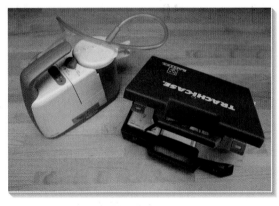

Emergency equipment

Essential equipment should accompany the child at all times.
This should be checked each shift:
- Spare tracheostomy tubes: one the same size and one a size smaller
- Suction apparatus and appropriate size suction catheters
- Scissors double round-ended, water-soluble lubricant
- Spare set of tracheostomy tapes and dressing
- Normal saline ampoules and gauze
- One-way resuscitation valve
- A cut suction catheter to act as a guide over which the new tracheostomy tube is placed in the event that the smaller size tube is unable to be passed. This has replaced the tracheal dilator in many centres
- ± Oxygen connection tubing for a tracheostomy
- ± Spare inner cannula
- ± Syringe to deflate the cuff
- ± Bag–valve mask (Ambu bag)

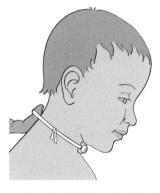

Securing the tube

- Cotton twill tapes (10 mm) securely tied are recommended for children less than 7 years
- Tapes are changed daily for children less than 1 year
- Tapes are changed on alternate days for older children
- Velcro tapes are considered in children over 7 years after a risk assessment
- It is essential that tapes are kept clean and dry as wet tapes may provide medium for infection and skin breakdown
- Rule of thumb! The tip of little finger should fit between neck and tapes with head flexed forward

The term tracheostomy refers to a surgically created opening in the anterior wall of the trachea, into which a tube is placed to provide an artificial airway. In paediatrics, a tracheostomy is performed in theatre under a general anaesthetic. Children with a newly formed tracheostomy are nursed in a paediatric intensive care or high dependency unit where staff are skilled in tracheostomy care and management. This is to ensure that children are continuously observed and monitored and early potential life-threatening events such as tube obstruction or accidental dislodgement are avoided. During surgery, the otolaryngologist will have placed 'stay sutures' at either side of the vertical incision in the trachea; these are secured on to the chest wall and clearly labelled. The purpose of the stay sutures is to assist with an early or difficult tube change. Once the first tube change has occurred, and a safe tract has been deemed by the otolaryngologist, the stay sutures are removed, after which children may transfer to a ward.

Most children have a tracheostomy placed when they are infants. The tracheostomy tube can be removed once the underlying pathology has been surgically corrected or has improved with growth. This occurs by the age of 18 months to 2 years.

The approach to care is multidisciplinary. The clinical nurse specialist acts as a resource for both parents and staff. Children who have a tracheostomy may need additional psychological support to assist them to cope with its presence. This support can be provided by the clinical nurse specialist, the play therapist or, in some instances, a psychologist. Parental education is commenced during hospitalization and parents must demonstrate competence in caring for their child's tracheostomy before discharge into the community.

Stoma and skin care

Stoma care and the skin care under the tapes are attended to daily, on alternate days or as needed in an older child. Observe the skin and stoma site for redness, excoriation, granulation tissue and dryness.

Mucus or exudate lying on the skin can contribute to skin breakdown. The stoma is cleaned using gauze squares that have been dampened with sterile normal saline. A skin protector can be applied. A specifically designed keyhole dressing can be inserted under the flange of the tube which absorbs mucus and exudate and also provides padding. The skin under the tapes is washed with warm water and a pH neutral wash; it is then rinsed and dried thoroughly. If dryness is evident an emollient is applied. Avoid products that contain small fibres, powders, creams and cotton wool which could accidently enter the stoma.

Suctioning

Suctioning should only be performed if clinically indicated and is not performed routinely. Prior to the procedure the following information needs to be established:
• *Catheter size.* The diameter of the catheter should be half the internal diameter of the tracheostomy tube
• *Depth of insertion.* The catheter is advanced to 0.5 cm past the end of the tracheostomy tube
• *Suction pressure* recommended for children is 80–100 mmHg
• *Duration of suctioning:* 5–10 seconds is recommended.

Humidification

After a tracheostomy has been formed there is a loss of filtering, warming and humidification of inspired air. Lack of humidity can lead to thicker secretions, increased risk of mucus plugging, leading to blockage of the tracheostomy tube. In the initial post-operative period, humidification is replaced by the use of a heated humidity system. Children then progress to the use of heat and moisture exchangers (HMEs); these are changed once they become contaminated with secretions. Normal saline nebulizers are administered to liquefy and loosen secretions.

Tube changes

Changing a tracheostomy tube can be a daunting procedure and may be a source of anxiety for the child, his/her parents and the personnel involved. Once the child senses a calm environment, and gains the trust of the person changing the tube, the procedure should go smoothly.

The frequency of a tube change may vary from weekly to monthly depending on the material of the tube. Two people are recommended for a routine tube change. However, in an emergency, such as blockage or dislodgement of the tube, time is of the essence and one person may have to change the tube. Signs of a blocked tube include failure to pass a suction catheter, increasing respiratory distress, pallor and cyanosis; all of which may lead to eventual respiratory arrest if not recognized and acted upon promptly by staff or parents.

Safety

While a child with a tracheostomy is encouraged to live as normal and active a life as possible, some precautions are necessary. Care must be taken to avoid water going into the tracheostomy tube or into the trachea via the stoma during bathing and hair washing. Swimming is not allowed. Care must also be taken with sand. Clothing that does not cover the tracheostomy or shed fibres should be selected. Avoidance of inhaled irritants such as cigarette smoke, pet hair, powder and aerosol sprays is advised.

Communication

As the majority of airflow bypasses the upper airway, children with a tracheostomy may have an altered ability to vocalize. Early involvement of the speech and language therapist allows the use of aides appropriate to the child's needs and abilities to promote communication. Check with the otolaryngologist if the child has a patent upper airway and is suitable for the placement of a speaking valve.

Feeding

The presence of a tracheostomy tube does not preclude oral feeding. An assessment of the child's swallow is performed by the speech and language therapist. As the majority of airflow bypasses the upper airway children with a tracheostomy have a reduced sense of smell and taste.

Complications

Early complications include tube obstruction, haemorrhage, pneumothorax, false passage and accidental tube dislodgement.

Late complications include tube obstruction, accidental tube dislodgement, haemorrhage, chest infections, supra stomal collapse, granulation tissue and laryngotracheal stenosis.

Key points
• Children are at a greater risk of tube occlusion than adults because their airways are smaller.
• Paediatric tracheostomy tubes have a single lumen.
• A blocked tube is life-threatening and requires immediate action.
• Paediatric tracheostomy care must be implemented by competent personnel.

23 Infant resuscitation

Figure 23.1 Paediatric Life Support Algorithm

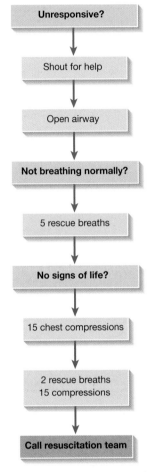

```
Unresponsive?
      ↓
Shout for help
      ↓
Open airway
      ↓
Not breathing normally?
      ↓
5 rescue breaths
      ↓
No signs of life?
      ↓
15 chest compressions
      ↓
2 rescue breaths
15 compressions
      ↓
Call resuscitation team
```

Reproduced with the kind permission of the Resuscitation Council (UK)

Figure 23.2 Correct neutral position of head for successful airway management

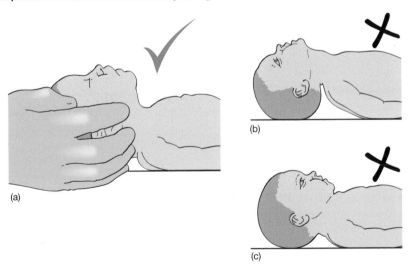

(a)

(b)

(c)

From Lissauer and Fanaroff (2011) Neonatology at a Glance, 2nd edition.
Reproduced with permission of Wiley

Children and Young People's Nursing at a Glance, First Edition. Edited by Alan Glasper, Jane Coad, and Jim Richardson.
© 2015 John Wiley & Sons, Ltd. Published 2015 by John Wiley & Sons, Ltd. Companion website: www.ataglanceseries.com/nursing/children

Cardiorespiratory arrest is an uncommon event for most child health nurses but the ability to perform the procedure effectively and efficiently is paramount. This section deals specifically with infant resuscitation (i.e. any child less than 1 year of age but not a newborn baby). This is a concise version of the full procedure offered by Resuscitation Council (UK) and all readers are strongly advised to read this guidance to ensure up-to-date practice while performing this procedure (Figure 23.1). The Paediatric Basic Life Support guidance does not include advice for the layperson and covers the actions of health care professionals with a duty of care (for the full guidance visit www.resus.org.uk).

Unresponsive – shout for help!

- Gently stimulate the infant by loudly asking 'Are you all right?' or calling the infant's name.
- If responsive, leave child in the position you find them unless the infant is in immediate danger or the airway is at risk.
- If there is no response, shout for help.

Open airway

- Turn infant on his/her back on a firm surface where you are able to be directly above the infant.
- Head tilt should be used initially by placing your hand on the forehead to gently tilt the head. While placing your fingertips on to the bony prominence of the child's jaw, lift the chin into a neutral position.
- If there is difficulty opening the airway or you are concerned about cervical injury, perform a jaw thrust.
- Place fingers either side of the infant's mandible (jawbone) and push the jaw forward.
- Do not place your fingertips on the soft tissue under the chin as you may block the airway.
    If breathing normally, place into the recovery position by:
- Placing in a true lateral position
- In a position that allows observation of the airway and drainage of any secretions
- Does not overly obstruct chest movements
- The infant should be easily positioned on to his/her back from this position if necessary.

Not breathing normally?

Once the airway is open, position the side of your face close to the infant's face.

LOOK   for chest movement
LISTEN for breath sounds
FEEL   air movement on your cheek

This should take **no more** than 10 seconds. If in doubt, assume breathing rate is abnormal and proceed with procedure.

Rescue breaths

If breathing is not normal or absent, clear the airway of any secretion or airway obstructions (do not use finger sweeps to remove obstructions) and give **five rescue breaths**.
    With the head in the neutral position:
- Take a breath and cover the nose and mouth with your mouth
- A good seal can be obtained by not overly opening your mouth and keeping your lips soft

- Blow steadily over 1–1.5 seconds until the chest visibly moves
- Maintain the neutral position while removing your mouth to watch the chest fall before applying the next breath
    If you are unable to get a good seal around the nose and mouth in the older infant you may:
- Attempt to just seal the nose or the mouth with the rescuer's mouth
- If using the nose, be sure to close the mouth while securing the airway to ensure air is not lost.

Signs of life
(should take no more than 10 seconds)
If you are confident in your ability to assess the brachial pulse, look for a pulse greater than 60 beats per minute.
    Look for signs of life:
- Movement
- Coughing
- Normal breathing not gasps, infrequent or irregular breaths.
    If you are confident that you can detect signs of circulation:
- Continue rescue breaths until the child shows signs of life
- When showing signs of life, place the infant into the recovery position and reassess.

No signs of life
Lone rescuers should:
- Compress the lower half of the sternum with the tips of two fingers. This equates to one finger breath up from the end of the sternum (xiphisternum)
- Depress the sternum by at least one-third the depth of the chest (do not be afraid to push to hard)
- Release the pressure to allow the chest to recoil
- During the cardiac compression stage you are looking for a rate of 100–120 per minute
- Compression to breath rate of 15:2
- Reassess after 1 minute, looking for signs of life.
    If **there are two or more rescuers**, then the encircling technique may be utilized:
- In the same position, compression pressure and rate as a single rescuer, place two thumbs on the lower sternum
- Thumbs should be pointing towards the infant's head.
    You must continue resuscitation until:
- The infant shows signs of life
- Further qualified help arrives
- You become exhausted.
    Get help as quickly as possible:
- If only one rescuer is present, undertake resuscitation for **1 minute** before going for assistance
- With an infant it may be possible to carry them to further assistance to minimize interruptions.

> ### Key point
> This chapter reproduces the basic life support guidance published on the Resuscitation Council's website. Practitioners are strongly advised to visit this site regularly to ensure their technique is up to date (www.resus.org.uk).

24 Young person resuscitation

Figure 24.1 Advanced Paediatric Life Support Algorithm

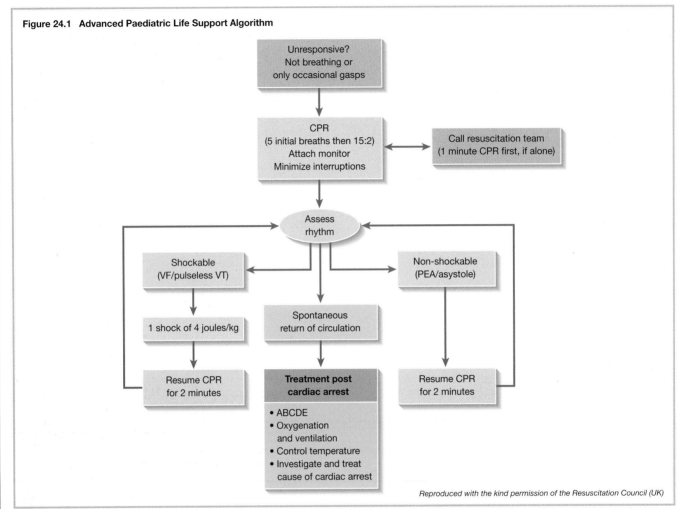

Reproduced with the kind permission of the Resuscitation Council (UK)

Children and Young People's Nursing at a Glance, First Edition. Edited by Alan Glasper, Jane Coad, and Jim Richardson.
© 2015 John Wiley & Sons, Ltd. Published 2015 by John Wiley & Sons, Ltd. Companion website: www.ataglanceseries.com/nursing/children

When involved in resuscitation it must be noted that there are differences to the resuscitation algorithm that are dependent on whether the patient is an infant (under 1 year of age), a child or young person (over 1 year of age) or if they are an adult. For the purposes of this section resuscitation is focused on a young person who is over 1 year of age.

Safe to approach

Always ensure that it is safe to approach the patient and that there are no obvious hazards.

Stimulate

Try to gain a response from the patient. This can be by calling their name or stroking their forehead or ears. If they respond, keep them comfortable and call for help. If they are unresponsive, continue with the young person resuscitation algorithm.

Shout

Shout for help and ensure that someone contacts the paediatric arrest team so that further assistance is provided.

Airway

Ensure that the mouth is clear from obstruction and then place the head into a 'head tilt chin lift' position so enable the airway to be fully opened. If there are concerns that the young person has been involved in a trauma then a jaw thrust should be performed to ensure that the head remains in a neutral position and is in alignment with the cervical spine.

Breathing

Once the airway has been opened it is important to look, listen and feel for breathing for 10 seconds. Look to see the rise and fall of the chest, listen for any breath sounds and feel for breath being expelled from the mouth and/or nose. If there is no breathing or ineffective breathing then **five effective rescue breaths** must be given. If any of the breaths are not effective then they must be repeated until the young person has received five effective breaths.

Circulation

When the five rescue breaths have been delivered, the next step is to palpate a central pulse. In the case of the young person a central pulse can be palpated at the site of the carotid artery. A pulse must be counted for 10 seconds. If there is no pulse or there is a pulse of less than 60 beats a minute then chest compressions must be commenced at a ratio of 15 compressions to two breaths. The landmark for chest compressions is two finger breadths above the xiphisternum; using the heel of the hand or both hands interlocked to deliver the chest compressions depending on the size of the child.

While cardiopulmonary resuscitation (CPR) is being carried out it is vital that a monitor is attached to the young person to determine what rhythm their heart is in and therefore if it is a shockable or unshockable rhythm.

Shockable rhythms: pulseless ventricular tachycardia and ventricular fibrillation

Unshockable rhythms: pulseless electrical activity (PEA) and asystole.

If the young person requires defibrillating the amount of energy that should be used is 4 joules per kilogram.

If the young person is in cardiac arrest, the pulse and heart rhythm must be rechecked every 2 minutes and the appropriate course of action taken.

Definitive care

It is important to note that while not all young people have a spontaneous return of circulation, some do make a very good recovery from a cardiac arrest. If a young person responds to the treatment then plans should be made for them to be admitted to either an intensive care unit on site or to another hospital where they have the expertise and facilities to care for them.

If the young person does not survive the cardiac arrest it is imperative that support services are put into place for the family to offer comfort during their bereavement and also that a debrief is carried out for all staff who were involved in the resuscitation to allow them an opportunity to discuss their feelings and the situation.

Key point
• The primary cause of cardiopulmonary arrest in young people is hypoxia. For this reason, if a young person is found unresponsive and not breathing the first action to be taken is for the rescuer to deliver five rescue breaths before seeking further help.

Red flag
• Effective ventilation and oxygenation may prevent a cardiac arrest from occurring in young people.

25 Resuscitation drugs

Figure 25.1   Uses and doses of resuscitation drugs

Adrenaline

Uses: cardiorespiratory arrest, bradycardia of <60 beats per minute after initial steps to improve oxygenation have been taken and anaphylaxis with hypotension

Dose: 10 μg/kg (0.1 mL/kg of 1:10000 solution) This can be repeated every 3–5 minutes as needed

If anaphylaxis: intramuscular adrenaline should be given (1:1000 solution)
   <6 years 150 μg (0.15 mL)
   6–12 years 300 μg (0.3 mL)
   >12 years 500 μg (0.5 mL)

Atropine

Uses: bradycardia as a result of vagal stimulation

Dose: 20 μg/kg (minimum dose 100 μg)

Oxygen

15 L via bag valve mask if not breathing or ineffective breathing or via non-rebreather mask if breathing not compromised

0.9% Sodium chloride

Uses: children in cardiac arrest or circulatory failure, or with hypovolaemia causing a circulation compromise must be given fluid resuscitation

Dose: 20 mL/kg

Glucose

Uses: hypoglycaemia

Dose: 2 mL/kg of 10% glucose followed by an infusion to prevent rebound hypoglycaemia once child has been successfully resuscitated

Amiodarone

Uses: refractory ventricular fibrillation (VF) or pulseless ventricular tachycardia (VT). If VF or pulseless VT remains after the third defibrillation shock, amiodarone should be given with adrenaline. This should then be given again after the fifth shock if defibrillation is unsuccessful

Dose: 5 mg/kg

If defibrillation was successful but VT or VF recurs, the amiodarone can be repeated and a continuous infusion commenced

Adenosine

Uses: supraventricular tachycardia (SVT). It is safe because it has a short half-life (10 seconds). Give it intravenously via upper limb or central veins to minimize the time taken to reach the heart. Give adenosine rapidly, followed by a flush of 3–5 mL normal saline

Dose: 100 μg/kg (maximum dose 6 mg) for first bolus. Second bolus can be doubled up to a maximum of 12 mg

Children and Young People's Nursing at a Glance, First Edition. Edited by Alan Glasper, Jane Coad, and Jim Richardson.
© 2015 John Wiley & Sons, Ltd. Published 2015 by John Wiley & Sons, Ltd. Companion website: www.ataglanceseries.com/nursing/children

When a child is in cardiorespiratory arrest it is imperative to ensure effective oxygenation and ventilation because the primary cause of arrest in children is hypoxia. If the child then requires drugs during the resuscitation it is important that vascular access is gained. However, the most important drug in the resuscitation of a child is oxygen.

Vascular access is essential to enable drugs and fluids to be given during resuscitation. However, venous access can be difficult to establish during resuscitation of an infant or child. If venous access is not readily attainable, early intra-osseous access should be considered, especially if the child is in cardiac arrest or decompensated circulatory failure. If attempts at obtaining intravenous access are unsuccessful after 1 minute, an intra-osseous needle should be inserted. It is also possible to administer medication via the tracheal tube, although intravenous and intra-osseous routes are much preferred. The tracheal route can be used to administer medications such as adrenaline, atropine and naloxone as they are lipid-soluble.

It is not advisable to use scalp veins during resuscitation because of the increased risk of extravasation injury. The largest possible intravenous cannula should be sited in a large peripheral vein such as in the back of the hands or feet or in the antecubital fossa. The antecubital fossa is preferred for the administration of adenosine as it is close to the heart and therefore will not take as long for the adenosine to reach the heart as it would if it was given in a vein in the hands or feet. This is particularly important because of the relatively short half-life of adenosine.

The preferred route of access in cardiorespiratory arrest in an intra-osseous needle as it is very easy and fast to insert, it allows for bone marrow to be aspirated which can be sent to the laboratory for analysis and it can be used to deliver all resuscitation fluids, medications and blood-based products.

In the event of cardiac arrest, the child or young person will require fluids as well as medications so it is imperative that they are delivered swiftly via an appropriate route of access.

The drugs and their indications for use are provided in the figure and their actions discussed here.

Adrenaline

Adrenaline is an endogenous sympathomimetic amine with alpha and beta adrenergic activity. The adrenaline causes vasoconstriction, which causes an increase in cerebral and coronary perfusion pressure. It also increases myocardial contractility, which is essential during resuscitation.

Amiodarone

Amiodarone is an anti-arrhythmic medication that increases the duration of the action potential and refractory period in the myocardium of both the atria and the ventricles. The conduction of the artioventricular node is also slowed. Amiodarone causes peripheral vasodilatation.

Atropine

Atropine blocks the effects of the vagus nerve on the sinoatrial and atrioventricular nodes which therefore increases sinus automaticity which subsequently increases the heart rate.

Adenosine

Adenosine is an endogenous nucleotide that causes atrioventricular block of a very short duration. It also prevents bundle re-entry at the atrioventricular node which is particularly useful as it is this bundle which usually causes supraventricular tacchycardia (SVT) in children.

Glucose

Glucose is the energy required by all cells in the body. Low glucose levels mean that the contractility of the heart muscle can be decreased which in turn reduces cardiac output. It is important that during resuscitation attempts the glucose level of the child or young person is recorded and appropriate action taken.

Other drugs that can be given during resuscitation include naloxone, magnesium, calcium and sodium bicarbonate; however, these are not first line drugs and therefore they are not discussed here.

26 Emergency care

Nursing children and young people requiring emergency care is a unique and challenging area of paediatrics. The emergency children's nurse has to be equipped to manage a broad spectrum of presentations ranging from a critically ill or injured child to those with more minor illnesses or injuries.

Standards for Children and Young People in Emergency Care settings (RCPCH 2012) provides health care professionals, providers and commissioners with clear standards of care applicable to all urgent and emergency care settings across the United Kingdom. Roles, responsibilities and competencies required in nursing teams are included within this paper.

Prior to the RCPCH (2012) paper, Why Children Die: A pilot study (CEMACH 2006) delivered important recommendations that can be applied to emergency children's nursing. Problems in recognizing serious illness in children were one of the key findings of the study.

The emergency children's nurse requires knowledge of other specialities in paediatrics. Many of these areas are covered in greater detail in other chapters of this book (e.g. fever, asthma, fractures, plaster care, resuscitation, PEWS, physical assessment, safeguarding, head injury and coma management).

This chapter provides a snapshot of common presenting complaints to an emergency department in relation to the developmental stages of childhood.

Nursing competency

To deliver the agenda set by the RCPCH (2012) and learn from the CEMACH (2006) report, the emergency children's nurse must have specific core competencies.

> **Core competencies required to nurse children requiring emergency care**
>
> 1 Physiological and psychological development
> 2 Taking and interpreting vital signs
> 3 Pain management
> 4 Medicines management
> 5 Management of the sick child
> 6 Management of the injured child
> 7 Mental health
> 8 Safeguarding the child and young person
> Source: Grant and Knight (2008); Royal College of Paediatrics and Child Health (2012).

The unwell baby

The unwell baby is a common presentation to an emergency department. Babies present a different challenge to the emergency nurse, and this can range from the 'worried parent', minor viral illnesses to a severely sick baby requiring critical care or resuscitative management. The children's nurse is crucial during the assessment of these babies with the assistance of a paediatric early warning score to identify severe illness and prompt escalation to the appropriate senior clinician.

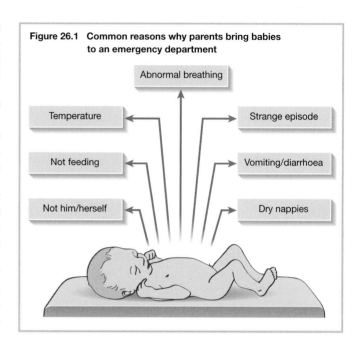

Figure 26.1 Common reasons why parents bring babies to an emergency department

Abnormal breathing

Temperature

Strange episode

Not feeding

Vomiting/diarrhoea

Not him/herself

Dry nappies

Parents are very aware of the careful balance between breathing, feeding and production of wet nappies. A change in one of these will lead to the baby being brought to an emergency department. These concerns can also be accompanied with a fever, rash or 'strange episode'. There is no way of predicting at what stage in the baby's illness they will present. Bronchiolitis, viral-induced wheeze, gastroenteritis, febrile convulsion, and oesophageal reflux are commonly diagnosed.

Common presentations in preschool children

The preschool child has endless adventures seeking out their environment during a time of rapid physical and intellectual development. Socializing with other children both aids their development and can lead to injury. Their immunity is developed by the daily sharing of minor infections. There is a predictable pattern of illness and injury of preschool children.

> **Common presentations in preschool children**
>
> - Foreign body to ear, nose or swallowed
> - Toddler's fracture
> - Clavicle fracture
> - Fingertip injury
> - Head injury
> - Minor wounds to head
> - Pulled elbow
> - Torus fracture to distal radius
> - Supracondylar fracture
> - Burn
> - Accidental ingestion
> - Fever
> - Otitis media
> - Otitis externa
> - Viral illness or rash
> - Asthma
> - Febrile convulsion

Children and Young People's Nursing at a Glance, First Edition. Edited by Alan Glasper, Jane Coad, and Jim Richardson.
© 2015 John Wiley & Sons, Ltd. Published 2015 by John Wiley & Sons, Ltd. Companion website: www.ataglanceseries.com/nursing/children

Common presentations in school-aged children

The school-aged child is more aware of their personal safety and that of others around them. They develop more responsibility for themselves and have some independence in their activities away from their parents. It is a stage when regular physical activity becomes embedded into their daily lives which influences their pattern of injury.

Commons presentation in school-aged children

- Head injury
- Clavicle fracture
- Torus fracture to distal radius
- Long bone fracture
- Metacarpal and phalangeal fracture
- Ankle injury (soft tissue and bony injury)
- Wound
- Foreign body in wound
- Animal bite
- Transient synovitis
- Septic arthritis and osteomyelitis
- Legg–Calvé–Perthes disease

Common presentations in adolescents

It can be a challenge to meet the needs of the adolescent in health care. Nursing the adolescent in the emergency department, the nurse must be aware that the 'vices' of adulthood creep into this age groups presentations.

Common presentations in adolescents

- Muscular skeletal injury
- Head injury
- Assault
- Alcohol intoxication
- Illicit drug use
- Fever
- Rash
- Abdominal pain
- Headache
- Mental health problems including deliberate self-harm and overdose
- Sexual health – including emergency contraception
- Concealed pregnancy
- Gynaecological problems
- Osteoarthritis or septic arthritis
- Slipped femoral epiphysis

Safeguarding

Safeguarding children and young people in an emergency department is core to all nursing practice. Nursing children and families not previously known, in a short period of time, requires a thorough and rapid assessment for 'red flags' to identify any safeguarding risks relating to their presentation. These are shown below.

Red flags

- Inappropriate delay in presentation
- Injury and mechanism of injury mismatch
- Immobile children with long bone fractures
- Head injury in children under 1 year old
- High frequency of attendances
- Domestic violence, alcohol, substance misuse or mental illness in the family
- Other concerns: home safety, supervision, bullying, child–parental interactions

Key points

- Receive the child to the department with warmth and allow them to play and relax.
- Get to the child's level and include them in the nursing assessment.
- Listen to the history given by the parents – they know the child better than anyone.
- Clarify with parents what the their main concern is – do not assume to know why they have come.
- Consider safeguarding risks on all children and young people.

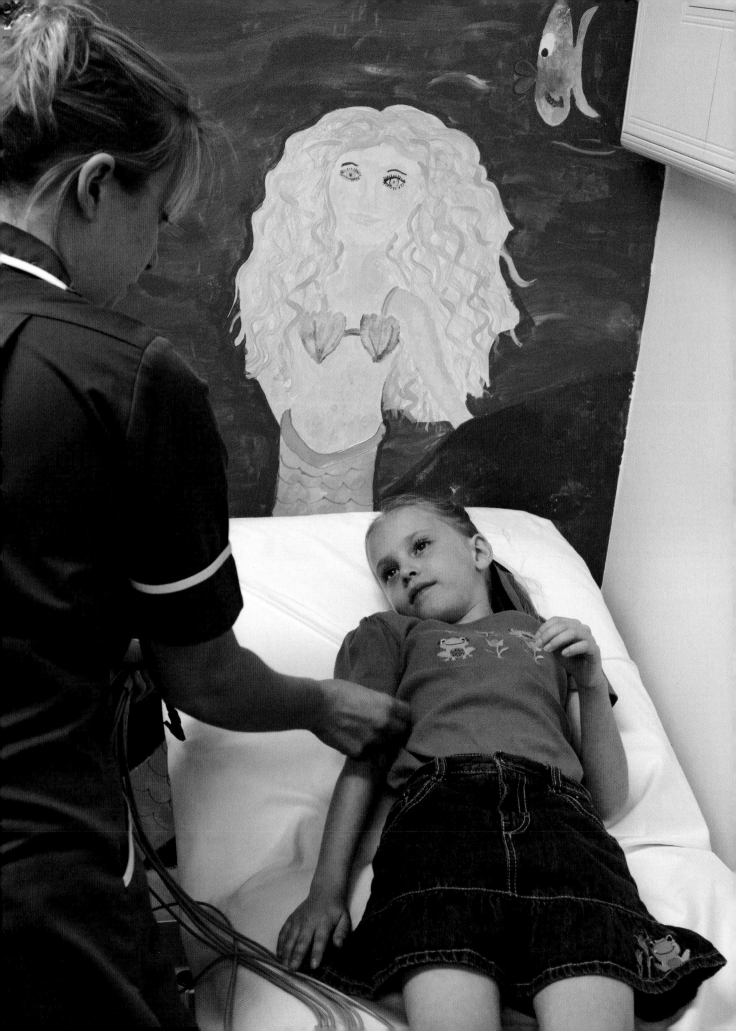

Working with families

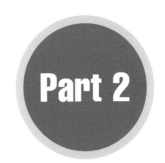
Part 2

Chapters

 Don't forget to visit the companion website for this book at www.ataglanceseries.com/nursing/children where you will find over 500 interactive multiple-choice questions to supplement your learning.

27 Partnership

Figure 27.1 Effective partnership

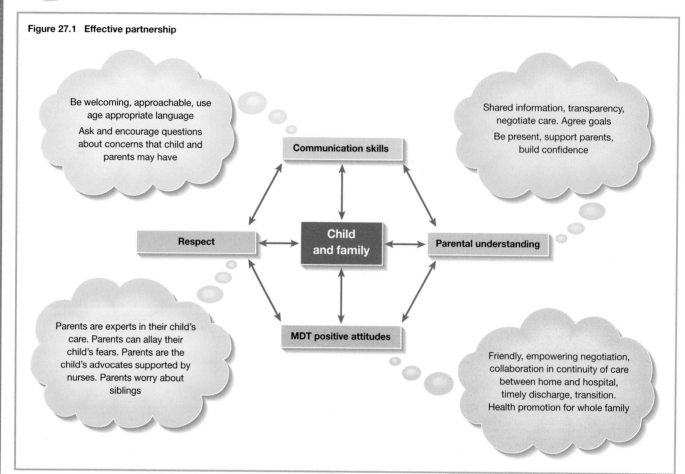

Be welcoming, approachable, use age appropriate language
Ask and encourage questions about concerns that child and parents may have

Shared information, transparency, negotiate care. Agree goals
Be present, support parents, build confidence

Communication skills

Respect

Child and family

Parental understanding

MDT positive attitudes

Parents are experts in their child's care. Parents can allay their child's fears. Parents are the child's advocates supported by nurses. Parents worry about siblings

Friendly, empowering negotiation, collaboration in continuity of care between home and hospital, timely discharge, transition. Health promotion for whole family

Children and Young People's Nursing at a Glance, First Edition. Edited by Alan Glasper, Jane Coad, and Jim Richardson.
© 2015 John Wiley & Sons, Ltd. Published 2015 by John Wiley & Sons, Ltd. Companion website: www.ataglanceseries.com/nursing/children

It is vital that nurses and the multidisciplinary team (MDT) realize that parents are the experts with regard to their child and that valuable knowledge and skills can be gained from parents regarding their child's routines.

The partnership model of care recognizes that the family are expert carers with regard to their child (Casey and Mobbs 1988). Care of the child needs to be negotiated with the child, family members and the nurse. The nurse's role is supporting, teaching and assisting the family to make informed decisions about their child's care (Casey 1995).Parents are the child's advocate and nurses provide support to ensure that the child's wishes and feelings are taken account of.

A plan of care is discussed and agreed. Direct care is carried out as planned. The nurse shares information, provides support, monitors progress and, with the family's consent, coordinates care with other professionals (Casey 1995). Parents will be concerned about the effects that hospital admission will have on the child and his/her siblings.

Effective partnership

For partnership care to be effective, nurses must have a positive attitude, respect for the family, good communication skills and an understanding of the complexity of the parents' role (Lee 2007).

Partnership and the multidisciplinary team

Nurses and members of the MDT have to be non-judgemental and work together with the family to discuss options, participate in negotiation and decision making. Noyes (2002) found that negative staff attitudes could result in the delayed discharge of children with complex care needs. Carers may feel that they are parenting in public (Darbyshire 1994) and that staff might disapprove of their family set up, cultural differences or parenting styles.

Parental stress and partnership

Nurses need to recognize that parents will have additional stressors when their child is admitted to hospital. These may be financial, personal or time pressures. Information is shared with parents to make them aware that there may be financial support available and this knowledge can reduce some anxieties (Coyne et al. 2011).

Mothers and fathers

Parents will engage in a collaborative partnership with the MDT to ensure continuity between hospital and care at home. This provides an opportunity for parents to share their concerns about how the admission of a child will affect their siblings (Shields 2001). Parents' fears can be allayed by the nurse, ensuring that the child is involved in decision making regarding his/her care. Nurses can also work in partnership with the family to ensure a timely discharge for the child as well as initiate health promotion for the family. When a child is admitted to hospital, parents can feel lonely and unsupported. Nurses need to provide emotional support before parents reach crisis point.

Parental needs

Effective partnership may be hindered by the lack of recognition of parental needs (Coyne 1995). Staff need to respect the family's social, religious and cultural beliefs (Casey 1988) and this can reduce negative interpretations. The child and parents may need to be prepared and supported to engage in partnership care prior to admission (Heimann 2000). This must be done without making the parents feel as though they are being forced to take part in the child's care. Nurses must realize that partnership is not always easy (Mountain et al. 2006). Working in partnership means that care does not have to be shared equally between the family and the nurse (Coyne and Cowley 2007). It is important that nurses realize that the amount of family participation will vary (Smith et al. 2002).

Communication

Excellent communication with the child and family is vital for partnership in care to be successful. When communicating with children, professionals need to communicate in a manner that is age appropriate and suitable for the child's intellectual ability (Hopwood and Tallett 2011). Parents need to be part of the decision-making process which keeps the child at the centre of care (Shields 2010). The MDT need to ensure that the child and family are listened to (Smith and Coleman 2010) and that they participate in the negotiation of care. Sharing information, reviewing the care plan with the family and maintaining a presence helps achieve this.

Smith and Coleman (2010) suggest that the partnership model of care continues to evolve and when effective partnership care is achieved, the child, family and nurse express satisfaction with the care that has been received.

28 Family centred care

Figure 28.1 Principles of family centred care

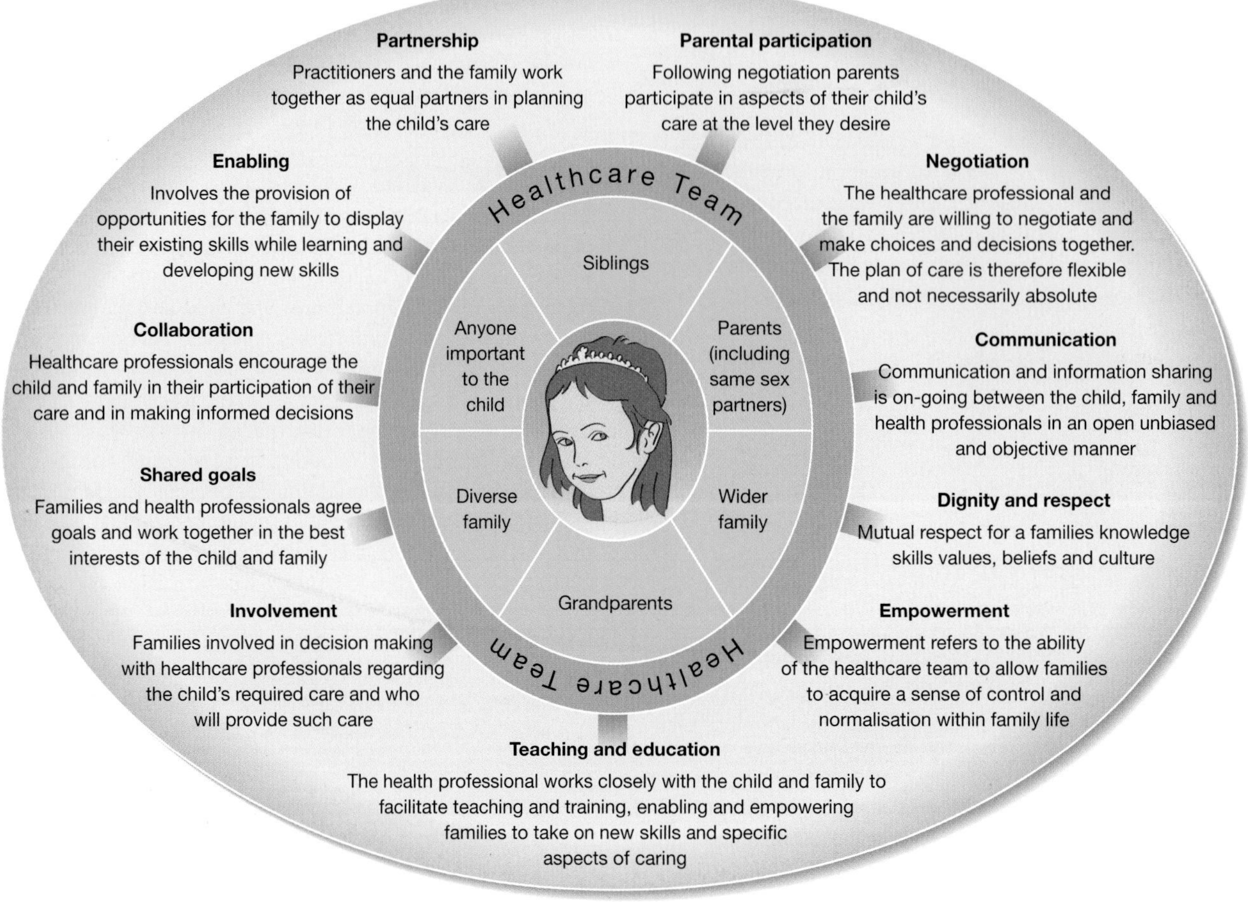

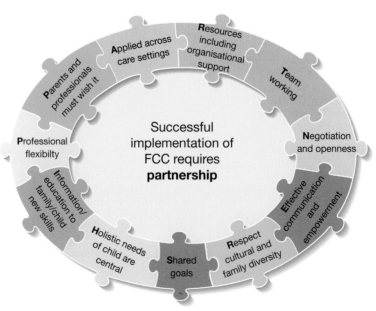

Partnership
Practitioners and the family work together as equal partners in planning the child's care

Parental participation
Following negotiation parents participate in aspects of their child's care at the level they desire

Enabling
Involves the provision of opportunities for the family to display their existing skills while learning and developing new skills

Negotiation
The healthcare professional and the family are willing to negotiate and make choices and decisions together. The plan of care is therefore flexible and not necessarily absolute

Collaboration
Healthcare professionals encourage the child and family in their participation of their care and in making informed decisions

Communication
Communication and information sharing is on-going between the child, family and health professionals in an open unbiased and objective manner

Shared goals
Families and health professionals agree goals and work together in the best interests of the child and family

Dignity and respect
Mutual respect for a families knowledge skills values, beliefs and culture

Involvement
Families involved in decision making with healthcare professionals regarding the child's required care and who will provide such care

Empowerment
Empowerment refers to the ability of the healthcare team to allow families to acquire a sense of control and normalisation within family life

Teaching and education
The health professional works closely with the child and family to facilitate teaching and training, enabling and empowering families to take on new skills and specific aspects of caring

Healthcare Team

Siblings

Anyone important to the child

Parents (including same sex partners)

Diverse family

Wider family

Grandparents

Figure 28.2 Successful implementation of family centred care (FCC)

Parents and professionals must wish it

Applied across care settings

Resources including organisational support

Team working

Professional flexibilty

Negotiation and openness

Information/ education to family/child new skills

Effective communication and empowerment

Holistic needs of child are central

Shared goals

Respect cultural and family diversity

Successful implementation of FCC requires **partnership**

Children and Young People's Nursing at a Glance, First Edition. Edited by Alan Glasper, Jane Coad, and Jim Richardson.
© 2015 John Wiley & Sons, Ltd. Published 2015 by John Wiley & Sons, Ltd. Companion website: www.ataglanceseries.com/nursing/children

Over the past six decades in the United Kingdom, family centred care (FCC) has become firmly established as a cornerstone of children's nursing practice. However, concern exists regarding FCC due to misunderstandings about what FCC is and how it can be implemented.

FCC is perceived as a philosophy of caring for children in partnership with their families, ensuring that care is planned around the unique and individual needs of the whole family. A family centred approach recognizes the family as central in a child's life and should also be central in the child's plan of care. Within children's nursing therefore, not only the child is viewed as a recipient of care, but also other family members.

While FCC embraces diversity in family structures, cultural backgrounds, choices, strengths and needs, acknowledgement exists that no single approach is right for all families.

Families and the health care team need to collaborate and work as partners in planning the child's care. Policies and organizational structures also need to be in place to successfully implement a true family centred approach. Families should be involved in decision making about who will provide the required care and negotiate whether they want to participate in care and if so at what level. Figure 28.1 shows the various components of FCC, illustrating how the health care team work in partnership with families around the child.

What is family?

At the core of FCC is the understanding that the child's family offers a primary source of support and strength, while upholding the child's best interests at all times. Family can be viewed as anyone who is important to the child and must recognize the ever-changing structure of families in society. Families can be big, small, extended or multigenerational. Families can include parents, siblings, grandparents, extended families, foster families, step families and same sex parents.

Models that facilitate a family centred approach to care

Two examples of models of nursing that help facilitate a family centred approach to care are listed here.

Casey model

Casey (1988) developed the partnership model of care, which was based on the assumption that: 'The care of the children, well or sick, is best carried out by their families, with varying degrees of assistance from members of a suitably qualified health care team whenever necessary.' Care is planned in negotiation with the families, who are considered as equal partners in their child's care. The model comprises of five components: child, family, health, environment and the nurse.

Nottingham model

The Nottingham model, developed by Smith (1995), is based on partnership and negotiation of care. Pivotal to this is the notion that the family is the client and acknowledges that care is given within the framework of the child's constant interaction in the family unit.

Advantages of family centred care
Advantages for the child
- Can improve clinical outcomes
- Reduces child's anxiety
- Promotes familiarity in an unfamiliar environment
- Reduces impact of separation in short and long term
- Supports the child in learning about and participating in their care and decision making
- Promotes an individual and developmental approach
- Supports transition to adulthood.

Advantages for the family
- Acknowledges that the family is the constant in the child's life
- Supports and empowers the family to work in partnership and make decision in relation to their child's care
- Reduces feelings of anxiety and guilt
- Increases confidence and control
- Honours cultural diversity and family traditions
- Encourages family-to-family and peer support
- Builds on family strengths and resources
- Recognizes different methods of coping
- Promotes holistic care.

Advantages for professionals and organizations
- Greater job satisfaction
- Parental insight can help in planning individualized care
- Reduced inpatient stay and associated costs
- Potential for fairer allocation of resources
- Recognizes the importance of community-based services
- Assurance that the design of the health care delivery system is flexible, accessible and responsive to family need.

Challenges of family centred care
- Individual attitudes/anxieties, knowledge and understanding
- Staff shortages/skill mix
- Surrounding environment
- Communication issues
- Lack of understanding and/or practical guidance
- Situations when family intention is not focused on best interests of child (e.g. issues relating to safeguarding)
- Limited support from organizations/policies to support FCC.

Summary
FCC has inherent advantages for child, family and health care professionals. Implementing successful FCC in practice requires **partnership**. The key prerequisites to success are summarized in Figure 28.2.

29 Family health promotion

Figure 29.1 Family health promotion

Scenario: Sue, a community children's nurse, visits Anika, a 7-year-old girl who is recovering from recent elective surgery. During the visit, Sue realizes that all the family members appear to be overweight and do very little physical activity. She therefore decides to consider how their health could be promoted. The family comprises of mum, dad, three children (aged 6 months, 7 and 9 years), their pet cat and dog. The children's maternal grandparents live approximately 2 miles away. Initially, Sue considers the positive aspects of the family's life and the things they enjoy (these are identified in the figure and discussed further in the text)

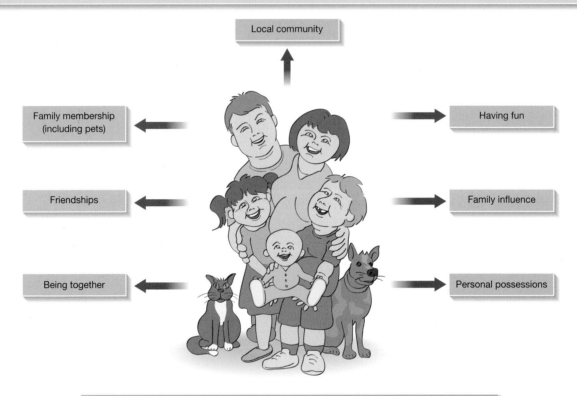

Local community

Family membership (including pets)

Having fun

Friendships

Family influence

Being together

Personal possessions

Next Sue considers the tools and approaches that she will utilize to promote the family's health

Tools for promoting family health

- Leaflets
- Posters
- Games, toys
- School, work presentations
- Magazines, comic books, newspapers
- Radio, television
- Bulletin boards
- Internet, including government and social media sites

Sue decides to visit her local health promotion unit to collect some games that the family can play together to help to promote health messages about diet and exercise

Being positive

- Encouraging family participation
- Making achievable suggestions that are engaging and fun for everyone, such as:
  1. The identification of parks where the family can go together to play and walk the dog
  2. Identification of low-cost activities such as family swim sessions
  3. The use of computer games that have a physical activity component
  4. Cooking together and learning new recipes
  5. Doing activities with other family members and friends

Benefits of a family approach

- The opportunity for the family to spend more time together
- The family works together to enhance everyone's health and well-being
- Positive reinforcement for all family members
- A healthier environment is created for the whole family, not just the person who is at risk

Acknowledgement. The authors would like to thank Rebecca Fleming and Renè Olivier for their helpful contribution to this chapter.

Children and Young People's Nursing at a Glance, First Edition. Edited by Alan Glasper, Jane Coad, and Jim Richardson.
© 2015 John Wiley & Sons, Ltd. Published 2015 by John Wiley & Sons, Ltd. Companion website: www.ataglanceseries.com/nursing/children

Most families want to be proactive in terms of enhancing health and well-being; therefore, for children's nurses, health promotion is 'about working with individuals – children, young people and their families' (Moyse 2009: 64).

The family has a fundamental role in the lives of children, not just in relation to children's growth, nurturing and development, but the family's everyday activities can influence children's health and well-being. This includes diet, exercise, alcohol consumption, smoking as well as family relationships and the impact they can have on a child's emotional health.

There can be no doubt that family structure in the twenty-first century is more diverse and complex than ever, with many children no longer living within a 'traditional' family unit. Nevertheless, children continue to be strongly influenced by the people who they have close relationships with.

Traditionally, health promotion has focused upon specific poor health behaviours – particularly areas that have the potential to be resource intensive in the long term, such as obesity and lack of physical activity. In other words, there has been a tendency to wait for a problem to develop, rather than working towards the general enhancement of health and well-being. This has been illustrated by the range of Public Service Agreements (PSAs) that have been formulated over the years (e.g. HM Treasury 2002; HM Government 2007).

Promoting family health not only provides the opportunity for a more holistic approach, but offers the opportunity to enhance the health and well-being of all family members.

What is important to the family?

There are a number of key issues that need to be considered when promoting family health; these can be termed as 'assets' as they are positive factors within family life. Morgan (2006) suggests that health assets are resources that people have that can be used to promote health and protect against ill health – this is why it is crucial to spend time identifying the areas that are particularly important to people. The following list provides some core examples.

Family membership

Family membership relates to the structure of the family and includes both blood relatives and step family members. This can mean that the family is large and complex, but it is important to identify the close relationships so that the relevant family members can work together to promote each other's health, with professional support – for example, children often have very close relationships with grandparents. In addition, family members may extend beyond the human element to embrace pets. These animals have the potential to enhance both physical and emotional aspects of health.

Being together

Families enjoy undertaking activities together so if these can be identified it will help to facilitate family engagement in health promoting activities. It is important to note that family health promotion is concerned with overall quality of life enhancement, so opportunities for families to eat meals together can be enormously beneficial from a psychological as well as a physiological perspective.

Family influence

Parents and grandparents positively influence children in relation to a range of activities. This sometimes results from their own personal interest (perhaps, for example, a father has always been an avid football supporter), motivating the parent to identify suitable sports or activity venues, the payment of the child's lessons or training and taking the child to and from the relevant classes. In addition, parents can influence their children's activities through the purchase of play equipment, toys and games consoles. Understanding both parental and the child's interests is therefore an important consideration in terms of promoting family health.

Being busy

Family life is busy and this needs to be considered if realistic suggestions are to be made (and achieved) in terms of the enhancement of family health. School, work and personal commitments all have a impact upon the family. However, a busy life has the potential to be positive as it means that there is often a clear routine, it fosters a family teamwork approach and can mean that parental work responsibilities generate more material resources, such as holidays and personal possessions – these can then promote emotional as well as physical health and well-being in the long term.

Local community

The local community has been recognized as being influential in terms of health and well-being. The proximity of other family members and friends, as well as physical resources (such as parks, swimming pools, clubs), mean that children develop a knowledge of their community. This in turn gives children self-assurance, but also allows parents to give their children some freedom within a defined set of boundaries.

Friendships

Children tend to form friendships easily, and these are highly valued across the age spectrum. Friends can be particularly influential in terms of activities undertaken, common interests can be developed and children, and their families, are able to share these. Friendships can also facilitate independence as children and young people are more likely to be allowed freedom if in the company of their peers. Positive relationships through friendships will enhance confidence and overall well-being.

Personal possessions

Our lives are undoubtedly influenced by the availability of physical resources and possessions, many of which are not only important to us, but can enhance our physical and emotional health. Identifying the possessions that families have access to will naturally influence the health promotion advice provided.

Having fun

Having fun is important to all of us and therefore there is more likely to be engagement with health promotion activities that are enjoyable. It may be more appealing for a family to attend a 'fun' swim session than a lesson. Likewise, playing 'hide and seek' in the woods may be of more interest than a running session.

The use of the areas identified could be drawn upon when working with families to facilitate understanding of different family situations. For example, Sue, the community children's nurse, had a goal to enhance the diet and physical activity levels of the family she visited. Sue could gain understanding of the family's circumstances before providing advice that is tailored to their specific needs.

Challenges to family health promotion

This chapter highlights positive approaches to health promotion within a family unit. However, it is important for the health care professional to be aware of individual challenges that a family could be facing. These could include the single parent or complex family, a family with minimal financial means, the family where one or more member has special needs or the family that simply does not wish to engage with health promotion.

However, family health promotion provides the opportunity to adopt a more holistic and positive approach that embraces the needs of several family members.

30 Communicating with children

Figure 30.1 Aspects to consider when communicating with children

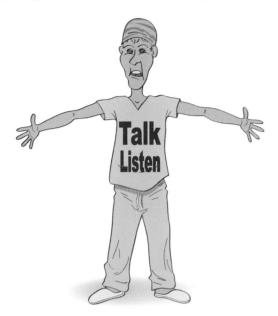

Purpose

- Sometimes it is just about talking to and interacting with children
- Establishing a therapeutic relationship
- Supporting children
- Eliciting and giving information
- Explaining procedures
- Listening to what they want to tell us
- Obtaining information about how they 'are feeling' to help with diagnosis

When to talk and when to listen

- Circumstance will dictate when to talk or listen but being aware of the child's needs are paramount
- Talking and questioning may be needed to elicit information
- Adopting an active listening approach is important when working with young people with mental health or social problems
- Active listening when hearing disclosures about abuse

Children and Young People's Nursing at a Glance, First Edition. Edited by Alan Glasper, Jane Coad, and Jim Richardson.

Communication with children and young people is both simple and complex, requiring the nurse to have a repertoire of skills to interact effectively. Many factors influence how, when and why the practitioner will communicate with children and much of this is equally influenced by the presence of parents or other main carers. Nurses use a range of skills in providing care for children but communication is the crux of much that we do and is the basis for demonstrating compassion. The wide range of arenas in which children's nurses work means that an equally wide range of skills and techniques are needed to meet specific situations and some of these are considered here.

Factors influencing communication

One of the most obvious and crucial aspects of communication is the age of children, which determines their level of development. These two issues clearly determine how children communicate and understand those communicating with them.

Children

Until they are about 8 years old, children differ markedly in how they understand and communicate, ranging from the cry of babies to the more complex language of a school-aged child. Communication abilities emerge through psychomotor and cognitive development such that the nurse should have a grasp of when and in what format children will usually communicate. Reference to speech and language charts can help to identify at what age a child can achieve certain skills such as pronouncing their first words through to when they can formulate sentences. This knowledge would be helped by an awareness of the stages of development theorized by Piaget, Vygotsky and Kohlberg. Thus, when communicating with children, the following principles are useful:

• Reflect on your professional style, attitude and behaviour when communicating with children and their families.
• Infants rely on cry as their communication but respond to touch, voice and facial gestures, particularly from the mother. Responding to these forms in a similar way enables communication directly with the infant and this can be important when the parent is not present.
• Non-verbal communication and cues are important to children and they will identify and respond to these so the nurse should be aware of how they project what it is they are trying to say and do.
• As children develop verbal language there is increasing use of words, phrases and sentences. However, they may not understand what these mean so testing these out can help in communicating with children.
• Being aware of developmental concepts to understand what children are likely to understand at specific ages.
• Children need time and clear appropriate explanations in order to understand communications, which can often be about doing things to them.
• Recognizing the impact of the situation and the status of the child on their ability to understand what you are trying to communicate.

• Be aware of children's inability to communicate verbally because of disabilities, developmental delays or traumatic scenarios and adjust your approach to meet their needs.
• Children may change their style of interaction, being passive or active, which the nurse needs to be aware of when communicating.
• Adopting the SOLER approach (face people Squarely; Open body shape; Lean forward slightly; Eye contact; Relax).
• Be prepared to come down to the child's level (e.g. sitting on the floor) when communicating directly with them.
• Use different approaches such as play, humour or drawing to engage with children.

Young people

Communicating with young people over the age of 12 years requires not only a different approach, but the use of specific skills suited to their circumstance and the way in which they talk. This is particularly important for the 16+ age group who may be adopting adult behaviours and language. Young people often communicate using their own codes of language, through different media and in a style which 'adults' do not understand. This is deepened through the influence of peers, the media, subcultures and, more recently, gang membership. Despite all this young people have the same needs for communication as other age groups but a crucial issue for them is to be listened to. We should listen to how they want to be communicated with and also the nurse sometimes needs to just listen – active listening is thus a crucial skill. Not attempting to adopt their language style is preferable, as communication can then become meaningless. In addition, the young person's sense of self means that the nurse should be aware of respecting personal space and adopting non-oppressive body language when interacting. The need for careful, clear and informative explanation is important as they may portray an attitude that suggests they understand when they do not.

Communicating in specific environments

While these approaches are useful when communicating with most children, there will be circumstances where this has to be altered to specific situations:

• Children undergoing procedures may be anxious, frightened and defensive so verbal and non-verbal communication is aimed at providing appropriate, supportive and calming explanations.
• Undergoing surgery is a frightening prospect for children and their families. Preparing them through age and developmentally appropriate language as well as using alternative methods such as play, puppetry, drawing and music may be needed.
• Children involved in trauma may be frightened as a result of the injury, what is happening and being movement restricted where spinal injuries are concerned. Non-verbal behaviour is crucial in supporting the child and here therapeutic touch can be important. Explaining clearly and within eyesight of the child enables them to understand some of what is occurring.
• Young people with mental health issues may require communication that is therapeutic while inquisitive in terms of establishing problems and adverse situations.

31 Hospital play

Figure 31.1 Hospital play

Having a Health Play Specialist or another member of staff dedicated to leading and facilitating play in hospital offers many benefits to the child, family and hospital staff

Play provides a link to home, aids normality and enables the child to fulfil medical requirements in an enjoyable way, reduces stress and anxiety, and facilitates communication

The National Association of Health Play Specialists is a charity that promotes the physical and mental well-being of children and young people who are patients in hospital

An appropriate method of play should be selected, depending on the age and ability of the child

When children or young people are admitted to hospital, they are at their most vulnerable. They are not only ill, but are also separated from their friends and familiar surroundings. Play can really make a difference

Play is at the very centre of a healthy child's life. From the earliest age, playing helps children to learn, to relate to other people and to have fun

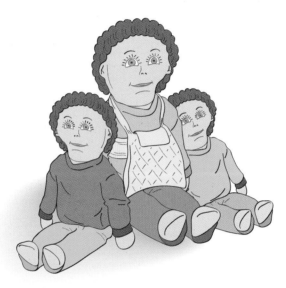

Timing of play preparation should be carefully considered. Younger children may not be able to retain the information if given too far in advance whereas young people may benefit from preparation a few days before the procedure to allow them time to process it and develop any coping strategies

The role of the Play Specialist is to help children master and cope with anxieties and feelings using a variety of techniques, use play to prepare children for hospital procedures, support families and siblings, contribute to clinical judgements through their play-based observations and to act as the child's or young person's advocate

It is important to gain as much information from parents as possible at admission with regard to the child's special toy and any special vocabulary they may have. In addition, it is important to take into account any previous experiences the child may have had in hospital

All children's nurses should be able to assess a child's stage of development and level of understanding which should be taken into consideration when giving a child information they need to be able to cope with a hospital procedure. This is because, for children, hospitals are filled with strange sights and sounds

Children and Young People's Nursing at a Glance, First Edition. Edited by Alan Glasper, Jane Coad, and Jim Richardson.
© 2015 John Wiley & Sons, Ltd. Published 2015 by John Wiley & Sons, Ltd. Companion website: www.ataglanceseries.com/nursing/children

What constitutes hospital play?

Therapeutic hospital play techniques can be hugely beneficial to all members of the multidisciplinary team. However, the techniques used are not often understood and therefore rarely used unless a Health Play Specialist is present to provide or facilitate such techniques. Play is essentially the language of children; through play they are able to learn about their environment and themselves.

Hospital play provides opportunities to:
• Provide a link to home – by allowing 'normal' play, children are able to act out scenes from home (i.e. role play) and remember things from home that they may not have seen for some time (i.e. photos and sound games). This is particularly important for long-stay patients or babies who have never been at home
• Aid normality
• Boost or regain confidence and self-esteem and allows children to take some control back into their life. This could include giving the child an active part in their treatment; for example, choosing to have oral medication in liquid or tablet form.
• Minimize regression
• Improve concentration skills
• Enable the child to fulfil medical requirements in an enjoyable way
• Act as an outlet for emotions – gives children the opportunity to express their feelings, frustrations and tension in an appropriate manner. For example, a child in traction might like to play with balloons, Velcro darts or play dough to release tension
• Reduce stress and anxiety
• Facilitate communication
• Enable information to be passed on in an appropriate and enjoyable manner – empowering the child and enabling informed consent
• Adapt games and activities for all children, whatever their needs
• Aid all areas of development
• Encourage parents and siblings to be involved
• Provide often much needed boundaries. Without a 'normal' routine and in unusual circumstances boundaries are slackened or lost completely leaving children feeling unsure and out of control
• Aid compliance with medical procedures
• Help to divert thoughts which occupy and stimulate minds (distraction therapy), and provide fun – escapism!

Effects of a hospital admission

Every child responds to hospitalization in a different way, some will sail through, seemingly unaffected, while others will experience high levels of anxiety, distress and other long-term effects. Hospital Play and Health Play Specialists can help avoid the negative aspects of hospitalization:
• Loss of concentration
• Affect on relationships with peers and siblings
• Temperament changes due to loss of boundaries and control

• Loss of 'normal life' and what it entails (e.g. home, school, friends)
• Loss of confidence and self-esteem
• Possible regression educationally and socially
• Poor coping techniques when faced with strong feelings of fear and anxiety
• Development of phobias.

Children are likely to be concerned about a hospital admission. Not only are they worried about physical pain they may have to endure, but they are also being confronted with a situation they are likely to know little about. Fear of the unknown will play a major part in the child's anxiety levels and illustrates the importance of preparation, sharing information and addressing any misconceptions at the earliest opportunity.

Role of the hospital play specialist

• Ensure a child friendly environment
• Organize suitable activities and events
• Promote child development and minimize regression
• Develop and execute individual play programmes
• Work as a part of the multidisciplinary team
• Promote and teach others the value of hospital play
• Contribute towards clinical judgements
• Work with child psychologists as required
• Facilitate informed consent and assent
• Use therapeutic play techniques to support children and their families – such as preparation, distraction and post procedural play
• Help children master and cope with anxieties
• Be a child's advocate.

Stages of hospital preparation

• *Pre-admission.* Preparation for hospital should begin in the home and there are many books and multimedia formats to help parents. Hospitals should ideally offer pre-admission visits and preparation programmes. Some of these can be in the format of online virtual tours which take the child through the stages of the hospital admission.
• *On admission.* At this stage it is important to develop trust with the child and to ascertain what toys, games or hobbies the child has and any special vocabulary they may have. In addition, it is important to take into account any previous experiences the child may have had in hospital. This period can be used by the Play Specialist to assess the child before any procedures are carried out, for example, dolls can be adapted and used to prepare children for procedures. Dolls made from calico are easy to make.
• *During and after procedures.* Distraction techniques can be used to divert attention, help children to cope and aid compliance. Post procedural play is important and this should always be offered to the child routinely and can take practically any form and should include praise, certificates and or stickers. This form of play allows children to evaluate the procedure or experience by examining the positive and the negative aspects.

32 Role of the community children's nurse

Figure 32.1   Role of the community children's nurse

- The changing epidemiology of child health has resulted in a reduction in infectious disease and an increase in the numbers of children who live with a chronic illness
- Children with a chronic illness are more likely to be hospitalized, and repeated hospital admission can be detrimental to their psychological and physical health
- Provision of care at home by community children's nurses (CCNs) is less stressful to children and facilitates normality for the child and family
- The CCN is a knowledgeable practitioner who supports and empowers children to become competent to manage their chronic illness at home

- CCNs need good communication skills when working with children and families
- The CCN needs to develop a relationship with the child and family
- Children want CCNs who are kind, happy and show an interest in their lives
- The CCN teaches children technical skills so that they can maintain their own health

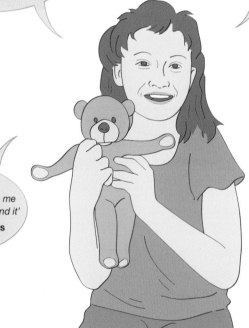

'I do my injections since the start X (CCN) taught me and she gave me a bear and I was squirting water into it'
Rhianon aged 11, diabetes

'I get the nurses every week they talk to me and say did you have a nice Christmas and what did you have for Christmas?'
Ellie aged 8, leukaemia

'I can tell her anything and anything and she will give me solutions of how I can get around it'
Rhianon aged 11, diabetes

Prevalence of chronic illness in childhood

There is no definitive definition of chronic illness in childhood. However, there are certain aspects that are included in most definitions: a condition that has lasted for longer than 3 months that affects the child's physical, cognitive, emotional or social well-being, and incurs periods of exacerbations that require hospitalization.

There remains a lack of robust and comprehensive data on the prevalence of chronic illness in childhood. The most common chronic illness in childhood is asthma. It is estimated that there are 1.1 million (1 in 11) children receiving treatment for asthma in the United Kingdom. Diabetes is also regarded as a significant chronic condition which can lead to disability and premature death if it is not managed well. The current estimate of type 1 diabetes in children in the United Kingdom is 1 per 700–1000. Cystic fibrosis is the most common genetic condition affecting Caucasian children. The incidence is 1 per 2500 births. Childhood cancer is relatively rare, affecting 1 in 10 000 children in the United Kingdom each year. The most common diagnosis is leukaemia.

Benefits of home care for children with a chronic illness

Home care is an alternative to hospitalization where children can receive nursing care at home provided by suitable qualified community children's nurses (CCNs). Compared with hospitalization, receiving care at home is less stressful for children, more conducive to family life and provides a better environment for children to recover. Home care is more convenient for children and their families as it can fit in with their daily routines. Home care is also less restrictive and costly for families compared with care in hospital as less time is spent travelling to hospital.

When receiving care at home children with a chronic illness can maintain normality within their lives by attending school, and going out with friends and family. Children prefer to be cared for at home as they find hospital boring, and suffer from homesickness. However, in their own home they can play with their own toys, sleep in their own bed, eat family meals, and be surrounded by their family and friends.

Receiving care in the familiar surroundings of their own home supported by the CCN, family, and friends improves children's quality of life.

Role of the community children's nurse

CCNs are registered children's nurses with a community nursing qualification. It was recommended by the Royal College of Nursing in 2009 that the provision of holistic care to a child population of 50 000 requires 20 full-time CCNs. However, research shows that there are still children in the UK who are unable to access care from a CCN. The provision of nursing care to children in their own homes by the CCN facilitates early hospital discharge, promotes independence and aims to provide continuity of care for sick children and their families.

The skills of the CCN are complex and multifaceted and incorporate clinical nursing skills such as administering medication, for example giving intravenous drugs, taking blood samples, wound dressings and teaching. The CCN also needs to possess more tacit skills so that they can listen, support and empower children and their families to manage chronic illness at home.

There are certain characteristics that children look for in a CCN: a happy disposition, respectfulness and empathy. Children want to be cared for by CCNs who provide more than just clinical care, they expect them to be interested in their everyday lives, and be willing to listen about issues that are important to them. Children want to be valued for who they are, they want to be seen as individuals in their own right and to be cared for by professionals who do not provide care that is solely based on their nursing needs. The initial contact with the CCN is of particular importance as it provides the foundations for the development of a trusting supportive relationship between the child, family and the CCN.

Vital aspects of the role of the CCN include assessment, teaching, management, advocacy and the facilitation of independence in children with a chronic illness. To gain independence, children require education about their condition and to learn the skills necessary to maintain their health. The CCN has the knowledge and expertise to teach children the skills they require to become self-caring. For example, children with type 1 diabetes need to master injection techniques, and take blood samples to record blood sugar levels. However, to become self-caring children also need to assimilate knowledge and understanding about normal blood sugar levels, what constitutes a healthy diet and how to manage diabetes in the event of a hypoglycaemic or hyperglycaemic attack if they are going to successfully manage their illness and make autonomous decisions about their health.

The CCN also supports and educates parents to care for children with a chronic illness. Effective partnership working between the CCN and parents is essential. Caring for a sick child can have physical and social implications for parents such as tiredness, stress and social isolation. However, the CCN can support parents by coordinating the child's care, providing them with information about their child's needs and ensuring that parents are aware of all the services that are available to them.

To become self-caring, children with a chronic illness need to go through a period of transition. This means that the day-to-day responsibility for the child's health needs transfers from the parents to the child.

Receiving care from a CCN can be seen to empower children to become self-caring individuals who can manage their condition themselves with the help and support of their family. Children with a chronic condition and their families have a better quality of life when cared for at home supported by CCNs with the relevant expertise.

33 Collaboration with schools

Figure 33.1 Hints and tips when engaging with schools and colleges

- Engage other local health professionals: GPs, school nurses, ambulance service, emergency department staff, play specialists. It is helpful to offer variety of professional experiences to share with the children and young people
- Introduce professionals to children and young people and encourage the children and young people to introduce themselves too
- Find out what the children and young people already know about health and health services – listen and value their experiences and contributions. Many will have either personal experiences or family members and friends who use health services
- Use the available resources (e.g. NHS Institute Primary or Secondary School Lesson Plans) which include interactive activities such as the NHS song, films and scenario cards (www.institute.nhs.uk)
- Signpost to other NHS services (e.g. NHS Choices, www.nhs.uk; and NHS Careers, www.nhscareers.nhs.uk)
- Gather and encourage feedback about local NHS services to assist in improving local services. Introduce websites such as www.patientopinion.org.uk
- Follow up with a letter of thanks to maintain links to secure assistance for future engagement and participation activities

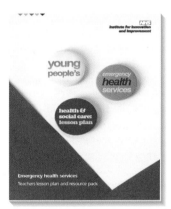
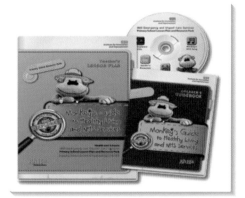

Examples of national resources available to support collaboration between health and education

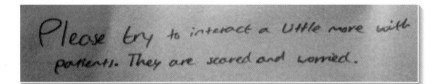

Children and young people repeatedly feedback that no-one shares information or educates them about the NHS until they are unwell, yet when they are given information and education they can make informed decisions about their health and health care. The NHS is seeing an ever-increasing and, some would argue, unsustainable demand on its services. For example, there is increased attendance at emergency departments (ED) and it is estimated that 40% of ED attendances could be avoided but there is limited public awareness about the range of health care services and alternatives available (NHS Institute 2010a). Engagement with children, young people and families identified that schools would be the ideal location to address these challenges. Schools offer an environment to educate and engage children and young people regarding health, while also informing education staff about NHS services. The Children's Outcomes Forum (Department of Health 2012) reinforced this, highlighting that schools are very important places in which children's and young people's health and well-being can be supported and improved, publishing a guide for school governors to assist them in holding schools to account regarding the physical and emotional health and well-being of their pupils.

The NHS cannot expect children and young people to come to the NHS to share their views and experiences. Health care providers need to be innovative and go to them in environments where they are comfortable and secure. Partnerships with schools provide an ideal environment, and offer input from education professionals who are experts in communicating and engaging with a wide range of children and young people.

The health agenda sits within the personal, social, health and economic (PSHE) element of the curriculum, which aims to help children and young people deal with the real-life issues they face as they grow up. The issues that PSHE education covers are central to children and young people's well-being: nutrition and physical activity; drugs, alcohol and tobacco; sex and relationships; emotional health and well-being; safety; careers; work-related learning; and personal finance.

Collaboration between education and health professionals within the PSHE curriculum therefore offers a perfect opportunity to extend current health input:
• Help children and young people understand personal actions they can take to promote their own health and well-being
• Encourage children and young people to identify how to access the different health services available to them
• Enhance the knowledge of education staff regarding health and well-being and health services
• Help health professionals develop a culture of continuous involvement with existing and potential young service users.

Children's Outcomes Forum (Department of Health 2012) states that schools should draw on the support of health services and engage with local health partners. Active engagement of health professionals in secondary and primary schools in addition to the contribution of school nurses can result in enhanced relationships with local GPs, pharmacists, practice nurses, emergency services, community and acute paediatric teams. Positive engagement and dialogue with children and young people about health services and the choices available to them can help encourage a change in their health care seeking behaviour and relieve the strain on an over-burdened NHS (NHS Institute 2010b).

The NHS Institute for Innovation and Improvement has co-produced Emergency and Urgent Care Lesson plans and suites of resources for 5- to 11-year-olds and 11- to 14-year-olds to support health and education in embedding this information in schools. Children and young people, health and education have all been partners in the design, testing and implementation of these resources to ensure they are fit for purpose, addressing acute and chronic health care, emotional and well-being needs. The lessons contain health information about self-care, community services and using emergency services wisely. They contain a range of activities about common scenarios aiming to stimulate discussion about personal experiences regarding health care and prompt further investigation about local health care services. Evaluation of the resources demonstrates that children and young people highlight the value of relationships with visiting health professionals and education about health and well-being, stating that until this point nobody had taught them about the various health services available and when to use them. Demonstrable benefits of close collaboration include the development of high quality signposting information to children and families, in school diaries, which highlight the range of services available to families, such as the role of the local pharmacist and ChildLine in promoting emotional health and well-being (NHS Institute 2010b). Structured resources such as these introduce children to language of health care, local services and mechanisms for providing feedback to the NHS about their experiences while within a familiar environment.

The NHS Constitution (2012) stresses that patient and public involvement should be part of the fabric of the NHS. Collaboration between health services and education can ensure that children and young people are actively engaged and participate in enhancing their own health and use NHS services appropriately. The influence of children and young people within their own families and also as future parents and users of services should not be underestimated, to do so would be at our peril.

34 Family information leaflets

Figure 34.1 Developing family information leaflets

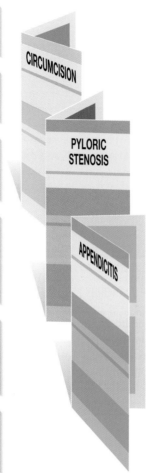

The children's nurse has a critical role in ensuring that children and their families have access to adequate high-quality information

Written communication has major advantages over verbal information because verbal information is quickly forgotten

Four key information points in the journey for the family with a hospitalized child have been identified: pre-admission, on admission, during hospitalization and after discharge

Writing a patient information leaflet at first glance appears easy, but it cannot just be written during a lunch break on a laptop computer and printed out. Although design is made easier with commercially available desktop publishing software, the contents require rather more skill

Readability formulae that allow writers to orientate their productions, such as information leaflets, at the right level, should be utilized. Remember, the average reading age in the UK is the level of a 9-year-old child (i.e. Key Stage 2, primary-school level)

Information should be based on the best and most up-to-date evidence and, importantly, be offered to families as a summary of the evidence in a way that is comprehensible to them

The internet has now become a significant resource for the dissemination of information, especially for children and young people

The dramatic increase in households with access to the internet will inevitably change the information-seeking behaviour of individuals and families. The rapid pace of change will challenge health care providers to seek new and innovative ways of harnessing the internet to meet the growing aspirations of health care consumers

The Children First for Health website, developed by Great Ormond Street Hospital and available through hypertext links on many other hospital websites, is a very good example of a kite marked one-stop information shop for families, children and young people (www.childrenfirst.nhs.uk/)

Multimedia methods of giving information (SMS messaging, Facebook, etc.) especially via the internet are invaluable. Information about treatment and care should therefore be offered in a selection of media formats, be given in individual stages and reinforced over time. Written information is still crucial to family empowerment but may not answer all the questions the child or family member may have about a condition or hospital stay, particularly if not well designed

The 'frequency of grammar' (Fog) Index is one of the best known readability formulas. It measures the level of reading difficulty of any document. The formula for the index is as follows: (find the average number of words per sentence by dividing the total word count by the number of sentences) + (number of words of three syllables or more) multiplied by 0.4 = Fog index. The Fog Index level 'translates' the number of years' education a reader needs to understand the material. The 'ideal' score is 7 or 8; anything above 12 is too complicated for most people

Children and Young People's Nursing at a Glance, First Edition. Edited by Alan Glasper, Jane Coad, and Jim Richardson.
© 2015 John Wiley & Sons, Ltd. Published 2015 by John Wiley & Sons, Ltd. Companion website: www.ataglanceseries.com/nursing/children

Families need information to help them make informed decisions about the care of their children. Efforts should be made to ensure that consistent advice and information is given to parents and carers, children and young people across different care settings and agencies, and in forms that are accessible. Good quality health information and education enhances patient cooperation and compliance with health care regimes. Additionally, good information may reduce their stress and anxiety, making it possible for the child and family to cope better with the procedure or experience.

Printed information may not answer all the questions the child may have about a condition or hospital stay, particularly if they are not well designed.

Giving information to some family groups can be especially challenging:
• Those with low literacy
• Young children and adolescents
• Those whose first language is not English
• Individual children with learning disabilities and special needs may require materials that have been specially developed.

Writing patient information leaflets

• Who is it aimed at (child or carer or both)?
• Know the setting under which the target audience will read the leaflet
• Know your purpose: ensure the information is relevant
• Know your subject
• Involve your audience
• Get support in order to produce the leaflet.

Consider the content and style of the leaflet

Make sure the title of the leaflet is clear.
• Use friendly everyday language and plain English
• Use clear and concise writing, keeping things brief and to the point
• Use short sentences (an average of 15–20 words)
• Avoid jargon or abbreviations
• Translate or explain essential terminology
• Use friendly language and give the reader a sense of ownership by using words such as 'we', 'you', 'your'
• Ensure information is accurate and up to date
• Be evidence based where appropriate
• To ensure a 'shelf-life' for the leaflet, avoid the use of names of staff where possible and use job titles instead
• Be sensitive to religious, cultural, ethical and gender issues
• Explain where the reader can obtain more information such as useful websites, organizations, PALS, etc.
• Always give contact numbers
• Think about the questions that the reader is likely to ask. Have you answered them?
• Clearly state the date the information was produced and when it will be reviewed.

Use the 10 principles of clear writing

1 Keep sentences short
2 Use simple, rather than complex explanations
3 Use familiar words where possible
4 Avoid unnecessary words
5 Put action into verbs used
6 Write like you talk
7 Use terms your reader can picture
8 Link in with your readers' experience
9 Use a wide variety of writing techniques
10 Write to express, not impress.

If your leaflet includes treatment information it should contain the following information:
• An explanation of the procedure: remember parents may be very anxious
• An explanation of the reason for consent
• An explanation of the risks as well as the benefits
• An explanation of any of the alternatives including non-intervention; if there are no alternatives that would be as effective, this should be stated
• Any areas of uncertainty surrounding the treatment
• An explanation of the effects of treatment on the quality of life of the child
• An invitation to ask questions about any areas of uncertainty.

Consider the order of the information in your leaflet

The order of your information is very important. It should reflect the child's health care journey and events and experiences the child or young person will encounter. For example, include what will happen before and after a procedure. Test the text of your leaflet by asking for peer review from critical friends and ensue that the leaflet complies with the Disability Discrimination Act of 1999.

Producing the leaflet

The leaflet should look professional and reflect a high standard of care provided. It should also be accessible to parents and children. T are a number of ways this can be achieved:

Pay attention to the layout of your leaflet:
• Use plenty of spaces so the page looks clean and uncluttered
• Avoid large blocks of text: use short separated blocks
• Use headings to break up text
• A question and answer format can help to divide up text
• Use bullets or numbering to make important information stand out
• Use bold type for headings and for emphasis. Use UPPER CASE letters
• Use italics and underlining sparingly as they make the text more difficult to read
• Align all text and subheadings to the left (justified text is harder to read)
• Font size: minimum 12 point. Use 14 point if you are writing information for visually impaired people
• Use Arial or Frutiger font only. Times New Roman is particularly hard to read by visually impaired people and therefore should not be used
• Do not write text over pictures or a design.

Key point

If the leaflet is for NHS purposes, the NHS organization has specific guidance or standards for producing patient information in line with the standards set for the NHS brand (see www .nhsidentity.nhs.uk).

35 Safeguarding

Figure 35.1 Timeline of legislation and guidance on legislation

- Children and Young Persons Act 1933
- Sex Offenders Act 1997
- Children Act 1989
- The Children Act (1989) England and Wales
- The Children (Northern Ireland) Order 1995 and the Children (Scotland) Act 1995 share the same principles and have their own Guidance
- Department of Health (2000) Framework for the assessment of children in need and their families (non-statutory guidance)
- Department of Health, Social Services and Public Safety 2003 Cooperating to Safeguard Children
- Female Genital Mutilation Act 2003
- Domestic Violence Crime and Victims Act 2004
- Sexual Offences Act 2004 (2008 for Northern Ireland, 2009 for Scotland)
- Serious Organized Crime and Police Act 2005 set up (Child Exploitation and Online Protection; CEOP)
- HM Government (2006) What to do if you're worried a child is being abused
- HM Government (2010) Working together to safeguard children: a guide to interagency working to safeguard and promote the welfare of children (currently under review)
- Scottish Government (2010) National guidance for child protection in Scotland
- Domestic Violence Crime and Victims (Amendment) Act 2012

Figure 35.2 Events surrounding safeguarding legislation

Pre Children Act
- Victoria Climbie died 2000
- Laming Inquiry DfES 2003 'Keeping Children Safe' led to
- 'Every Child Matters Green' paper which led to
- Children Act 2004 (which does not replace or amend Children Act – just sets out processes for integrating child services)

Post Children Act
- UN Convention on the Rights of the Child (UNCRC) (1989) ratified in 1991. Recognized by all UK but so far only Wales has embedded this into law (Rights of Children and Young Persons (Wales) Measure January 2011 – enacted from May 2012 and May 2014
- The Human Rights Act 1998 incorporates the UNCRC into UK law
- Children and Adoption Act 2006
- Forced Marriage Act (Civil Protection) 2007
- Criminal Justice and Immigration Act 2008
- Children and Young Person Act 2008 (legislates on 'Care Matters' White Paper DfES 2007
- Borders Citizenship and Immigration Act 2009
- Apprenticeship Skills Children and Learning Act 2009 (two lay members from community to sit on LRSC or equivalent in Scotland and Northern Ireland)
- Education Act 2011 (changes to provisions on school discipline with restrictions on public reporting of allegations made against teachers)

Children's Commissioners
- Children's Commissioner for Wales Act 2001 the first Child Commissioner in UK
- Commissioner for Children and Young People (Northern Ireland) Order 2003
- Commissioner for Children and Young People (Scotland) Order 2003
- England: created from Sections 1–9 of the Children's Act 2004
The English Commission is unique in the United Kingdom in not having the remit to promote children's rights

Children and Young People's Nursing at a Glance, First Edition. Edited by Alan Glasper, Jane Coad, and Jim Richardson.
© 2015 John Wiley & Sons, Ltd. Published 2015 by John Wiley & Sons, Ltd. Companion website: www.ataglanceseries.com/nursing/children

From Maria Colwell (1973) to Peter Connolly (2007)

Protecting children from adults is a social and legal imperative and a raft of legislation produced both within and outside the United Kingdom reflects this sad fact. Many different laws exist to shield children from physical, sexual and emotional harm, whether it be in the home environment or from the wider community or cyberspace. There is no single piece of legislation but there are laws amended by new legislation passed by Westminster for England and in devolved governments; the Welsh Assembly, Northern Ireland Assembly and the Scottish Parliament. Not all laws cover the whole of the United Kingdom and legal systems vary in the different countries (Figure 35.1)

The Laming Report 2003 following the death of Victoria Climbie in 2002 led to Every Child Matters and subsequently the 2004 Children Act amendment of the integration of children's services.

Following the tragic events at Soham in 2002, the Bichard Inquiry (2004) set up the Safeguarding Vulnerable Groups Act (2006). Reviewed in 2011, this saw the Protection of Freedoms Act set up in May 2012 which deals with vetting, barring and disclosure. This covers England and Wales only. The equivalent legislation in Northern Ireland is Safeguarding Vulnerable Groups (Northern Ireland) Order 2007, and in Scotland Safeguarding Vulnerable Groups (Scotland) Act 2007.

Munro Report

Following the death of Peter Connolly in 2007 there was an independent review of child social work and child protection in England (2010) which led to the Department for Education and Skills' (2011) Munro Review of child protection: final report, and the Department for Education's (2011) A child-centred system, the Government's response to the Munro Review. The five main headings are to develop:

1 A system that values professional expertise
2 Clarifying accountabilities and improving learning
3 Sharing responsibility for the provision of early help
4 Developing social work expertise
5 The organizational context: supporting effective social work practice.

Northern Ireland

The Regional Safeguarding Board for Northern Ireland (SBNI) was created under statutory provision (Safeguarding Board for Northern Ireland Regulations (Northern Ireland) 2011). The SBNI is hosted and supported by the the Public Health Agency (PHA) and replaces the Regional Child Protection Committee (RCPC) and its five Trust Panels (TCPPs) (www.safeguardingni.org).

Rest of the UK

There is no equivalent regional body in England, Scotland or Wales. The nearest equivalent bodies are local safeguarding boards in England and Wales and the area child protection committees in Scotland.

Disclosure and Barring Service

In the UK since 1 December 2012, Criminal Records Bureau (CRB) merged with the Independant Safeguarding Authority (ISA) to become the Disclosure and Barring Service (DBS) established under the Protection of Freedoms Act 2012. This is an executive non-departmental body sponsored by the Home Office.

Key point

Everyone, everywhere:
- Has a duty to protect children
- Should be aware of the risks of child abuse
- Should be aware of the signs and symptoms
- Should be aware of their responsibilities and action required

The welfare of a child is paramount

36 Fabricated or induced illness

Previously known in United Kingdom as Munchausen syndrome by proxy, the term 'fabricated or induced illness in children' (FII) was coined by the Royal College of Paediatrics and Child Health (RCPCH) in 2001, further refined in 2009 and reviewed in 2012–2013 to describe a spectrum of disorders where the carer, usually the mother, presents a child for medical attention having either fabricated or induced the child's symptoms. This spectrum transcends boundaries of social class and other known deprivations.

Presentation

- Males and females similarly affected
- Main carer is the perpetrator (usually but not always the mother)
- Usually, the child is under 5 years of age though can be older
- The older age groups may seem to collude with the perpetrator
- Repeated medical attention and investigations may mean medical staff unwittingly cause unintentional harm
- Can result in neurological damage, illness, disability and, in some cases, death
- Sequalae of emotional and psychological problems and behaviours for the affected child into adulthood
- Difficulties in reaching a diagnosis or a decision on FII being the cause

Problems are compounded when staff may be aided by an unusually helpful perpetrator and the therapeutic trust built up between staff and perpetrator becomes damaged as staff begin to realize the potential for FII to be a cause for the child's illness. Mothers may have an need for attention, recognition of their 'good' parenting' or may have themselves been a victim of FII in their early years. There may be altered or interrupted attachment such as death of a previous child. There seems to be no mental disorder as such.

Recognition of fabricated or induced illness

- Repeated or unexplained symptoms in a child that cannot usually be corroborated
- Medical notes may show different attendances at a variety of settings
- Symptoms only occur when the perpetrator is present and resolve when absent
- Perpetrator has some level of medical or nursing knowledge
- Perpetrator may seem either overly concerned or rather unconcerned at the child's plight
- Perpetrator is usually the mother; unusual to be the father
- Perpetrator may contaminate specimens or fluids or wounds or poison the child with medications or inappropriate substances
- Perpetrator may semi-suffocate child in order to simulate respiratory or cardiac problems
- Perpetrator may falsify accounts or results of tests

There are major problems with establishing whether FII exists in a case, not least of which is 'thinking the unthinkable'. Obtaining evidence of FII is difficult without disclosing medical concerns and may cause the FII to stop – in itself a concern. Catching the perpetrator in action may be impossible without some sort of observation in secret; however, there are ethical and legal concerns over the controversial practice of using covert video surveillance (CVS) as an aid to generating 'evidence' on which to challenge the perpetrator. RCPCH (2009) caution that CVS should only be used in extreme cases and only under certain strict circumstances. CVS should not be instigated by health care staff. This is a matter for the police and social services following set policy and procedures around safeguarding the child and other children in the family.

Treatment options are to ensure the welfare of the child first and foremost and to manage the perpetrator behavior by therapeutic interventions ensuring that any return to the parent does not put children at risk.

Children and Young People's Nursing at a Glance, First Edition. Edited by Alan Glasper, Jane Coad, and Jim Richardson.
© 2015 John Wiley & Sons, Ltd. Published 2015 by John Wiley & Sons, Ltd. Companion website: www.ataglanceseries.com/nursing/children

37 Gaining consent or assent

In the United Kingdom there is no set legal age at which children are determined to be competent to make decisions about their health care. The 'best interests' of the child apply in decision-making processes and should reflect a careful consideration of the rights of the child and reflect the wishes of that child. The ability to consent is currently based on the child's developmental stage and his/her expression of understanding of what it is he/she is consenting to.

Informed consent is a process and not a single event and it is considered good practice to invest time, effort and care into ensuring that all decisions to be made are 'informed' choices and the individual has an understanding of both the risks and benefits of any proposed treatment or intervention and also of not receiving that treatment or intervention.

Refusal of consent occurs for varying reasons. It is particularly important to ensure that the 'informed consent' process had been respected and that sufficient time is given for the individual to consider the consequences of selecting various options – including refusal.

When a child refuses treatment in his/her 'best interests', then **parental consent** may take precedence over the child's refusal. Courts can also intervene when it is considered to be in the best interest of the child to have the treatment and also in cases where both the child and the parent refuse treatment.

Persons aged 18 years or over can always give consent for themselves unless they are deemed not competent to do so (England Wales and Northern Ireland).

Persons 16–18 years old are presumed in law to be competent and therefore can consent to treatment in the absence of parental consent. However, it is considered good practice to involve the family in decision making unless there is reason to believe that it may not be in the best interest of that child to do so ((England Wales and Northern Ireland).

Persons under 16 years of age cannot give consent unless deemed Gillick or Fraser competent – and this is a contentious area for some practitioners (England Wales and Northern Ireland). In Scotland, children of any age can consent to treatment unless they lack the capacity to do so (Larcher 2005).

The age of the child is not the sole indicator of whether he/she can make a decision. Information should be developmentally appropriate and delivered in a way that best suits the needs of the child (*Gillick v. West Norfolk and Wisbech AHA* (1985) 3 All ER 402 1985).

Parental responsibility: when a child is not competent to give consent for him/herself then the practitioner should seek consent from a person deemed to have 'parental responsibility'. This may, or may not, be the child's parents. Legally, consent is required from one person with 'parental responsibility' but it is considered good practice at all times to seek the views of the child or those close to the child affected by the decision-making process.

Parental responsibility ends when the child is 18 years old (England Wales and Northern Ireland) and at 16 years in Scotland, though parents can still give 'guidance' (Larcher 2005).

Children and Young People's Nursing at a Glance, First Edition. Edited by Alan Glasper, Jane Coad, and Jim Richardson.
© 2015 John Wiley & Sons, Ltd. Published 2015 by John Wiley & Sons, Ltd. Companion website: www.ataglanceseries.com/nursing/children

38 Clinical holding

Figure 38.1 Holding a child in a supportive manner

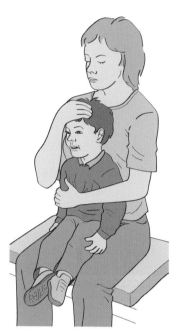

Children and Young People's Nursing at a Glance, First Edition. Edited by Alan Glasper, Jane Coad, and Jim Richardson.
© 2015 John Wiley & Sons, Ltd. Published 2015 by John Wiley & Sons, Ltd. Companion website: www.ataglanceseries.com/nursing/children

Many terms are used to describe restricting a child's movement, depending on the perceived degree of force used; for example, restrictive physical intervention, restraint, immobilization, clinical holding, therapeutic holding and holding. These terms are based on presumptions of force, and suggest that nurses have a common understanding of what constitutes the use of force in the clinical setting. Children, parents and children's nurses find many types of procedures stressful and sometimes traumatic, and often have questions around why, when and how restriction happens.

Restricting a child's movement for routine clinical procedures is distressing for the child and may have an impact on their later psychological development. Parents have also expressed feelings of helplessness and powerlessness when their child was restricted for a clinical procedure. They are in a very vulnerable position, often unable to adequately comfort or care for their child, and not questioning practice because they feel disempowered in an unfamiliar environment.

There are a number of considerations for the nurse when caring for a child that needs to be held still for a clinical procedure, relating to the care of the child, care of the parents and self-care for the nurse. There are three main phases: the lead in to the procedure, care during the procedure and the post-holding phase.

Considerations

Caring for a child undergoing a clinical procedure requires the nurse to consider the individual needs of the child and family. This includes questioning the necessity for restriction, considering alternatives to restriction, establishing the potential of parent's involvement, considering the child's physical and emotional needs and affording the child and parent(s) the opportunity to debrief after the procedure if they wish. It is possible that younger children are more likely to be restricted for a clinical procedure because of the nurse's anticipation that such children are more difficult to keep still.

Children need to have some sense of control when undergoing a clinical procedure, in order to help them cope. Addressing the child's comfort and need for control may encourage greater compliance from the child, thus enhancing the delivery of safe care. This is supported by the work of many theorists on child development who identified the need for young children to have a sense of control in their environment, to have a sense of participation and to trust those caring for them.

Pre-holding considerations

In the lead in to holding the child, the nurse should consider the needs of the child, the parent, and their own professional needs as follows.

Child-focused considerations

- Is it necessary for this child to be held still for this procedure?
- Is this decision influenced by the procedure to be performed, the child's age or the child's cognitive ability?
- Is the procedure urgent or necessary?
- Are there any alternatives to holding the child still that are appropriate to the child's stage of development? What are they (e.g. distraction, imagery, sedation)?
- What will it mean for this child to be held still?
- How are they likely to react and how will I manage and support them through that?
- What is the child's understanding of what will happen? What are their information needs?

Considerations for the nurse

- How do I feel about holding a child still?
- Do I have the education, experience and skill to do this safely?
- Is there any policy that should guide my involvement in this?

Parent-focused considerations

- Are the child's parents present?
- What is their understanding of what will happen?
- Do they have an expectation of being involved? If so, how will this work in practice?
- What guidance do they require?
- Is there a named person to care for their needs if I am involved in holding their child?

Care during clinical holding

If a decision is made to hold the child still for a clinical procedure it is important that the child is very clear on who their lead person is, what they can do if they are distressed and where their parents are.

Some questions for your consideration:
- Who is giving direction to the child?
- Is the child being held for the shortest time possible?
- Are the child's and parents' physical and emotional needs being met?

It is very likely that a child will object to being held still, when this happens the focus in always on gaining cooperation through de-escalation. This can evoke a wide variety of feelings for you, so it is worthwhile to consider what this might mean for you. Did you agree with the need for clinical holding? Are you in a hurry to complete the procedure due to time pressures? Do you feel you have enough support? Is the child or parent not cooperating to the extent you would wish? Why do you think this is? It is very important to think about these issues as you may communicate your feelings through your verbal or non-verbal actions to child and parents.

In the event of non-cooperation it is essential to try to establish what the child's motivation for his/her behaviour is. Think back to the earlier prompt questions. Were all information and comfort needs of the child and parent addressed? What has changed? What are their needs now, and who is best placed to address them?

Post-holding considerations

The aftermath of clinical holding is an opportunity for the nurse to consider what went well and what aspects of the care could be improved on. Consideration should be given to the following:
- Was there an appropriate rationale for clinical holding?
- Was the method and length of holding suitable in this situation?
- Are there any potential effects for the child or parents?
- Were they addressed and how can this be addressed in future?
- Documentation: it is very important that notes on all of the above are documented to enhance continuity of care and to communicate the child's particular preferences, and the coping strategies employed that were found to be particularly useful.

39 Breaking bad or significant news

Figure 39.1 Factors influencing the process of breaking bad or significant news

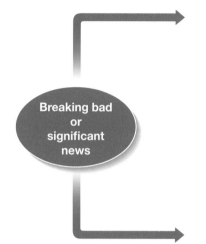

Barriers for the family

- Poor or inappropriate communication skills of professionals
- Lack of appropriate support
- Being given too much, conflicting or confusing information
- Being given inadequate information
- Not understanding language or terms used
- Feeling uncomfortable in expressing emotions
- Not having time to ask questions

Barriers for professionals

- Lack of experience in breaking bad news
- Previous bad experiences in giving bad news
- Unsure of role in the process
- Poor or inexperienced communication skills
- Inadequate preparation for the event
- Having to use an inappropriate environment
- Not feeling able to respond appropriately to the family's emotion or subsequent behaviour
- Feeling inadequate in supporting the family after the news has been given

(Breaking bad or significant news)

For most health care professionals one of the most challenging and stressful elements of their role is when they are required to give news to children, young people, their parents and carers that they are likely to perceive as significant or bad. This is further exacerbated if they feel unprepared (Harrison and Walling 2010). This chapter offers a guide to the principles underpinning best practice for health professionals when breaking bad news to families.

Preparing to break bad news

Before giving bad or significant news to a child's family careful preparation is needed. Prior to the meeting it is vital that the professionals involved discuss and plan their contribution together in delivering this news. In most cases, when the news is significant, such as the confirmation of a diagnosis or the news of a child's worsening illness or death, the news will be given by a doctor and the role of the children's nurse is to accompany the doctor and support the family (Price et al. 2006).

It is imperative that the health professionals involved feel prepared with appropriate knowledge and skills and have any necessary information or evidence to share with the family that may be required at the time. If you are asked to accompany a doctor to do this, it is important to consider whether you feel you have the appropriate skills and experience to support the family. Ideally, if the family have already established a rapport or trusting relationship with another member of the nursing team they would be the preferred professional to accompany the doctor.

Sometimes, the need to break bad news has some urgency (e.g. in the case of an emergency). However, whenever possible, the optimum time and appropriate place to give this news should be considered. The environment should be selected in advance, ideally in a quiet room, never in the middle of a public place such as a corridor or busy practice area, with consideration given to the arrangement of furniture and ensuring water and tissues are discreetly placed in the room. It is important to ensure you will not be disturbed by distractions such as undue noise, a ringing telephone or interruptions from other professionals.

When planning to deliver the bad news it is important to ensure parents or carers will not be alone, that partners will be together to support each other and lone parents or carers have a family member or significant other with them. Every child has the right to be involved in decisions about their health but in preparing parents to receive bad news it is important to establish whether they wish their child to be present at the disclosure. It should be remembered that children will respond to the emotions of their parents or carers and for this reason parents often prefer their child not to be present at the initial interview. If this is the case, ensure the child is occupied and not left alone while the family is receiving the news.

Supporting the family when bad news is given

Good communication skills are pivotal to the process of breaking bad news. One of the strongest memories parents often have of when the news was broken is not what was said, but *how* it was said, particularly when told of their child's impending death (West Midlands Paediatric Macmillan Team 2005). When talking to parents use the child's name. It is important to explain the news clearly using jargon-free language, giving the correct facts and not withholding information, but balance this with not overloading the family with too much information.

It is important never to assume what the initial responses of parents or family members will be at the time of hearing bad news. The emotions they experience may be very complex and those they reveal may be very different from those they are feeling. Cultural and familial factors have a major influence on our public display of emotion and depend on factors such as personality, coping strategies, gender, role in the family and the relationships with the professional breaking the news.

Emotions that may be demonstrated through their actions at the time include anger, disbelief, confusion, shock, denial or, conversely, a lack of emotion or apparent acceptance. Depending on the circumstances prior to the disclosure (e.g. if the family have been worried about their child's unexplained illness, the diagnosis has been anticipated, the child or young person has a life-threatening or limiting illness or has been receiving palliative care for a long time), the news may come as a sense of relief, sometimes followed by a sense of guilt. The emotions experienced include outward displays of distress or grief ranging from crying or shouting to silence, or disengagement. It is important to remember cultural differences in the display of emotions and not to show surprise at any of these emotions or the subsequent behaviour of those receiving the news. On hearing bad news, family members may use different coping strategies. Some parents may be immersed in their emotional responses whereas others will want to do something practical.

In supporting the family, your own body language should convey compassion and empathy but also recognize the recipients' need for personal space and dignity. The use of appropriate non-verbal communication such as facial expressions and appropriate eye contact need careful consideration. Touch can be therapeutic but never assume it will be welcomed. In deciding whether to use this as a means of communication it is important to take cues from family members and be guided by their body language. Do say you are sorry but never say 'I know how you must feel'.

After the bad news has been broken

Give the family some time for the news to sink in. Silences are important and one should never feel the need to talk and fill the gap. Give the family an opportunity to ask further questions or reinforce the news if necessary. Ask if there is anyone you can call, anything they need, whether they would like some time alone or if they would like you to stay for a while. They may need further information or referral to other professionals or services.

Breaking bad or significant news and supporting families through the process of receiving it is a challenging element of the children's nurse's role. It is vital for all professionals to collaborate with the goal of achieving best practice if children and their families are to feel well supported through the ordeal.

40 Care of the dying child

Figure 40.1 Care of the dying child

Context of caring for the dying child

- Fortunately, childhood death is rare
- Losing a child is a life-altering event for the family and defies the expected order of life
- Home, hospital and hospice are potential locations for end-of-life care. Each family will have their own preference and their preference, where possible, should be facilitated
- The way a child dies has an impact on the family's response in bereavement
- Caring for a child at the end of life should centre on the individual needs of the child and family (including siblings and grandparents)
- Developmental factors influence the child's ability to understand illness and death as well as their capacity to communicate anxieties and preferences regarding care

Assessing and planning care

- Professionals should be open and honest with families when the end of life is recognized
- Joint care planning with families should take place as soon as possible
- A written care plan should be agreed and made available to the multidisciplinary team
- A pathway like that by ACT (2004) can provide the means of ensuring the end of life care needs and wishes of the dying child and their family are met effectively (see Figure 40.1)
- Ongoing assessment: care plans should be amended taking into account changes
- Provide clear and simple information and respect silences

Key components of care

- Compassionate child and family-centred care
- Good communication
- Supporting the parents in decision making
- Pain and symptom management
- Culturally sensitive care
- Care responsive to changing needs
- Access to clinical expertise
- Emotional, psychological and spiritual support for the child, the parents and the siblings including bereavement support
- Practical assistance with the care of the child including respite, equipment and financial support
- Privacy, comfort, rest, nourishment
- Trust and hope
- Team work

Principles of symptom management

- Listen to the child and the parents
- Remember that symptom management not only promotes the child's comfort, but enhances quality of life for child and family
- Adopt a team approach
- Know your limitations and ask for help
- Continuous reassessment and review
- Consider pharmacological and non-pharmacological approaches
- A written plan detailing what to do and who to call if symptoms worsen
- Important to anticipate symptoms, provide information and develop a plan
- Address parents' concerns and fears around morphine use

Symptoms experienced

Symptoms experienced depend on the child's underlying diagnosis. However, the following includes some commonly occurring symptoms:

- Nausea and vomiting
- Seizures
- Constipation
- Muscle spasm
- Fatigue
- Pain
- Agitation
- Dyspnoea
- Diarrhoea
- Anorexia

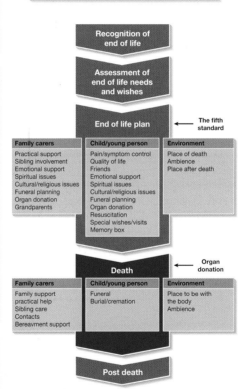

Needs of child and family

Last days of life

- Provide information: physical changes of the dying process, planning the funeral
- Perform regular mouth and eye care
- Attend to pressure area care
- Contact appropriate personnel: chaplain, social worker, family and friends
- Encourage sibling involvement
- Create memory opportunities: photographs, hand and foot prints (paint or plaster), memory book
- Cultural sensitivity is imperative when considering creative memories. Gain consent first

After the child dies

- Reassure the family there is no hurry – family can spend as much time with their child as they need
- Offer the family opportunity to bath and dress their child in favourite clothes
- Offer opportunity to take child home if in hospital
- Ensure legal procedures are followed (e.g. certification)
- Address parents' issues about organ donation if raised

Reproduced with kind permission of Together for Short Lives

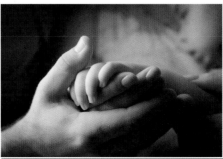

© Gavin Blue, Heartlfelt

Ethical considerations

Ethical issues abound when caring for a dying child. Fostering a culture of honest and sensitive communication where ethical dilemmas can be openly discussed is crucial. Ethical issues include:

- Communication issues around truth telling
- Withdrawing treatment
- Long-term ventilation
- Provision of hydration and nutrition
- Medical ethics in different cultures

Quality care for the dying child and family

Fortunately, childhood death is rare. However, when it does happen the death of a child represents a life-altering event for parents and the whole family. During the end of life period, the nurse has a key role within the multidisciplinary team providing care and in ensuring the ideal of the good death is upheld. It is important to remember that nurse and family may have different ideas of what is a good death. The composition of the team will differ depending on where the child's end-of-life care is being provided, but the team will likely include professionals from both statutory and voluntary organizations. Care should be holistic and individualized, recognizing that the needs of each child and family at this time are different. In what follows we examine each of the main aspects of quality care in turn (i.e. physical, psychological, social and spiritual elements), recognizing that these are interconnected.

Physical needs

The physical care of a dying child and their family greatly influences the quality of their lives and the ability of the parents and siblings to cope with the child's death. Perceptions that a child is suffering impact greatly on the child and the family unit. Good symptom management should be viewed as a key component of care. The first goal should be to address all distressing symptoms. Frequent assessment and review is imperative. Commonly, one of the great fears for parents at end of life is that their child will suffer unrelieved pain. The assessment of pain in children, however, is influenced by the child's age and developmental stage. Underestimating pain, particularly amongst neonates and non-verbal children is common. Pain scales appropriate to the child's development stage, simple observation and parental reporting are fundamental in good assessment. A detailed symptom management plan is essential. This plan should outline what to do and whom to call if symptoms worsen and anticipate and plan for other potential symptoms. Management should include access to medical and nursing support 24 hours a day regardless of the place of care.

Nursing care in the last days and hours of the child's life influences the family's experience of death and impacts bereavement. Involving parents, siblings, extended family and friends in care can create a sense of order and help families exert some control on their situation. Information regarding the physical changes that can occur to the child as death approaches should be shared and normalized. Restlessness, agitation, noisy or rattly breathing, incontinence, eye changes and circulatory changes are common symptoms experienced during the dying process. Reassure the family that although noisy breathing is distressing for them, the distress to the child is thought to be minimal or non existent.

While many families will choose to care for their child at home on grounds of familiarity and family togetherness, it is important that families understand that they can change their mind. Plans should include options for seamless transition between home, hospital and hospice.

Psychosocial needs

The psychosocial needs of child and parents are inextricably linked and hence so is the resultant support. Knowing their child is dying can result in major emotional, practical and financial stressors for parents and the entire family circle. Parents report that they are often caught up juggling the competing demands of family life while attempting to remain focused on being there for their dying child. Parents find themselves overwhelmed by uncertainty, decision making, care giving, guilt and grief. Sharing time with other siblings is difficult. Each individual child, parent and family unit has their own ways of coping so the type and amount of psychosocial support required from professionals is unique to each individual and family. The focus of psychosocial support should be about quality of life for child and family, despite the nearness of death. Provision of reassurance, comfort, creating some sense of normality and making memories are fundamental aspects of providing care for a dying child.

Whether or not the child is aware of the fact that he/she is dying can further complicate the psychological care offered. While it is thought that many children, especially those who have lived through a long-term illness, have an awareness that they are dying, many parents often assume their child will not understand the issues surrounding death and are therefore reluctant to broach the subject in an attempt to protect their child. This can cause tensions between professionals and parents, because professionals may feel giving children the opportunity to communicate may allay their fears regarding dying.

Regardless of where the child's care is being provided, it is often the nurse who is most frequently with the child and family providing sensitive individualized care. The children's nurse should listen to the child and family's feelings carefully and respectfully, as well as their needs and wishes. Further, the nurse will need to ensure good levels of communication are maintained and that information is given in easily understood language and reinforced over time as required. This information will enable parents and, if appropriate, children, to make decisions regarding care. Given the complexity of such decisions, communication between parents and health care professionals should be characterized not as a one-off activity, but rather an ongoing process within which discussion takes place. Such support is essential in allaying fears, permitting a sense of control and facilitating anticipatory grieving. The use of play as a strategy to help the child express his/her feelings should not be understated. The nurse should identify his/her limitations and refer the child and family on for specialized support as appropriate.

Spiritual needs

Spirituality will have a different meaning for every family and, as with physical and psychosocial needs, requires ongoing assessment. More than simply ensuring a family's religious practices are upheld, spirituality is about expressing oneself, meaning and purpose, individual values, self worth and faith in self, others or in a higher power. Thus, spiritual care is care that is responsive to the human spirit and the nurse should endeavour to provide opportunities for what is important to the individual child and family. For some it may be arranging a visit from the chaplain or administering a sacrament. For others it could be creating some meaning through rituals or creative memories. Rituals provide the opportunity for the child, parents, siblings and other family members to express their love, sadness and remember precious memories.

41 Dealing with aggression

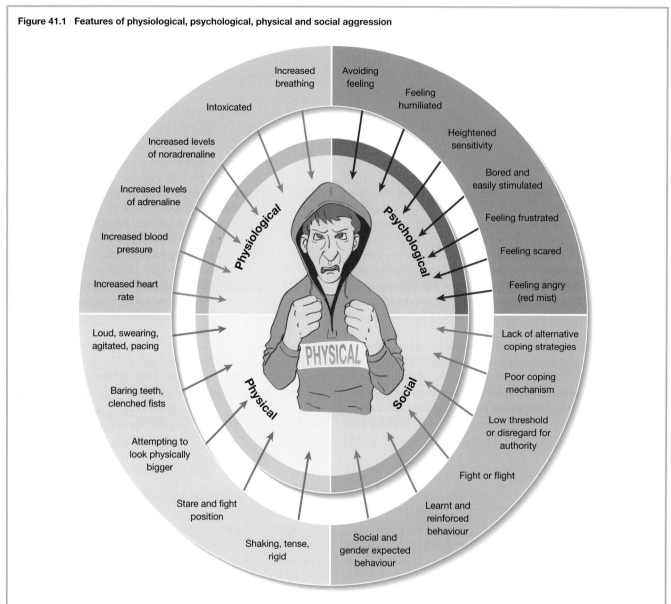

Figure 41.1 Features of physiological, psychological, physical and social aggression

What is aggression?

There are a number of competing theories about what aggression is and the purpose it serves. Social psychologists define aggression as *behavior that is intended to harm another individual who does not wish to be harmed*. Dealing with aggression can be scary for professionals and other service users working in young people's health care settings. Aggression in the theoretical sense has a number of subsets which range from all out 'violence' to 'verbal threats' and 'irritating annoyance'. Thus, not all acts of aggression are intended to cause physical damage, but rather serve as warning and a response to frustration. Quite often aggression is the result of 'hot headed' non-thinking reactions to either threatening or frustrating situations young people find themselves in. Examples ranging from road rage to temper tantrums serve to remind us that

aggression is a complex phenomenon which impacts on a number of domains and bodily systems (physiological, physical, psychological, and social; Figure 41.1). If you think about the times you have been aggressive, it would probably be when you were tired, angry, upset, frustrated, scared or feeling ill. You would remember feeling agitated, short tempered, tense, loud, and maybe tearful and later regretful. In the heat of the moment you would probably have little regard for other people and not be responsive to reason. Physiologically, your heart would be pumping fast; you would be breathing hard and in a state of fight or flight. These are the symptom of aggression and a result of aversive events, our thoughts (cognitions) and the release of and response to chemicals, including alcohol, but in particularly the male sex hormone testosterone.

Children and Young People's Nursing at a Glance, First Edition. Edited by Alan Glasper, Jane Coad, and Jim Richardson.
© 2015 John Wiley & Sons, Ltd. Published 2015 by John Wiley & Sons, Ltd. Companion website: www.ataglanceseries.com/nursing/children

What causes aggression?

Physiologically, aggression is caused by hormones and evolutionary factors. Physically, it is wired into the deepest and oldest parts of our brain and has the aim of protecting ourselves as much as giving us means of surviving. In the past 20 years or so, there has been a recognition of dietary factors and that some children are aggressive as a result of specific childhood psychological conditions such as attention deficit hyperactivity disorder (ADHD). Socially, aggression has been valued in some cultures and is often unwittingly reinforced in gender stereotyping and cultural variables. As children mature and develop it is through social learning that they begin to refrain from tantrum behaviour and gain a sense of self and cognitively begin to moderate their behaviour.

Dealing with aggression is a personal thing. Most children and young people display aggressive outbursts when they feel threatened by others or are frustrated and cannot get their own way. Thus, most aggressive outbursts are dependent on situation, circumstance, the cognitive awareness of the child and associated trigger factors. This means that much aggression can be planned for and strategically reduced. Personality variables that relate to perceived threat also predict aggression.

Emotional or impulsive aggression

Impulsive aggression occurs with no or only a small amount of forethought or intent. It is usually defined by a short loud outburst that has an obvious cause and can be easily contained. A typical example is the child who embarrassingly cries, screams in a fit of tantrum in a supermarket or the infant who never wants to go to bed. At this younger age aggression serves a purpose for the child of expressing unhappiness and desire of wants. Over a period of time with consistent reinforcement, routine and supportive parenting, most children can overcome these types of emotionally triggered aggressive outbursts.

For teenagers and the health care professionals who work with them aggression has different connotations related more to cognitive triggers that are characterized by more intentional planning, forethought and frustration. Aggression in this respect shows itself in at least two ways: as physical or as non-physical.

• **Physical aggression** is *aggression that involves harming others physically* – for instance spitting, hitting, kicking in more than self-defence. Physical aggression is immediate, violent and requires urgent de-escalation interventions to reduce arousal.

• **Non-physical aggression** is often referred to as *passive or verbal aggression*. It does not involve physical outbursts but rather verbal aggression such as threats, shouting, screaming, name calling and in some cases 'social aggression'. This is the active participation in the intentional harming of others' social relationships by spreading rumours and other behaviours such as blanking, silent treatment, name calling, racist and sexual stereotypical jokes and spreading gossip. Social aggression is becoming an increasing concern in cyberspace with cyber bullying.

Triggers of aggression

The best approach to understanding the triggers of aggression is prevention. This means planning ahead and also having a predetermined plan for dealing with aggression as a team when it occurs. This means being aware of policy, attending relevant training and knowing your clients. The primary triggers for most young people are when they are frustrated or disappointed or feel undermined or unfairly treated. Whether this is the case or not, if that is their perception and they have a 'nothing to lose' feeling and if the young person has a history of having a short fuse, then planning ahead and having strategies for dealing with potential outbursts needs to be a consideration. These include having a stringent routine, a full programme of activities to prevent boredom, a transparent sense of equity between all young people being cared for and rewards for good behaviour. Other strategies include role modelling expected behaviours towards disappointment, having a reward to work towards at the end of the shift, easily achievable small tasks and, in nearly all cases, the development of an authentic caring relationship to help the young person ventilate feelings appropriately.

De-escalating physical aggression

Aggression can be explained in terms of learning, reinforcement, modelling, punishment, arousal and cognition, but this is rarely relevant when a young person becomes physically aggressive in a health care setting. Dealing with physical aggression in a team approach requires the implementation of predesigned policy and training of all involved. The metaphor of the escalator serves well to emphasize that the quicker a team can prevent and then stop the escalator rising with the young person on it, the better the outcome of any incident. The following is an outline of the key points when dealing with a **physical aggressive** incident:

1 **Safety:** of self, the aggressor and others. Seek assistance and clear the immediate area. If the child is endangering him/herself or others, attempt to remove harmful objects safely.

2 **Wait:** if you try to engage in conversation with the aggressive person it will probably escalate the incident. Wait. They will run out of steam eventually. Then try to talk calmly about the issue.

3 **Gently engage:** deal with the immediate situation by remaining calm and employing non-verbal cues (pay particular attention to proximity, volume of voice, open posture and non-threating stance). Keep verbal clues simple to reduce stimulating and, for now, avoid judgement, moralizing or giving an opinion. Give reassurance and clear instructions as to your intentions and expectations. Offer compromise and limited alternatives. Only as a last resort grapple and attempt to physically restrain the child.

4 **Post incident issues:** apply consequences (remember to teach compromise). Consider the personal triggers for the child and work towards addressing creative ways of confronting these in the future.

Put into place an incident debrief and paperwork. Consult policy and guidelines. Ensure team training is in place.

42 Minimizing the effects of hospitalization

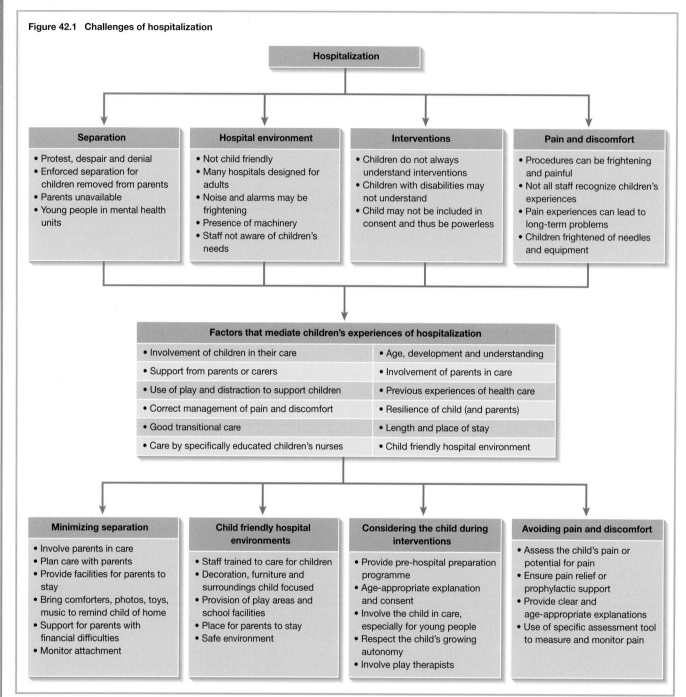

Figure 42.1 Challenges of hospitalization

Hospitalization

Separation
- Protest, despair and denial
- Enforced separation for children removed from parents
- Parents unavailable
- Young people in mental health units

Hospital environment
- Not child friendly
- Many hospitals designed for adults
- Noise and alarms may be frightening
- Presence of machinery
- Staff not aware of children's needs

Interventions
- Children do not always understand interventions
- Children with disabilities may not understand
- Child may not be included in consent and thus be powerless

Pain and discomfort
- Procedures can be frightening and painful
- Not all staff recognize children's experiences
- Pain experiences can lead to long-term problems
- Children frightened of needles and equipment

Factors that mediate children's experiences of hospitalization

- Involvement of children in their care
- Support from parents or carers
- Use of play and distraction to support children
- Correct management of pain and discomfort
- Good transitional care
- Care by specifically educated children's nurses

- Age, development and understanding
- Involvement of parents in care
- Previous experiences of health care
- Resilience of child (and parents)
- Length and place of stay
- Child friendly hospital environment

Minimizing separation
- Involve parents in care
- Plan care with parents
- Provide facilities for parents to stay
- Bring comforters, photos, toys, music to remind child of home
- Support for parents with financial difficulties
- Monitor attachment

Child friendly hospital environments
- Staff trained to care for children
- Decoration, furniture and surroundings child focused
- Provision of play areas and school facilities
- Place for parents to stay
- Safe environment

Considering the child during interventions
- Provide pre-hospital preparation programme
- Age-appropriate explanation and consent
- Involve the child in care, especially for young people
- Respect the child's growing autonomy
- Involve play therapists

Avoiding pain and discomfort
- Assess the child's pain or potential for pain
- Ensure pain relief or prophylactic support
- Provide clear and age-appropriate explanations
- Use of specific assessment tool to measure and monitor pain

Children and Young People's Nursing at a Glance, First Edition. Edited by Alan Glasper, Jane Coad, and Jim Richardson.
© 2015 John Wiley & Sons, Ltd. Published 2015 by John Wiley & Sons, Ltd. Companion website: www.ataglanceseries.com/nursing/children

Hospitals can be threatening, frightening and painful environments where children are faced with strangers who want to 'do' things to them. Illness, trauma and hospital care are often the most traumatic things children experience, even with the presence of their parents. In addition, hospitals present a conflict for children who are taught about ownership of their body and to be wary of strangers. Nonetheless, changes in the way health care is provided, giving rights to patients, improvement in staff knowledge and increasing knowledge of children and parents about medical issues, mediated through the internet, has impacted on how hospitalization is experienced. Similarly, the concept of hospitalization has changed with shorter bed stays, development of primary care, avoidance of hospital care and overall improved health of children.

The experience of hospitalization

Hospitals used to be places of long stays, routine, rigidity, restricted visiting, limited emotional care and often painful experiences for children. Much of this has changed; however, it does not necessarily alleviate how children experience what is happening to them. What is trivial to an adult can be a major stressor to a child.

Experience of the child

While much of hospital is anxiety-producing, one experience has the potential to cause trauma for children and this is separation from their parents. Parents can usually stay with their children but other responsibilities may prevent this and so the child becomes separated. The impact of separation is dependent on circumstances, age and development but may be displayed in specific stages:

1 **Protest.** The child actively searches for their parents and protests through clinging to them, crying, screaming, rejecting staff and may be aggressive.

2 **Despair.** The child is exhausting their ability to protest and so enters a stage of despair about the situation. This may result in withdrawal, sadness, non-communication and possible regression to earlier behavioural stages of development.

3 **Denial or detachment.** The child's attachment is focused on those around them rather than the parents. They seek out, interact and respond to staff and may even reject their parents. This stage is rarely seen now except in children who have been abused or neglected.

Experience of parents

Much research has identified the adverse experience of hospitalization on children. However, there can be impacts on parents that in turn affects the child:

- Anxiety when separated from their child
- Feelings of guilt
- Conflict between parents if they are not able to stay with their child
- Emotional impact of the ill child on their ability to cope
- Physical demands of maintaining life and being at the hospital
- Development of postnatal depression.

Interventions and adverse experiences of hospital

Experiencing hospital care can lead to a range of situations and interventions that are potentially traumatic for the child, although this is not always the case as children are resilient and cope with many stressors. Stressors for the child include the following factors.

The environment

- Strange, clinical and often frightening environment which may not necessarily be child friendly
- Adult-oriented environments
- Machinery and equipment that is large and frightening in comparison to the size of the child
- Noise, lights and alarms
- Loss of control as they are not in their usual environment.

The staff

- Having to interact with strangers
- Staff who are more oriented toward adults
- Not considering the specific needs of children and families
- Staff who do not understand the child's developmental needs for support, preparation and care.

Circumstance

- Emergency situations in which the survival needs override those of the child
- When the child has experienced trauma
- Safety of the child when there is a concern about abuse
- The child requires interventions that he/she does not want.

Interventions

- Loss of control resulting from the specific intervention
- Pain resulting from the intervention, lack of preparation, staff not following analgesia pathways
- Procedures over which the child has no control or input
- The child is restrained in order to undertake a procedure.

Interventions to alleviate the impact of hospitalization

Hospitals and children's units

Hospitals admitting children should have policies about their rights, issues of consent, safeguarding, and nursing and medical procedures so that the deleterious impacts of hospital are minimized.

Staff

Children should be cared for by professional staff who have in-depth knowledge of children, development and conditions that affect them. Staff must provide care that is child-centred while being sensitive to their rights and wishes. Nurses particularly must advocate on behalf of children in order that no harm is done and the child does not suffer, particularly when painful procedures are performed.

Interventions

Throughout all interventions children's needs must be the central concern and the aims to appropriately prepare them, obtain their consent, ensure analgesia or anaesthetic is provided, communicate effectively about what is happening and support them, bearing in mind the child's age, development and status.

43 Transition

Figure 43.1 Care issues for consideration when the family with a child with complex care needs are transitioning from the acute hospital setting to home

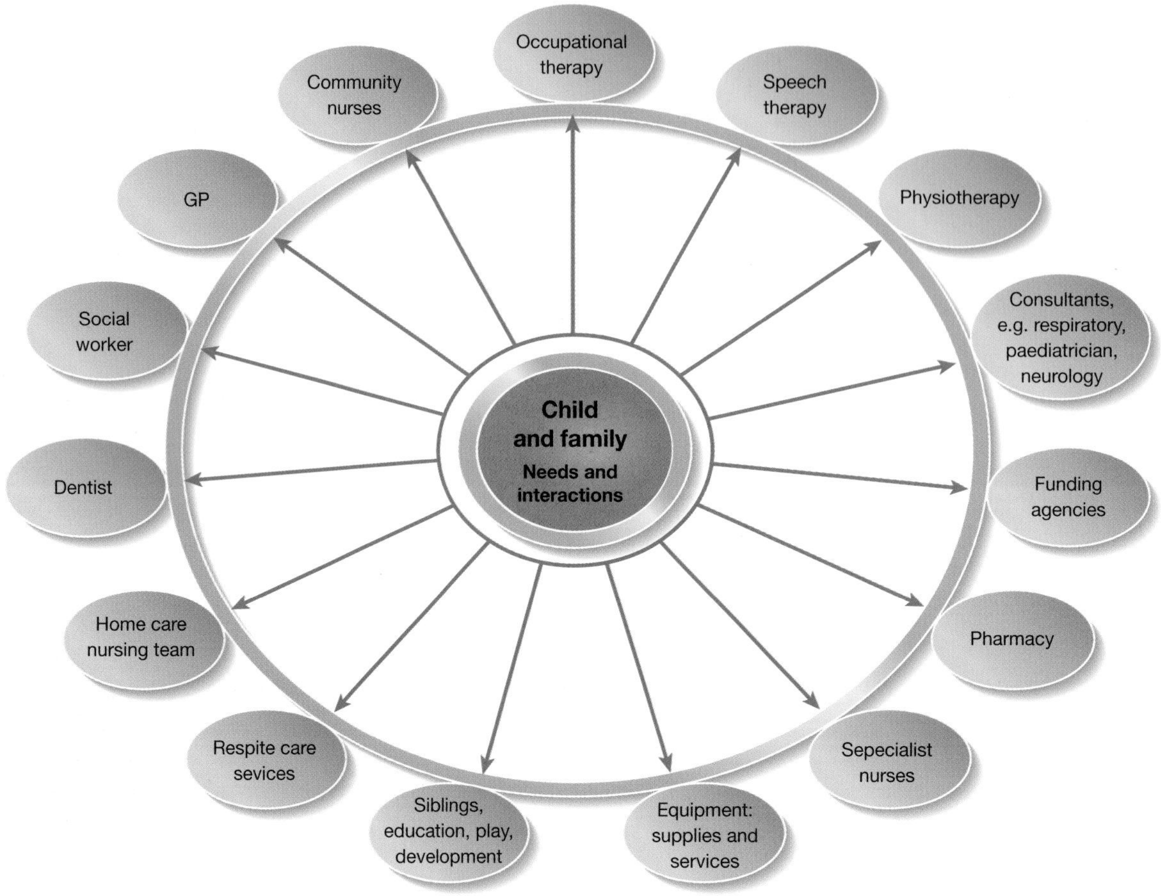

Children and Young People's Nursing at a Glance, First Edition. Edited by Alan Glasper, Jane Coad, and Jim Richardson.
© 2015 John Wiley & Sons, Ltd. Published 2015 by John Wiley & Sons, Ltd. Companion website: www.ataglanceseries.com/nursing/children

This chapter presents care issues that emerge for consideration when the family with a child with complex care needs are transitioning from the acute hospital setting to home. This includes children with chronic conditions and those who are technology dependent, where ongoing care necessitates the involvement of multiple providers. Figure 43.1 identifies many of the needs and interactions of the family with a child with complex care needs.

Children should be cared for, where possible, with their family, in their own home. However, if the family are to cope with being the primary carers, then a number of structures need to be in place to ensure a dynamic partnership between service providers and the child's family. Knowledge of the needs of each individual family is required to identify the strengths of each family and to identify and address their specific physical, emotional, financial and social needs, to ensure they can adapt their lives in a positive way to their changing circumstances.

Challenges to transitioning to home

Many children and their families may wait protracted periods of time in acute hospitals while negotiation ensues between the acute and community services over a wide range of transitional care needs:

• Absence of a coordinated vision for discharge in the tertiary care setting and no clear time frame for discharge
• Lack of leadership and clear negotiation and communication between with the parents, primary, secondary and tertiary care services
• No clear funding arrangements
• Absence of organized home care service delivery
• Delayed modifications to the child's home
• Procurement of adequate technology for home care
• Parents' financial challenges in changing work patterns
• Preparation of parents for the physical care of the child at home.

Assessing needs for discharge to home

There is a need for a thorough and accurate assessment of the needs of the child and family. Ideally, planning the discharge home of a child with complex care needs begins once it is established that the child, with some accommodation, could be cared for in their own home. This initially requires the tertiary care centre, together with the family, to widely consult with the multidisciplinary team to identify the extent of support services required for the child's care at home. This consultation phase is key to beginning the process of planning for home care and begins the process of establishing a trusting relationship between the parents and the primary, secondary and tertiary care services, as the parents begin to transition to being the primary carers.

Specific needs

Education needs. Parents need to know how to care for the child, how to identify changes in the child's condition, how to respond to any changing conditions, and how to access relevant support services in relation to equipment.

For example:
• Airway management and dealing with airway emergencies
• Care of a tracheotomy
• Care of the ventilated child and care of associated technology
• Care of the immobilized child including cleansing and dressing and pressure sore prevention or management
• Drug therapies, dosage and adverse effects
• Communication – specific aids required
• Pain assessment and management.

The family may require:

Care support. Home care nursing, respite services and access to ongoing health support services such as GP, community nurses physiotherapy, speech therapy, psychological support to help parents cope.

Social needs. Housing modifications may be required; parents will require financial advice and support in relation to the cost of caring for a child with complex needs at home; support to access education and developmental care needs.

Integrated care pathway

An agreed discharge plan and a specific care package should emerge from the assessment phase. The implementation of this plan requires a key worker or named coordinator, who has responsibility for acting as a dynamic service coordinator for the family. This means that they will have oversight of the family's interaction with hospital and community services, financial advice, procurement and servicing of equipment, and the ongoing review and refinement of the family's needs. This should include maintenance of a record of all appointments, funding plans and budget allowances, with responsibility for identifying and accessing services to support any changing needs of the family.

Key points

• A wide range of supports need to be in place to ensure a dynamic partnership between service providers and the child's family.
• Planning for transitioning to home should start very early.
• Parent's have education, social, emotional and financial needs.
• An integrated care pathway guided by a named coordinator can support the child and parents through their transition to home.

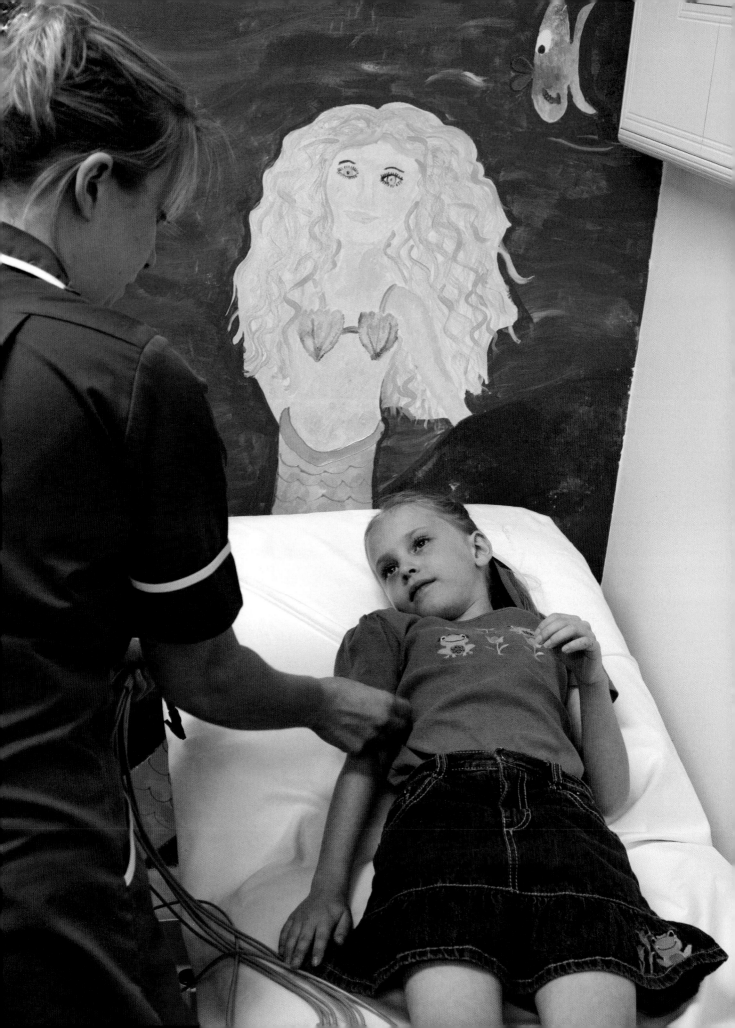

The newborn infant

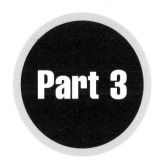

Chapters

Don't forget to visit the companion website for this book at **www.ataglanceseries.com/nursing/children** where you will find over 500 interactive multiple-choice questions to supplement your learning.

44 Fetal development

Figure 44.1 Fetal circulation

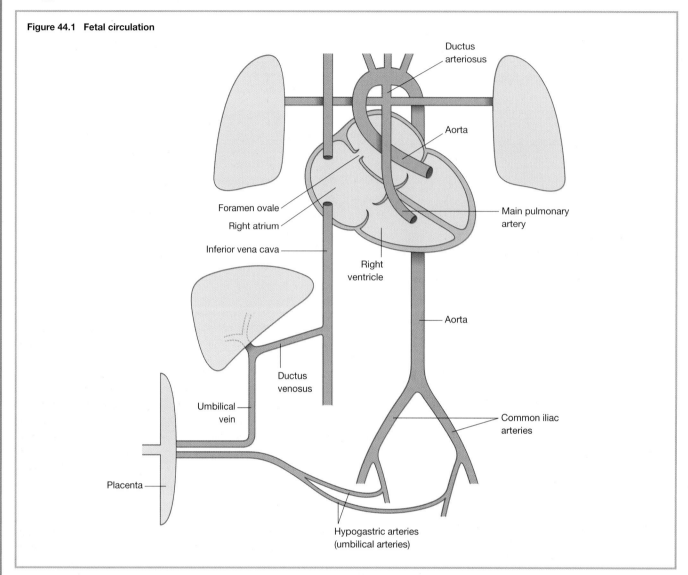

Pre-embryonic development

The fertilized ovum undergoes mitotic division resulting in a zygote then a morula. Within 4 days it becomes a blastocyst which implants into the uterine endometrium.

Embryonic development

Three germ layers – the ectoderm, mesoderm and endoderm – form the main tissues and organs in the developing embryo. By 4 weeks the embryo has a head, a trunk and tiny limb buds. Blood is also circulating around embryonic body at this stage. By 4–8 weeks, the embryo measures 2.5 cm and has recognizable facial features and major sensory organs are developing such as eyes, ears, nose, lips and tongue. The cardiovascular system, kidneys and liver are functional and the lungs are developing. Skeletal growth is cartilaginous and the limbs begin to lengthen.

Fetal development

8 weeks. The embryo becomes the fetus.

9–12 weeks. The eyelids close, the oral palate fuses, urine is produced and genitals are established. Red blood cells are produced in the liver. The fetus measures approximately 6.5 cm and weighs around 18 g.

13–20 weeks. Ossification of the skeleton begins and limbs reach their final proportions. Head hair is visible and lanugo is present over the body as is vernix. The liver and pancreas secrete enzymes and the fetus is capable of sucking. The fetus measures around 15 cm at this stage.

21–28 weeks. Lungs mature with alveoli visible. Fat deposits increase and lanugo begins to disappear. There is rapid brain growth at this stage.

28–32 weeks. Skin is pink but lacking in subcutaneous fat, but brown fat deposits increase. The main organs are functional and cerebral development increases as the brain grows. Length is approximately 38 cm and weight around 1800 g.

34–37 weeks. Fat deposits increase and the fetus becomes 'chubby'. The fetus 'practices' breathing movements – the lungs are now capable of breathing spontaneously. Genitalia are visible on ultrasound scan and the fetus is seen sucking and swallowing fluid. Fine tuning of the brain and neural system continues till birth. Length is approximately 45–50 cm.

37–40 weeks. The fetus is now capable of surviving at birth without intensive care. Movements felt by the mother are less intense as the growing fetus has less room to move around and the fetal head descends into the mother's pelvis. Lanugo has disappeared and the lungs are fully functional. The fetus will be able to breathe, suck milk, digest, absorb and excrete products. The central nervous system is fully functional, exhibiting numerous reflexes and behaviours. Length is approximately 50 cm and weight 3–4 kg.

Fetal circulation

The main differences between fetal and adult circulation:

Low pulmonary blood flow → pulmonary vascular resistance (PVR) high

Low placental resistance → systemic vascular resistance (SVR) low

Shunting of blood from right to left side of circulation through fetal shunts.

Fetal blood flow

Blood containing nutrients and oxygen flows from the placenta into the umbilical cord via the umbilical vein which goes to the liver where it branches off to the left lobe and receives the venous blood from the portal vein. This mixed blood bypasses the liver via the ductus venosus to enter the inferior vena cava where it travels to the right atrium of the heart. Approximately 75% of this mixed blood is diverted through an opening in the septum called the foramen ovale → into the left atrium. The remaining 25% of the blood is pumped into the right ventricle → pulmonary artery → some will go to the lungs but most will go into the ductus arteriosus which bypasses the lungs to deliver blood to the aortic arch. All of this is influenced by the high resistance in the right ventricle and pulmonary artery. The blood from the left atrium passes into left ventricle then enters the aorta passing along its branches to supply head, neck and arms before travelling through the vessels in the chest and abdomen. The aorta divides into the common iliac arteries, small streams passing down into the legs but the main streams pass into the hypogastric arteries. These arteries arise in the pelvis and pass through the umbilicus and enter the cord as the two umbilical arteries which return deoxygenated blood back to the placenta for oxygenation. In the fetal circulation, the right side of the circulation is dominant due to high PVR so any shunting will be from right to left. The left side is less dominant due to low SVR because the placenta is a low resistance organ.

Adaptation at birth

Once the umbilical cord is clamped the umbilical vein ceases to pump blood and collapses – the umbilical arteries and veins constrict → low resistance from placenta is removed. There is a rise in SVR → increased pressure (SVR) in the left atrium as well as a fall in pressure in the right atrium results in blood trying to move from left to right across the septum → closure of the foramen ovale. The baby breathes, the airways open and pulmonary circulation improves → increased oxygen levels close the ductus arteriosus (a reduction in prostaglandin levels also assists) → greater blood flow to the lungs. Blood flow in the hypogastric arteries ceases and these become ligaments.

Other factors

Baby breathes: air is drawn into alveoli and blood into the capillary networks surrounding them → lung fluid pushed into lymphatic system and pulmonary circulation → PVR falls. (Lungs do not fully expand for a few hours after birth.) Rising PO_2 constricts PDA (15 minutes–3 weeks). Surfactant – produced by type II cells in lungs – reduces surface tension and prevent alveoli from collapsing. Circulating catecholamines (adrenaline) reduces secretion of lung fluid and increases absorption through the lymphatic system. They also increase heart rate and contraction as well as coronary perfusion.

Adaptation of other systems at birth

Haematology – deficiency of vitamin K. Haemoglobin F initially. Physiological jaundice due to breakdown of red blood cells

Regulation of body temperature – utilization of glucose and fat stores to maintain body heat

Digestive system – feeding, absorption, excretion (meconium)

Renal – should pass 3 mL/kg/hr within the first 24 hours

Central nervous system – sensitive to stimuli – poor motor development

Immature immune system – breastfeeding provides IgA

Neonatal examination

Figure 45.1 Examination of the neonate

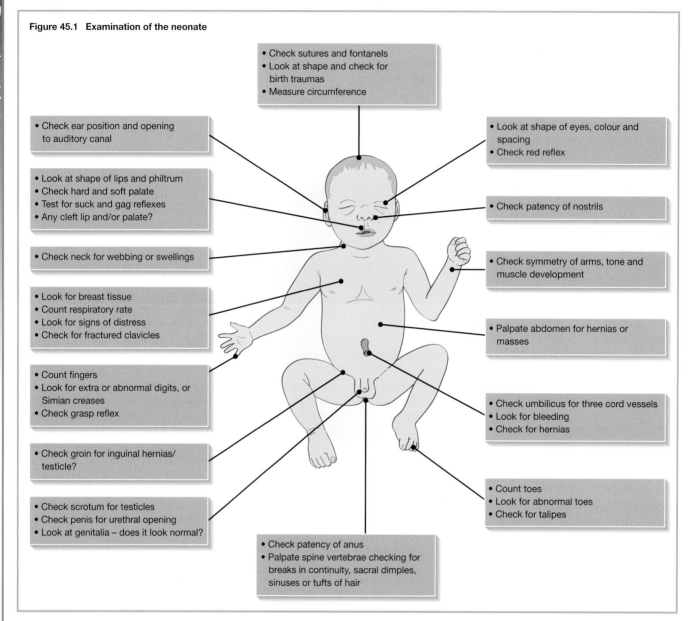

- Check sutures and fontanels
- Look at shape and check for birth traumas
- Measure circumference

- Look at shape of eyes, colour and spacing
- Check red reflex

- Check ear position and opening to auditory canal

- Check patency of nostrils

- Look at shape of lips and philtrum
- Check hard and soft palate
- Test for suck and gag reflexes
- Any cleft lip and/or palate?

- Check neck for webbing or swellings

- Check symmetry of arms, tone and muscle development

- Look for breast tissue
- Count respiratory rate
- Look for signs of distress
- Check for fractured clavicles

- Palpate abdomen for hernias or masses

- Count fingers
- Look for extra or abnormal digits, or Simian creases
- Check grasp reflex

- Check umbilicus for three cord vessels
- Look for bleeding
- Check for hernias

- Check groin for inguinal hernias/testicle?

- Count toes
- Look for abnormal toes
- Check for talipes

- Check scrotum for testicles
- Check penis for urethral opening
- Look at genitalia – does it look normal?

- Check patency of anus
- Palpate spine vertebrae checking for breaks in continuity, sacral dimples, sinuses or tufts of hair

Children and Young People's Nursing at a Glance, First Edition. Edited by Alan Glasper, Jane Coad, and Jim Richardson.
© 2015 John Wiley & Sons, Ltd. Published 2015 by John Wiley & Sons, Ltd. Companion website: www.ataglanceseries.com/nursing/children

The initial examination carried out after birth is to identify any deviations from normal but it should be pointed out to parents that some conditions only become apparent days and weeks after birth and so this examination cannot rule out problems later on. A general physical examination of the baby is carried out by the midwife or paediatrician soon after birth. At this time the weight, head circumference and length are measured and recorded in the baby's Personal Child Health Record book. These measurements are plotted on a centile chart. Average head circumference for a term baby is in the range 35–38 cm; length is usually 46–55 cm in term babies.

Term babies normally lie in a flexed position, moving their arms and legs occasionally. The practitioner should look for symmetry when looking at movement, posture and the overall appearance of the baby. Each part of the baby is examined systematically.

• **Skin**: look at colour. Term babies have thicker skin which looks creamy pink; preterm babies have thinner skin which looks more reddish in colour and may be covered in vernix (a white waxy substance) or lanugo (fine hairs). Check for rashes or birth traumas.

• **Mouth**: feel the hard and soft palate for clefts and also look for premature teeth or tongue ties. Check suck and gag reflexes are present.

• **Head**: feel around the skull for the suture lines as well as the anterior and posterior fontanels, checking for normality of these. Often there is moulding (overlapping). Check for large swellings which can either be cephalhaematoma (bleeding between two layers of bone) or caput succedaneum (oedema), both of which can be painful and require analgesia. Measure head circumference.

• **Eyes**: make sure eyes are present; look at spacing, shape, and iris for deviations from normal. Check colour of sclera for jaundice, blueness (osteogenesis imperfecta) or infection. Red reflex should be checked for presence – also that pupils are reactive to light.

• **Nose**: check for shape and bridge configuration – also patency of nostrils.

• **Ears**: tops should be level with eyes. Look for rotation: low set, rotated ears can be indicative of chromosomal abnormalities. Check for an opening to the auditory canal. Lack of cartilage suggests prematurity. Hearing should be tested prior to discharge.

• **Neck**: look for webbing (chromosomal defect) and cystic hygromas (swellings) which can block the airway.

• **Arms and hands**: check for symmetry in length and shape as well as the range of movement of arms. Count the fingers and look for webbing, extra or overlapping digits, which may indicate genetic defects. Look for simian crease (single deep crease on palm), which is linked to trisomy 21 (Down's syndrome). Check the colour of fingernails – blueness may indicate cardiac disease.

• **Chest wall**: look for symmetry, breast tissue and nipples (absence indicates prematurity). Observe breathing rate (40–60/min) and look for respiratory distress (indrawing, tachypnoea). Check clavicles for fractures – common in large babies or difficult deliveries.

• **Abdominal wall**: gently palpate for any lumps (hernias), particularly around the umbilicus or groin areas. Check umbilicus for three cord vessels before shortening the cord and applying the Hollister clamp.

• **Legs and feet**: check for symmetry in length and shape as well as the range of movement. Count the toes and look for webbing, extra or overlapping digits, which may indicate genetic defects. Look for inverted feet (talipes), can be positional or true talipes, both of which will require treatment with physiotherapy or orthopaedic treatment.

• **Genitalia**: girls: look for labia majora and minora, clitoris and urethra. Labia majora covers these structures in term babies but gapes open exposing them in preterm babies. Boys: check penis for urethral opening (abnormal opening on the underside – hyposadias) and the scrotal sac for two testicles – may be undescended. Both these conditions require referral and follow-up.

• **Spine**: feel the spine from the base of skull right down to anal sphincter. Check for breaks in continuity of spinal column. Look for tufts of hair or sinuses, all of which may be indicative of occult spina bifida.

• **Anal sphincter**: check that it is patent. The baby should pass meconium within 24–48 hours after birth. Failure to do so may indicate meconium ileus, bowel obstruction or imperforate anus. The baby should also pass urine – 3 ml/kg/hour.

The baby should have colour, heart rate, respiratory rate and temperature checked before leaving the delivery suite to ensure that these fall within the normal parameters. Colour should be cream–pink but the baby may still look a little blue in the hands and feet (acrocynaosis) for up to 24 hours. Heart rate should be 110–160/min; Respiratory rate should be 40–60/min. Temperature should be 36.4–37°C. The umbilical cord should be checked at intervals for bleeding. Normally, the heart sounds, femoral pulses, neurological reflexes, red reflex and hips are checked when the baby is having the final examination prior to discharge home. Hearing tests are carried out within the first week of life.

46 Neonatal screening tests

Figure 46.1 Neonatal screening tests

To allow early diagnosis of rare, severe diseases and start treatments as early as possible

Features

- Easy to perform, low cost
- Early diagnosis can change prognosis
- A specific treatment protocol is available
- As specific and sensitive as possible
- Not operator-dependent
- On large populations

Methods

- Capillary blood drawn by heel prick
- Collected on special filter cards
- Between 24 hours and 7 days after birth
- Child must have been fed at least once
- Voluntary or mandatory according to local regulations
- Preterms may need further samples
- Tests for specific metabolites or enzymes or genetic mutations

PKU

- Phenylalanine concentration in blood
- Mental retardation, microcephaly, severe learning disabilities, seizures
- Phenylalanine-free formulas for new borns and infants, reduce foods that contains a source of phenylalanine plus amino acid supplementation

SCD

- Presence of abnormal haemoglobin in blood
- Vaso-occlusive episodes, acute pain, infections, anemia, haemolysis
- Antibiotic prophylaxis, blood transfusion, pain killers, immunosupressants, folic acid, dehydration prevention

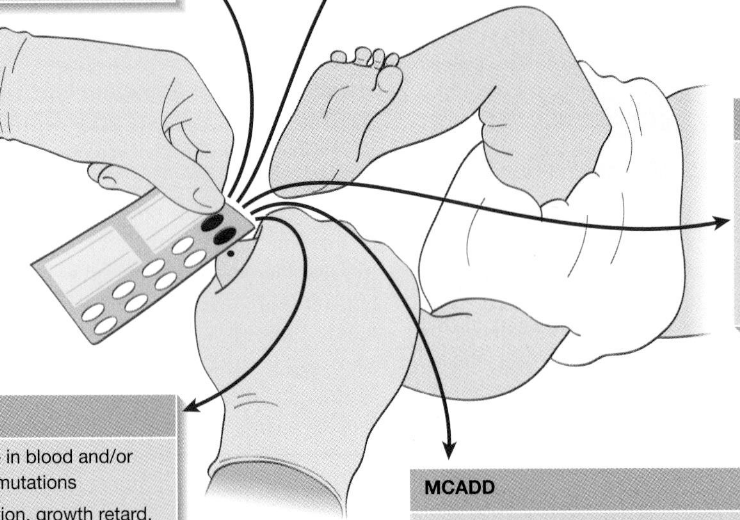

CHT

- Thyroxine or thyreotropin concentration in blood
- Lethargy, hypotonia, growth failure, mental retardation
- Oral administration of thyroxine for life

- Test performed
- Clinical manifestations if untreated
- Treatment that can improve prognosis

CF

- Immunoreactive trypsine in blood and/or specific genetic (CFTR) mutations
- Malabsorption, dehydration, growth retard, chronic lung infections, respiratory impairment
- Strict treatment regimen including panceatic enzymes, respiratory PT, antibiotics, airway infections prevention

MCADD

- Carnitine (C6, C8 or C10) in blood
- Fatigue, lethargy, hypoglycaemia, breathing difficulties, liver disorders, brain harm
- Prevention of fasting, maintain caloric intake during illnesses

Children and Young People's Nursing at a Glance, First Edition. Edited by Alan Glasper, Jane Coad, and Jim Richardson.
© 2015 John Wiley & Sons, Ltd. Published 2015 by John Wiley & Sons, Ltd. Companion website: www.ataglanceseries.com/nursing/children

Neonatal screening programmes

Neonatal screening programmes (NSPs) are performed on newborn infants to allow the early detection of uncommon and severe congenital diseases that are not clinically evident at birth but in which the prognosis can be significantly influenced by starting specific treatments very early in life of a subject. An NSP is not intended to provide the diagnosis of a specific disease but to identify within a population those subjects who are at higher risk of being affected by such disease. The newborn babies who have positive results to the screening test (usually about 1%) undergo further diagnostic tests to exclude or confirm the diagnosis.

Ideally, an NSP should be easy to perform, not operator-dependent and low-cost; it could be easily performed on large numbers of people; it should be run only where a specific treatment protocol is available that can change the outcome for those diagnosed. Moreover, an NSP should be acceptable to the public and determine as little psychosocial harms to false positive families as possible. Finally, an NSP should be as specific and sensitive as possible, in order to reduce both false positive results and false negative results to the lowest level. However, a relatively small number of false negative results are always present. Recently, tandem mass spectrometry scanning allowed a huge expansion of potentially detectable congenital disorders of metabolism.

NSPs are usually funded by public health systems. The diseases included in an NSP vary across countries, depending on the resources available and on the incidence of the diseases. According to local regulations, undergoing an NSP may be on a voluntary basis or mandatory for all newborn babies.

Sample collection and analysis

Neonatal screening tests are usually performed on the newborn infant's capillary blood drawn by heel prick. A number of blood spots are collected on special filter cards and allowed to dry. The cards also contain information regarding the newborn baby. Collection of blood spots is usually performed between 24 hours from birth and before the seventh day of life, with the child having been fed at least once. In preterm infants, a supplemental blood sample may be required later. Blood is analysed for the presence of specific metabolites, enzymes or genetic mutations.

Conditions commonly screened

Phenylketonuria (PKU)

PKU is an autosomal recessive genetic disease that prevents metabolization of phenylalanine (Phe), an amino acid introduced in the body with several proteic foods (incidence 1 in 9000). At birth children are normal but if untreated they develop mental retardation, microcephaly, severe learning disabilities, EEG alterations and seizures. Children with PKU have a tendency to hypopigmentation of hair and skin and a characteristic musty odour of sweat and urine. Treatment consists in reducing foods that contains a source of Phe (e.g. eggs, fish, dairy products, meat, nuts, legumes, some artificial sweeteners) and in administering amino acid supplementation. Special Phe-free formulas are administered to infants. The screening test measures Phe concentration in blood.

Congenital hypothyroidism (CHT)

CHT is an endocrinopathy that affects 1 in every 3000–4000 newborn babies and is mainly caused by a defect of development of the thyroid gland. If untreated, within a few weeks from birth the child develops growth failure and irreversible mental retardation. Typically, an infant with CHT appears sleepy, hypotonic, colder than normal and uninterested in feeding. The treatment is oral administration of thyroxine for life, which is sufficient to prevent the onset of symptoms. Regularity in thyroxine administration and adherence to a follow-up programme is paramount. Body weight and heart rate should be periodically checked. The onset of fatigue may indicate the need to adjust the drug dosage. There are different screening strategies for CHT; they are usually based on the measurement of thyroxine or thyreotropin in blood.

Cystic fibrosis (CF)

CF is an autosomal recessive disease (incidence varies in ethnic groups 1 in 2500–100 000) that determines a malfunction of mucous cells membrane ion exchange, resulting in an excessive thickness of all exocrine secretions. Babies with CF present with malabsorption due to exocrine pancreatic insufficiency, chronic lung infections with progressive respiratory impairment and a large number of other clinical manifestations that reduce life expectancy. However, CF may remain asymptomatic long after birth. No cure is currently available but an early treatment regimen has shown to be effective to reduce disease progression, delay lung infections and increase lifespan. CF screening is based on dosing immunoreactive trypsine (IRT), which is higher in children with CF, and/or on the research of a panel of genetic mutations coding for CF. Children found positive by screening undergo the sweat test (titration of chloride in sweat) to confirm diagnosis.

Sickle cell disease (SCD)

SCD is an autosomic recessive disease of blood, with higher incidence in tropical and Mediterranean populations. It is caused by defective haemoglobin; red blood cells assume a sickle shape and lose elasticity causing acute vaso-occlusive episodes with acute pain, infections, anaemia, haemolysis and several other manifestations and long-term complications. Treatment is complex and includes blood transfusions, antibiotic prophylaxis, immunosuppressants, pain killers, folic acid, preventing cold and dehydration and many other measures. Early detection of SCD reduces the risk of some complications (in particular pneumococcal infections) and may improve patients' quality of life. A screening test investigates for the presence of abnormal haemoglobin in the newborn infant's capillary blood. If the test is positive, a second blood test is performed to confirm the diagnosis within the second month of life. SCD screening may also detect subjects with beta-thalassaemia disorders.

Medium-chain acyl-CoA dehydrogenase deficiency (MCADD)

This is an autosomal recessive disease (incidence 1 in 4000–17 000) that impedes the conversion of some body fats into energy, in particular during fast. This may cause fatigue, lethargy and hypoglycaemia. Symptoms appear early in life and left untreated MCADD can lead to severe complications such as seizures, breathing difficulties, liver disorders, brain damage, coma and death. Early diagnosis improves prognosis as it allows prevention of risky situations, such as fasting – in particular during illnesses– and other circumstances where body energy production requires fatty acid oxidation.

47 The premature baby

Figure 47.1 Characteristics of the premature baby

Skin

- Red or ruddy in colour
- Thin skinned, lacks keratin, skin is transparent and leaks water with visible blood vessels, little if any subcutaneous fat
- Covered with lanugo or a soft downy hair
- Soles and palms are smooth, creasing increases with gestational age
- Nails are soft

Head

- Large head, large surface to body weight ratio
- Fine hair is present from 22 weeks, eyebrows and eyelashes evident from 23 weeks
- Eyelids are fused until 25 weeks
- Retina is avascular until 16 weeks; retinal vessels grow concentrically from the optic nerve. From 32 weeks the vessels develop towards the vascular edge of the retina
- Cry is weak or feeble
- Initially the ear is shapeless, pinna is soft and lacks shape; cartilage formation increases with gestational age

Posture

- Extended posture as a result of underdeveloped muscles. Tone and flexion increases with gestation

Breast tissue

- Areolar is raised by 34 weeks and breast tissue is evident by 36 weeks

Genitalia

Boys: testes undescended, scrotum smooth and small

Girls: prominent clitoris, labia majora widely separated, labia minora protruding

Breathing

- Irregular respirations, pliable thorax, weak respiratory musculature

Photograph
From Lissauer and Fanaroff (2011)
Neonatology at a Glance, 2nd ed.
Reproduced with permission of Wiley.

Table 47.1 The premature baby

Definitions	Incidence
Preterm: <37 completed weeks' gestation *Moderate or late preterm:* 35–37 completed weeks' gestation *Very preterm:* 29–34 completed weeks' gestation *Extremely preterm:* <28 completed weeks' gestation	About 5–10% of deliveries in developed countries are preterm According to the Office for National Statistics (2005), the incidence of premature births in the United Kingdom is approaching 8% or 1 in 13 live births • 50% of twin births are premature • 93% of preterm births occur after 28 weeks' gestation • 6% occur between 22 and 27 weeks' gestation • 1% occur before 22 weeks' gestation

Causes of prematurity

- Maternal hypertension
- Intrauterine growth restriction
- Intrauterine infection
- Antepartum haemorrhage
- Cervical incompetence
- Maternal smoking

Outcome

Survival rate for the preterm infant has improved greatly over the last 30 years. Premature birth can result in a wide range of physical and cognitive deficits, such as cerebral palsy and learning difficulties. Mortality and morbidity are influenced by the gestational age at birth; the lower the gestational age, the greater the risk of death or disability.

Depending upon the degree of prematurity and wellness at birth, premature babies receive different levels of care:

- Transitional care
- Special care
- High dependency
- Intensive care.

The various levels of care are provided by different types of neonatal units: special care units (SCUs), local neonatal units (LNUs) and neonatal intensive care units (NICUs).

Table 47.2 Regardless of level of care or unit required, all premature babies should be kept 'PINK, WARM and SWEET' and the 'PARENTS TOO'

Nursing care of the premature baby anticipates the potential problems resulting from the infant's anatomical and/or physiological immaturity and presenting characteristics

	Problem	Aim	Nursing care
PINK	Potential problem of respiratory distress indicated by: • Chest recession, • Tachypnoea (respiratory rate >60) • Nasal flaring • Expiratory grunting • Cyanosis • Apnoea Due to surfactant deficiency, pliable thorax, weak respiratory musculature, immature respiratory centre	To maintain adequate gas exchange as indicated by • Normal arterial blood gas • SaO$_2$ ≤32/40 88–93% 　　　>32/40 91–94% 　　　>32 without CLD 　　　93–99% in O$_2$ Respiratory rate 40–60	• Monitor, observe and record respiratory rate and pattern, heart rate and blood pressure • Observe for signs of respiratory distress • Administer O$_2$/respiratory support to maintain SaO$_2$ within agreed limits • Position for best oxygenation and support • Monitor and record apnoeas • Ensure emergency equipment at hand
WARM	Potential problem of cold stress as indicated by: • Widening toe–core differential, and/or • Axilla temperature <36.6°C Due to lack of subcutaneous and brown fat, extended posture, immature skin/↑ transepidermal water loss and handling Four modes of heat loss/transfer and the order of magnitude for the premature infant: • *Evaporation*: heat is lost when water evaporates from the skin or breath • *Convection*: heat is loss to currents of air • *Radiation*: heat is lost by electromagnetic waves from skin to surrounding surfaces • *Conduction*: direct heat loss to solid surfaces	To maintain axilla temperature at 36.6–37.2°C and toe–core differential at 1.5–2°C	• Nurse in an incubator in a neutral thermal environment. Consider the four modes of heat loss/transfer • Maximum humidity (80–85%) if <1 kg or <28/40, 60% if <32/40 • Use heating aids appropriately • Monitor temperature continuously and/or 4–6 hourly • Position flexed to minimize surface area and heat loss • **MINIMAL HANDLING**
SWEET	Potential problem of altered nutrition including hypoglycaemia and inadequate intake to maintain hydration and meet body requirements as indicated by: • Weight loss >10% • Blood glucose <2.0 mmol/L Gastric tubes: Size 5 <1500 g Size 6 ≥1500 g Minimum size 8 should be used for gastric decompression regardless of baby's gestation or size Methods of feeding: breast, bottle, cup orogastric/nasogastric tube	• Infant remains hydrated • Blood glucose >2.5 mmol/L • Infant tolerates feeds and gains appropriate weight Signs of hypoglycaemia: hypotonia, feeding difficulties, abnormal cry, jitteriness, cyanosis, tachypnoea, irritability, temperature instability and convulsions	• Administer mL/kg/day • Maintain fluid balance and in–out chart • Give IV/oral fluids as prescribed • Ensure safety/patency of IV lines • Observe for clinical signs of hypoglycaemia • Choose appropriate oral method based on: wellness, maturity of suck/swallow reflex (usually develops around 34 weeks), parental feeding wishes • Monitor and record feeding tolerance (gastric aspirate or vomiting) • Encourage mother to express breast milk and/or breastfeed • Monitor blood glucose
PARENTS TOO	Actual problem of parental anxiety due to separation, infant's condition, unexpected prematurity, unfamiliar equipment and surroundings	To promote family relationships and reduce anxiety Parents participate in the care of their infant	• Good communication – listen, use parent friendly language, document visits • Inform parents of infant's condition, treatment and progress; repeat and clarify as necessary. Provide written literature • Encourage visiting, phoning and involvement in infant's care • Encourage positive parent and family interaction with infant (e.g. Kangaroo Care, touching, stroking, containment holding as tolerated by the infant) • Orientate family to neonatal unit • Offer support and advice to help mother initiate and maintain lactation

Premature infants are at risk of other problems including intraventricular haemorrhage, periventricular leukomalacia, patent ductus arteriosus, jaundice, sepsis – including necrotising enterocolitis (NEC), retinopathy of prematurity and chronic lung disease.

48 Neonatal transport

Common reasons for transfer

- Extreme prematurity
- Respiratory distress syndrome
- Meconium aspiration syndrome
- Hypoxic ischaemic encephalopathy
- Congenital anomalies including:
  - respiratory
  - surgical
  - cardiac

Types of transport

Internal:
- Admission from labour suite
- Transfer within the maternity department
- Transfers to departments for investigations

Inter-hospital transfer:
- Acute intensive care transfer
- Non-acute transfer
- Back transfer to referral unit
- Transfer to specialist department for investigations

Transport vehicles

- Specialized Neonatal Transport Service with dedicated neonatal ambulance
- Emergency services vehicle
- Air transport by fixed wing aeroplane, helicopter or Ministry of Defence aircraft

Mode of transfer: influencing factors

- Nature of the illness and urgency
- Distance
- Weather
- Geography
- Traffic conditions
- Cost of transfer

Figure 48. 1   Road transport

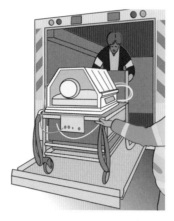

Figure 48.2   Air transport

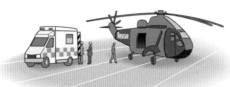
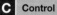

Figure 48.3   Sea King helicopter

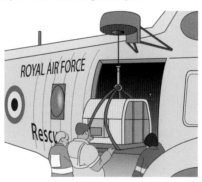

ROYAL AIR FORCE

Principles of safe transport

Systematic approach: **ACCEPT** model applied at each stage
- Assessment
- Control
- Communication
- Evaluation
- Preparation, packaging and pre-departure check
- Transportation

A   Assessment
- What is the problem?
- What intervention is required or, if already implemented, what is the effect?
- What further management is needed?

C   Control
Delegated team leader leads transport

C   Communication
- Parents
- Colleagues
- Documentation

E   Evaluation
- Is transfer appropriate?
- Identify problems at each stage

P   Preparation, packaging and pre-departure check
- Stabilization before transfer
- Equipment checks
- Pre-departure checklist

T   Transportation
- Mode of transport
- Safety of patient and staff during journey

Children and Young People's Nursing at a Glance, First Edition. Edited by Alan Glasper, Jane Coad, and Jim Richardson.
© 2015 John Wiley & Sons, Ltd. Published 2015 by John Wiley & Sons, Ltd. Companion website: www.ataglanceseries.com/nursing/children

Centralization of tertiary paediatric and neonatal services throughout the United Kingdom has influenced the provision of neonatal intensive care facilities. When a neonate requires additional care to that which is provided locally it may be necessary to transfer them to a specialized centre for assessment and ongoing care. This development has had an effect on the demands placed on local and regional neonatal transport services.

Neonates transferred by transport teams are frequently critically ill. They may be extremely preterm, require surgical assessment and intervention or have congenital heart disease. Ongoing innovations in clinical management during transport such as extracorporeal membrane oxygenation (ECMO), high frequency oscillation (HFO) and inspired nitric oxide therapy (iNO) have resulted in the need for highly technical and specialized transfers.

Transporting a sick neonate can be a complex procedure, involving preparing the neonate for movement into portable intensive care equipment, loading of the equipment into vehicles for transfer such as an ambulance, a helicopter, fixed wing plane or military helicopter. During transport, environmental influences such as fluctuations in temperature, noise, movement, vibration, G forces and barometric pressure can potentially be areas of stress, pain and discomfort to the neonate.

These innovations have necessitated the development of specialized teams of clinicians and nurses to manage these transfers safely and in a timely manner.

Planning a transport

Detailed local procedures for referral and transfer of a neonate are available regionally within the United Kingdom. However, the principles of a safe and effective transport are outlined in several publications (Jaimovich and Vidyasagar 1996; Barry and Leslie 2003) and are contained within a structured education programme to guide management of a transport (Byrne et al. 2008).

Organization and management of a transport

The stages involved in transporting a patient have been described within a systematic approach in order to facilitate a streamlined, safe and effective transport. One approach is the ACCEPT method described by Byrne et al. (2008), which is used in adults but can also be used in paediatrics and neonates and will be applied to summarize the process.

Assessment (A)

The first stage in the transport is assessment. In some situations the clinicians involved with the care of the neonate may undertake the transport. However, increasingly, regional transport teams are mobilized to facilitate the transport and will therefore have no prior knowledge of the neonate's clinical history. Communication and documentation is therefore paramount between the referring unit and the transport team.

The clinician who is responsible for the decision to transfer the neonate will liaise with the transport services and the receiving unit. A succinct summary of the problem should be relayed to the transport team. This will enable a decision to be made on the most appropriate mode of transport and receiving unit.

What information should be relayed to the transport team?
- **Description of the problem**: history, clinical condition, vital signs laboratory results.
- **Intervention**: what has been done or is needed, what has been the effect? This information will aid diagnosis and future management.
- **What further management is needed?** This will facilitate appropriate management during transport and on arrival at the receiving unit.

Control (C)

A transport lead is delegated to provide advice prior to and during transport and delegate tasks.

Communication (C)

At all stages of the transport communication is crucial.
- **Parents**: update on their baby's condition, reasons for transfer and information about the receiving unit such as location and visiting.
- **Colleagues**: concise information throughout the transfer relayed among the referral unit, transport team and receiving unit.
- **Documentation**: pre-transport, during transport and on arrival at the receiving unit. Including vital signs, all interventions, effects and changes in management.

Evaluation (E)

- Is transfer appropriate for the baby? Is the baby too unstable for transfer, or can a specialist review the baby in the referral unit?
- Identify and document problems at each stage of the transfer.

Preparation, packaging and pre-departure check (P)

- **Stabilization before transfer**: rapid assessment and management of life-threatening problems (ABC):
    Airway: must be patent and stable throughout the transfer
    Breathing: may be necessary to intubate prior to transfer
    Circulation: vascular access secured and dependent on intensity of patient
- **Equipment checks**: prior to departure
- **Pre-departure checklist**: includes final review of ABC.

Transportation (T)

- **Mode of transport**: select the most appropriate for the patient and circumstances.
- **Safety of patient and staff during journey**: safety is a priority throughout. Is it safe to move the patient? Is it safe for staff to move the patient?

Red flag
- Safe transport is crucial for an effective transport.

49 Jaundice and hyperbilirubinaemia

Figure 49.1   A baby nursed under a phototherapy unit with support rolls and eye covers

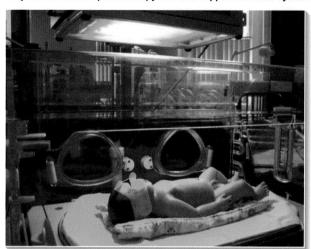
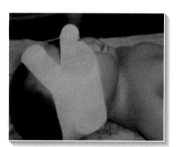

Physiology of bilirubin

All babies have high haemoglobin levels at birth but in the early days the red blood cells are destroyed in large volumes resulting in increased levels of bilirubin in the plasma. This is unconjugated bilirubin which is fat soluble and cannot be excreted by the body in this form so it travels to the liver for conjugation. The unconjugated bilirubin attaches itself to albumin binding sites and travels to the liver. If the bilirubin becomes detached it circulates as free unconjugated bilirubin and can cross the blood–brain barrier, resulting in encephalopathy or brain damage. (Certain drugs can displace bilirubin from its binding site, e.g. sulfonamides and lipofundin.) Once it reaches the liver the unconjugated bilirubin is acted on by liver enzymes glucuroneryl transferase and glucuronic acid but oxygen and glucose are required for this to happen. Once conjugated, the bilirubin leaves the liver as water-soluble bilirubin which can now be excreted by the body. Approximately 80% of this bilirubin travels down the common bile duct to the small intestine where it is excreted in the stools as stercobilinogen. Approximately 15% enters the bloodstream and travels to the gut and the kidneys where it is excreted as urobilinogen; the remainder continues to circulate in the enterohepatic circulation. Unconjugated bilirubin levels are reported in a lab result as the indirect bilirubin level; conjugated bilirubin is reported as the direct bilirubin level. Babies become jaundiced when the level of bilirubin in the plasma exceeds the albumin binding sites or the ability of the liver to conjugate and excrete bilirubin from the body by normal means.

Hyperbilirubinaemia

Hyperbilirubinaemia is an excess of bilirubin in the blood that results in serum bilirubin (SBR) levels higher than 300 µmmol/L in term babies and 200 µmmol/L in preterm infants. Babies appear yellow, particularly the skin, sclera of eyes and the mucous membranes of mouth, as bilirubin is deposited in the tissues. Normally, in the case of physiological bilirubin where there is delayed conjugation and excretion, the jaundice will usually disappear with 7–10 days. In pathological jaundice, the levels may increase and excretion will take longer. If left untreated it can lead to encephalopathy (brain damage) which can result in abnormal neurological function or death.

Causes

Physiological: normal breakdown of red blood cells resulting in high levels of unconjugated bilirubin in the first 3–4 days of life. The baby is fed more frequently and may require phototherapy treatment; usually resolves within 7–10 days.

Pathological: may appear within the first 24–48 hours of life and indicates ongoing haemolysis. Causes include rhesus or ABO incompatibility, congenital sepsis (TORCH viruses) and haemaglobinopathies such as sickle cell disease.

Pathological: occurring within the first week of life: acquired infections, breastfeeding jaundice, liver disorders, bruising (birth trauma).

Jaundice that persists for longer than 2 weeks

This is caused by metabolic conditions such as galactosaemia, hypothyroidism; infections such as urinary tract infections; breast-milk jaundice. High levels of beta glucuronidase slow down conjugation of bilirubin and so indirect levels may be high – this will resolve itself and there is no need for the mother to discontinue breastfeeding. Jaundice may persist for >3 months.

Obstructive jaundice or biliary atresia

This is caused by an obstruction of the common bile duct. Conjugated bilirubin cannot travel to the gut for excretion and so builds up in the liver. There will be a high direct bilirubin level (>20% of total SBR level), the baby's stools will be pale in colour, he/she will appear very jaundiced, may be sleepy and not feeding well. Any baby who remains jaundiced for >2 weeks after birth should have a repeat SBR level checked as well as liver function test to exclude biliary atresia which is a life-threatening condition.

Children and Young People's Nursing at a Glance, First Edition. Edited by Alan Glasper, Jane Coad, and Jim Richardson.

Investigations of jaundice

• Check the mother's history for details of other babies, pregnancy (blood group and rhesus factor), medications, labour/delivery and method of feeding. Check the baby's condition since birth (e.g. alertness, feeding method, stools).

• Look at the baby's skin colour, also the sclera of the eyes and mucous membranes – all may appear yellow.

• Check baby's state of alertness – dangerously jaundiced babies tend to become very sleepy and difficult to feed.

• Check colour of stools and urine – if stools are pale or grey it could be a result of biliary atresia. Urine may be a little darker than normal.

• Use transcutaneous bilirubin meter. If result is $>250\,\mu$mmol/L then take a blood sample for testing SBR.

• Check SBR levels – the indirect (unconjugated) + direct (conjugated) levels can be requested. Rule out anaemia and/or sepsis.

• Babies with prolonged jaundice should have fractioned SBR levels checked as well as liver function tests to rule out biliary atresia.

Management of jaundice

Depending on the cause, treatment varies from additional feeding and exposure to sunlight for physiological jaundice, to phototherapy, albumin transfusions or exchange transfusions for the more serious cases. Rhesus disease is less common as mothers who are rhesus negative are screened for rhesus antibodies during pregnancy and are given prophylactic anti-D immunoglobulin. In all cases of jaundice, the SBR levels must be monitored very closely with results being plotted on a graph to indicate the rate of increase; the graph also provides indicators as to how the condition should be managed. National Institute for Clinical Excellence (NICE 2011) Guidelines for Neonatal Jaundice (CG98).

Phototherapy

Phototherapy is the use of fluorescent lights to break down and begin the process of treating unconjugated bilirubin in the plasma reducing the workload of the immature liver. The lights are directed on to the naked baby's skin in an effort to conjugate the bilirubin in the subcutaneous tissues. Phototherapy can be administered via overhead lamps, spotlights, biliblankets or mattresses. Overhead lamps are the more common form used and normally consist of white and blue lights; the blue are more effective at reducing SBR levels. The lamp should be the recommended distance from baby and can be used over incubators or cots (as long as there is a plexiglass shield in place to reflect harmful UV rays from baby). Some units use covers over the incubator to keep the light inside the incubator, thereby increasing the effect.

Care of a baby having phototherapy

• The baby should be nursed naked except for a phototherapy nappy (very small thereby exposing as much of the skin as possible).

• Feeds and fluids should be calculated to ensure that adequate protein is given on a daily basis (albumin binding sites); this will mean more frequent feeds for babies feeding enterally. There is no indication for increasing intravenous fluids for phototherapy treatment.

• Eyes should be covered while under phototherapy to prevent retinal damage. Eyes should be cleansed regularly.

• Skin temperature should be recorded 3–4 hourly to prevent hypothermia as baby is nursed naked.

• Skin rashes can occur due to photosensitivity – no treatment is necessary. Check nappy area for excoriation as stools containing bile salts can burn the skin resulting in red sore areas which require specialized treatment.

• Ensure that the baby has time out of phototherapy for feeding when the eye pads are removed and eye contact with the parents is established.

• Baby may be more unsettled in an incubator with eye pads on – use soft rolls around the baby when positioning. Use tinted eye screens.

• It may be difficult to observe cyanosis when babies are nursed under blue lights so O_2 saturation monitors may be necessary for clinically unstable babies.

• Breastfeeding may be challenging because of the need to remove the baby from underneath lights but biliblankets may be used during feeds.

50 Congenital heart disease

Figure 50.1 Examination of the neonate

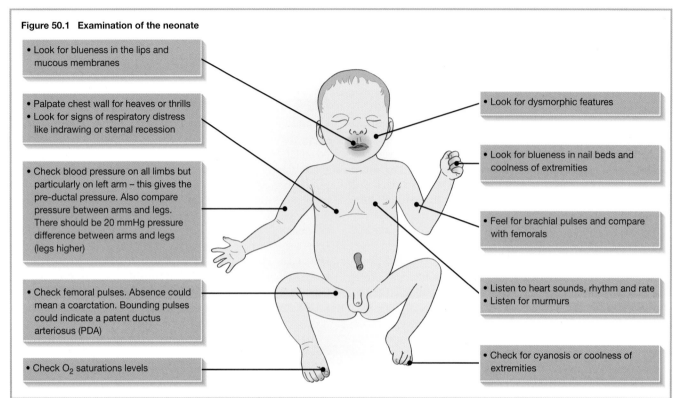

- Look for blueness in the lips and mucous membranes

- Palpate chest wall for heaves or thrills
- Look for signs of respiratory distress like indrawing or sternal recession

- Check blood pressure on all limbs but particularly on left arm – this gives the pre-ductal pressure. Also compare pressure between arms and legs. There should be 20 mmHg pressure difference between arms and legs (legs higher)

- Check femoral pulses. Absence could mean a coarctation. Bounding pulses could indicate a patent ductus arteriosus (PDA)

- Check O$_2$ saturations levels

- Look for dysmorphic features

- Look for blueness in nail beds and coolness of extremities

- Feel for brachial pulses and compare with femorals

- Listen to heart sounds, rhythm and rate
- Listen for murmurs

- Check for cyanosis or coolness of extremities

Children and Young People's Nursing at a Glance, First Edition. Edited by Alan Glasper, Jane Coad, and Jim Richardson.
© 2015 John Wiley & Sons, Ltd. Published 2015 by John Wiley & Sons, Ltd. Companion website: www.ataglanceseries.com/nursing/children

Pathophysiology

The embryonic cardiovascular system is functional by 21 days. Cardiac anomalies can be congenital or acquired, but this system is highly susceptible to abnormalities when exposed to teratogens in early pregnancy. Congenital heart disease (CHD) affects about 1 in 145 babies, but half of these will not require treatment; many will be treated with medication and/or surgery. Congenital heart defects are usually described as cyanotic or acyanotic.

Acyanotic: left to right shunting will not cause cyanosis because blood flows from the systemic to the pulmonary system.

Cyanotic: right to left shunting results in blood flowing from the right side of the circulation to the systemic circulation (i.e. de-oxygenated blood mixes with oxygenated blood causing cyanosis, even when nursed in 100% oxygen).

Diagnosis

Taking a detailed history is vital: family history (other siblings); prenatal history, any illnesses, medications, complications in pregnancy, labour or delivery; and the baby's condition since birth in relation to feeding, observations, weight gain and general health.

Cardiac problems can present in four ways: colour change (cyanosis), respiratory distress, collapse or the baby may be asymptomatic.

Genetic syndromes: babies with trisomy 21 (Down's syndrome) have a higher risk of multiple cardiac defects. Look for unusual features.

Colour: central cyanosis – blue lips, mucous membranes and nail beds. If colour improves with oxygen, the condition is more likely to be respiratory. Heart failure usually results in increasing pallor as the blood pressure falls, peripheries become cold.

Respiratory rate increases, as does effort. Flared nostrils, subcostal and intracostal retractions, grunting and/or wheezing sounds.

Capillary refill time (CRT): CRT of >3 s can be indicative of poor peripheral circulation. Babies may look mottled and pale.

Auscultation: listen for 'lub-dub' heart sounds, rhythm and regularity. Listen for murmurs, which indicate turbulence of the blood at some juncture in the heart. They can be classified according to their location, intensity, quality and timing (systolic or diastolic).

Palpation: pulses should be checked for presence and strength (brachial and femoral). Absence of femoral pulses may be indicative of coarctation of aorta or left ventricular outflow conditions. The chest wall should be palpated for precordial activity (heaves and thrills) which indicate reduced pulmonary or aortic outflow.

Blood pressure readings: four limb blood pressure readings can highlight differing pressures between upper and lower limbs. A systolic difference of 15–20 mmHg between upper and lower limbs is indicative of coarctation of aorta (pressure in legs should be higher).

Oxygen saturation levels: O_2 saturation readings should be >95%, so readings <90% indicate either cardiac or respiratory illness.

Chest X-ray: identifies respiratory disease or enlarged heart size.

ECG will assess atrial and ventricular function and should be interpreted by an appropriately skilled professional.

Echocardiogram provides information on cardiac structures, pressures and gradients within the heart and the overall function.

Cardiac catheterization: an invasive procedure that provides diagnostic or therapeutic treatment such as balloon septostomy.

Common conditions

There are over 30 types of CHD. Listed below are some of the more common cardiac conditions:

Patent ductus arteriosus (PDA)

Before birth, this fetal shunt (ductus arteriosus) enables blood to bypass the lungs as the fetus obtains its oxygen through the placenta. The ductus normally closes soon after birth, allowing blood to travel to the lungs and pick up oxygen. In PDA it remains open, resulting in potential respiratory and cardiac problems for the baby (most frequently in premature babies). Treatment with ibuprofen or indometacin during the early days of life often closes the ductus; failing that, surgery may be required.

Septal defects

A hole in the separating central wall (septum) between the two atria or the two ventricles causing blood to circulate improperly, so the heart has to work harder. Atrial or ventricular septal defects can be repaired by sewing or patching the hole.

Coarctation of the aorta

A narrowing of the aorta, usually occurring in the descending section results in a reduced flow of blood to the lower parts of the body. Femoral pulses may be absent. A surgeon resects the narrowed section, replacing it with man-made material or part of a grafted blood vessel. The narrowed section can sometimes be widened by inflating a balloon on the tip of a catheter inserted through an artery.

Management of cardiac disease

The infant should be nursed in a quiet comfortable environment with reduced stimuli or stress. Crying increases O_2 requirements.

Continuous monitoring of colour, heart rate, respiratory rate, blood pressure, oxygen saturations, TCO_2 and CO_2 levels as well as fluid intake and output.

Blood gas analysis: frequency depends on the baby's ongoing condition. Oxygen requirements altered according to results.

Daily blood tests including FBP, urea and electrolytes (U&E), and any other necessary investigations such as drug levels.

Temperature regulation: nurse in neutral thermal environment. Maintain normal temperature, minimizing use of oxygen and calories.

Calculation of IV fluids, feeds and nutrients to ensure growth, normal U&E levels, avoiding metabolic disturbances. Monitor blood glucose.

Feeding: deliver feeds (preferably breast milk) in a way that minimizes effort and calorie consumption. Tube feeds may be necessary.

Administration of medications must be timely with observation for effects and adverse effects recorded, particularly digitalis and inotropes.

Minimizing the risk of infection is vital because of the risk of sepsis in this vulnerable group. Prevention of infection protocols must be adhered to.

Family support is vital as cardiac conditions will result in anxiety for all concerned. Information and good communication are essential.

Follow-up and prognosis

Due to advances in heart surgery, 85% of children with CHD will survive into adulthood. All babies and young children will be reviewed by the surgeon who carried out their surgery or the cardiologist who will manage their condition into childhood or adulthood.

51 Neonatal resuscitation

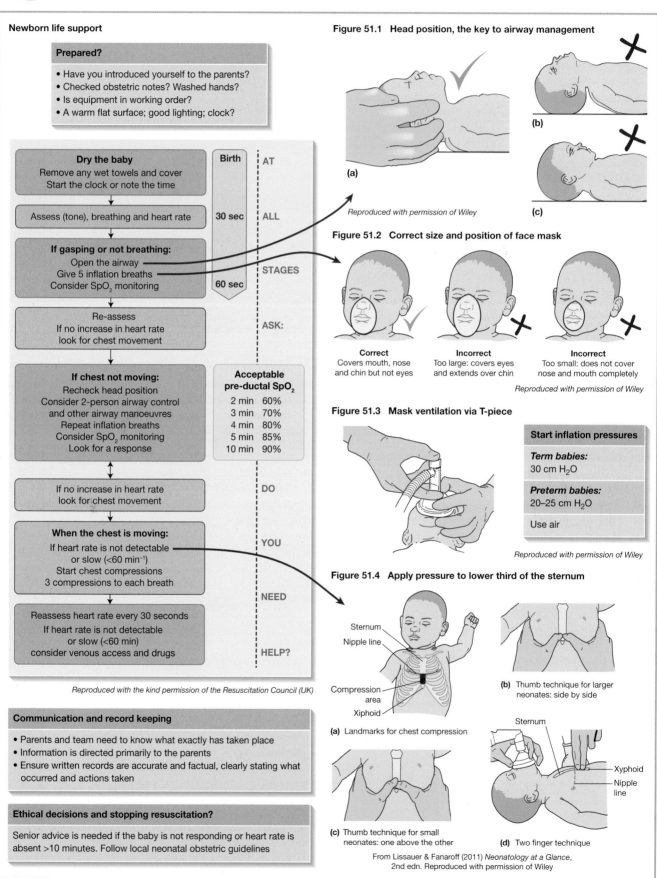

Newborn life support

Prepared?

- Have you introduced yourself to the parents?
- Checked obstetric notes? Washed hands?
- Is equipment in working order?
- A warm flat surface; good lighting; clock?

Dry the baby Remove any wet towels and cover Start the clock or note the time	Birth	AT
Assess (tone), breathing and heart rate	30 sec	ALL
If gasping or not breathing: Open the airway Give 5 inflation breaths Consider SpO₂ monitoring	60 sec	STAGES
Re-assess If no increase in heart rate look for chest movement		ASK:
If chest not moving: Recheck head position Consider 2-person airway control and other airway manoeuvres Repeat inflation breaths Consider SpO₂ monitoring Look for a response	**Acceptable pre-ductal SpO₂** 2 min 60% 3 min 70% 4 min 80% 5 min 85% 10 min 90%	
If no increase in heart rate look for chest movement		DO
When the chest is moving: If heart rate is not detectable or slow (<60 min⁻¹) Start chest compressions 3 compressions to each breath		YOU
Reassess heart rate every 30 seconds If heart rate is not detectable or slow (<60 min) consider venous access and drugs		NEED HELP?

Reproduced with the kind permission of the Resuscitation Council (UK)

Communication and record keeping

- Parents and team need to know what exactly has taken place
- Information is directed primarily to the parents
- Ensure written records are accurate and factual, clearly stating what occurred and actions taken

Ethical decisions and stopping resuscitation?

Senior advice is needed if the baby is not responding or heart rate is absent >10 minutes. Follow local neonatal obstetric guidelines

Figure 51.1 Head position, the key to airway management

(a)
(b)
(c)

Reproduced with permission of Wiley

Figure 51.2 Correct size and position of face mask

Correct Covers mouth, nose and chin but not eyes

Incorrect Too large: covers eyes and extends over chin

Incorrect Too small: does not cover nose and mouth completely

Reproduced with permission of Wiley

Figure 51.3 Mask ventilation via T-piece

Start inflation pressures

Term babies: 30 cm H₂O

Preterm babies: 20–25 cm H₂O

Use air

Reproduced with permission of Wiley

Figure 51.4 Apply pressure to lower third of the sternum

Sternum
Nipple line
Compression area
Xiphoid

(a) Landmarks for chest compression

(b) Thumb technique for larger neonates: side by side

Sternum
Xiphoid
Nipple line

(c) Thumb technique for small neonates: one above the other

(d) Two finger technique

From Lissauer & Fanaroff (2011) *Neonatology at a Glance*, 2nd edn. Reproduced with permission of Wiley

Preparation and readiness

Effective resuscitation of the newborn baby requires good organization and preparation. The following advice follows Resuscitation Council (UK) Newborn Life Support standards (2010). If a Resuscitaire is not available, you will need a warm flat surface with good lighting and a clock or watch to record the timing of events.

Check all equipment before use

- Resuscitaire with gas supply; pressure relief valve; T-piece circuit; Tom Thumb or T-piece device
- Self-inflating bag (500 mL) with pressure-limiting device
- Round soft silicone face masks – sizes 00; 0/1; 2
- Suction apparatus – Yankauer sucker; catheter sizes 12–14 French
- Guedel airways – sizes 000; 00; 0 and laryngoscope + Oxford blade
- Stethoscope – neonatal/paediatric
- Saturation probe and oximeter
- Warm towels and wraps.

Keep infants warm: avoid heat loss

Babies are wet at birth and have a large surface area : body weight ratio. Hypothermia and acidosis inhibit surfactant production which may lead to respiratory distress. It is crucial that newborn infants are dried and kept warm during resuscitation procedure. **Dry** and **cover** with warm dry towels. The action will also stimulate the baby. *Preterm infants* are placed **wet** into plastic bag, hat applied and then placed under radiant heater, immediately following delivery. Room temperature should be 26°C.

Initial assessment at birth

Start the clock and note the time. Assessment should note the baby's tone; colour; breathing; heart rate. Well babies have good tone and are flexed; have spontaneous regular breathing pattern, a good heart rate >100/min and pink; this usually occurs by 3 minutes of age. Babies who have inadequate breathing and slow (<60/min) heart rate are compromised and need resuscitation or help in transition to extrauterine life. APGAR scores are unreliable and not considered helpful.

> **Red flag**
> - Never be afraid to ask for assistance.

Follow ABC approach
Airway

Check the baby's airway is patent. Obstruction is usually caused by flexed head or tongue position rather than blood, mucous plugs or secretions. Only suction under direct vision. Figure 51.1 (a) shows the **correct head position**. Avoid overextension (b) or flexed position (c). If the baby is floppy, a jaw thrust may be needed to bring the tongue forward. Place one or two fingers under each side of the jaw angle and push the jaw forwards. Inserting an oropharyngeal airway (Guedel) under direct vision (laryngoscope) in the anatomically correct position is useful. Choose one that when aligned along the lower length of the jaw, the flange sits below the tip of the nose, and the end of the airway meets the angle of the jaw.

Breathing

If breathing or chest movement is absent, **inflation breaths** will be needed to aerate the lungs. Use mask and T-piece or mask and bag to inflate the lungs. Give **five inflation breaths of 3 s each** (use appropriate cm H_2O pressure). Reassess the baby's response – spontaneous breathing will usually occur. If not:

- Do you have airway control? Recheck head and airway position
- Ventilation technique – is the chest moving? Is there any obstruction?

Face masks: correct mask size should cover the mouth, nose and chin (Figure 51.2).

Mask ventilation via T-piece: connect to **air** using pressure limited circuit. Oxygen is rarely required but, if given, use blender and monitor the baby's response using pulse oximetry. **Avoid** SpO_2 >95% (Figure 51.3).

Self-inflating bags: useful if piped gas is not available. It is recommended that this skill is practised using infant manikins as the bags can be difficult to use. It is only on rare occasions that babies need endotracheal intubation.

Circulation

If the heart rate remains slow and fails to increase with effective aeration of the lungs, commence chest compressions. The aim is to move oxygenated blood from the pulmonary veins to the coronary arteries. Chest compressions will only be useful if the lungs have been aerated first. Ask for assistance.

Chest compressions (Figure 51.4) (a) Apply pressure to the lower third of the sternum. Avoid the xiphoid. Depress to reduce the anteroposterior diameter of the chest by one-third with no bounce. Thumb technique (b,c) is more effective than the two–finger technique (d), but is useful if you are alone or have small hands. Give **three compressions to 1 breath** (90 : 30/min). Allow the chest to recoil between compressions to allow blood to fill the heart. With good quality compressions the heart will normally respond quickly. Stop and recheck heart rate after every 30 s. When heart rate rises (>60 bpm) stop chest compressions. Monitor baby's progress. If the heart rate remains slow or undetectable then local senior advice is needed. Meanwhile do not stop resuscitation.

Drugs

On rare occasions the baby may not demonstrate the expected response. If effective ventilation and good quality cardiac compressions have been delivered yet cardiac output remains poor or absent, then drugs may be needed to reverse intracardiac acidosis. In such circumstances the prognosis is generally poor.

Sodium bicarbonate 4.2%   Dose = 2–4 mL/kg via UVC
Adrenaline 1 : 10 000   Dose = 0.1 mL/kg via UVC
Dextrose 10%   Dose = 2.5 mL/kg via UVC.

Central venous access for drug administration

Insertion of an umbilical catheter (UVC) provides a quick and effective means to administer drugs close to the heart.

Babies needing specialist neonatal care

A baby needing support in transition to extrauterine life may be transferred to a neonatal unit. Use local policy for admission criteria.

Parents, communication, record keeping

Direct information shoud be given, primarily to the parents of the baby. Once the baby responds and spontaneously maintains respiratory and cardiac output, hand the baby to the parents.

Structured clear factual information is required in any resuscitation event. The SBAR approach is useful. Avoid subjective statements. All resuscitation events need to be recorded in the notes. Include what time you were called and when you arrived; the baby's tone, breathing, heart rate; action taken and the baby's response; arterial/venous cord blood pH, base excess; who participated in the resuscitation; what was said to the parents.

52 Incubator/Babytherm care

Figure 52.1   Comparison of babytherm and incubator

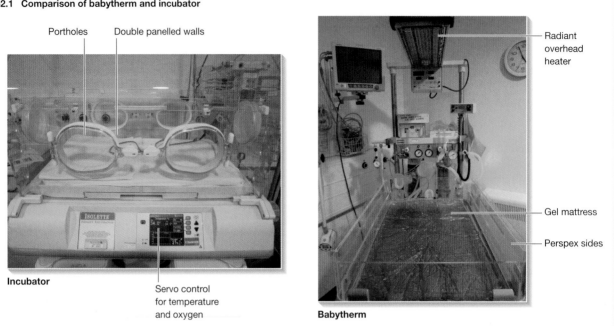

Portholes   Double panelled walls

Incubator

Servo control
for temperature
and oxygen

Radiant
overhead
heater

Gel mattress

Perspex sides

Babytherm

Children and Young People's Nursing at a Glance, First Edition. Edited by Alan Glasper, Jane Coad, and Jim Richardson.

Heat balance

The goal in controlling the infant or child's environment is to minimize the energy expended in order to maintain a normal temperature, and to eliminate thermal stress. With a normal body temperature, the infant or child has a minimal metabolic rate and minimal oxygen consumption which serves to ensure cardiac output is maintained.

Infants and neonates (under 36 weeks' gestation) rarely shiver when exposed to a cold environment and must rely on non-shivering, or chemical thermogenesis, to produce heat. Oxygen and glucose are consumed during non-shivering thermogenesis; therefore, the infant who already has low glucose and oxygen levels may become hypoxaemic or hypoglycaemic when faced with added thermal stress. Measures to keep the environment normothermic are paramount in order to maintain homeostasis.

Heat loss

It is vital that care providers understand the principles of heat balance in order to be able to provide a normothermic environment for the infant. The two key principles are: (1) to block avenues of heat loss (four mechanisms of heat transfer); and (2) to provide heat and environmental support to maintain a normal temperature.

Four mechanisms of heat transfer

Radiation

Heat loss is in the form of warm skin surface near to a cooler object which is not in contact with the baby – inside the incubator or window. Radiation is the main source of heat loss because of the infant's large surface area.

Conduction

The loss of heat due to a cooler object being in direct contact with the newborn baby (e.g. cold scales, stethoscope).

Convection

The loss of heat to moving air at the skin surface and is dependent on the air's velocity and temperature (e.g. cold drafts from vents).

Evaportation

Water from the skin or mucous membranes is lost to the air. The baby needs to be dried at delivery and management of insensible losses is vital.

Incubator and Babytherm management and care

Incubator

Incubators provide a controlled enclosed environment that is convectively heated with warm air. The temperature can be preset and control units gradually increase or decrease the heat output to maintain the temperature constantly and without significant fluctuations. An incubator is most likely to be used for neonates of <1.5 kg and/or gestational age of <30 weeks.

Babytherm

Babytherms are less enclosed and are radiantly heated by an overhead heater and gel mattress. Babytherms are beneficial for those infants who require multiple interventions and treatment, and who are slightly larger.

When considering which is the most suitable environment for the infant, careful attention should be paid to the following factors.

Incubators:
• Once switched on, it takes approximately 30 minutes for the optimum temperature to be reached.
• Care must be taken not to place the sensor over an area of brown fat (found mostly in the nape of the neck, axilla and between the scapula). Brown fat is a specialized type of fat that contains thermogenin, a key enzyme in regulation of non-shivering thermogenesis.
• Incorrect readings will take place if the sensor is covered or becomes disconnected.
• The portholes should not be left open for long periods.
• Accurate baby and air temperature monitoring and recording should be performed hourly.
• The incubator should be kept away from air conditioning ducts, direct sunlight and windows with a draft.
• If humidification is required, sterile water should be used; the water level should be checked hourly.
• Daily cleaning should be undertaken as per local policy and every 7 days the incubator should be changed for a clean one.
Babytherms:
• Once switched on, the mattress takes approximately 1 hour, and the overhead heater takes approximately 30 minutes, for the set temperature to be reached.
• Each level of the overhead heater is 10% higher or lower than the next so careful attention should be paid when adjusting the temperature of the overhead heater.
• As with incubators, regular monitoring and documentation of the baby's temperature should be performed.

Weaning from an incubator or Babytherm

Weaning an infant from an incubator to an open cot (bassinette) is important in preparing the baby and the family for discharge. The infant's temperature should be monitored regularly (up to every 15 minutes) for the first hour, and hourly thereafter, to ensure the baby is regulating his/her temperature satisfactorily. Care must be taken to ensure thermal stability during cares and interventions. Teaching and support should be given to the parents about the signs and symptoms of heat loss and heat retention and what to do if they are concerned. Furthermore, the importance of the parents maintaining an environment, at home, that prevents heat and cold stress should be discussed before the baby is discharged home.

53 Sudden infant death syndrome

Figure 53.1 Sudden infant death syndrome

Sudden infant death syndrome, or sudden unexpected death in infancy, is a term commonly used to describe an unexpected death in infancy:

- Uncommon under the age of 1 month
- Peaks at 2 months
- 90% occur by 6 months
- Very few occur over 1 year

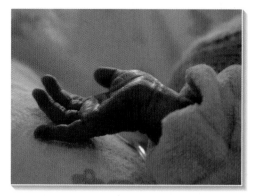

Cause of sudden infant death syndrome include:

- Accidents
- Infection
- Congenital abnormality
- Metabolic disorder
- Combination of factors
- Undiscovered causes

Risk factors

- Premature infants
- Low birth weight infants
- Male infants
- Infants born to mothers who are still young

Smoking

Smoking parents, or infants cared for in a smoky environment are at a much higher risk of a sudden infant death. Health promotion is paramount to help reduce this risk

Sudden infant death syndrome can occur:

- In a cot
- In a pram
- In a car seat
- In parent's arms
- In parent's bed

It usually occurs during a period of sleep

Reducing the risk of cot deaths

- Cut smoking in pregnancy
- Do not allow anyone to smoke in the same room as the infant
- Put the infant to sleep on his/her back and not on front
- Place the infant with his/her feet at the bottom of the cot to prevent wriggling down under the covers
- Never sleep with an infant on a sofa or armchair

Never sleep with an infant in bed

Children and Young People's Nursing at a Glance, First Edition. Edited by Alan Glasper, Jane Coad, and Jim Ryrichardson.
© 2015 John Wiley & Sons, Ltd. Published 2015 by John Wiley & Sons, Ltd. Companion website: www.ataglanceseries.com/nursing/children

Definition

Cot death is the sudden and unexpected death of a baby for no obvious reason. The post-mortem examination may explain some deaths. Those that remain unexplained after post-mortem examination may be registered as sudden infant death syndrome, sudden infant death, sudden unexpected death in infancy, unascertained death or cot death.

Incidence

The latest figures for sudden infant death syndrome were documented in 2010, when it was stated that 8% of infant deaths were a result of sudden infant death. This equates to 254 unexplained deaths in England and Wales at a rate of 0.35 per 1000 live births. In the United States, 2500 deaths on average occur every year.

There is a higher incidence in boys (0.4 deaths per 1000 live births), which accounted for 59% of unexplained deaths. In girls, the incidence is 0.3 deaths per 1000 live births, accounting for 41% of unexplained deaths.

Most deaths occur within the first year of life. It is very uncommon for an infant less than 1 month or over the age of 1 year to die of sudden infant death syndrome, 90% will die by the time they reach 6 months of age, with a peak incidence of 2 months of age, accounting for 72% of all unexplained deaths to have occurred in infants less than 4 months of age.

Infants with a low birth weight (<2.5 kg) are over four times more likely to die from sudden infant death syndrome than an infant born with a birth weight >2.5 kg.

Mothers less than 20 years of age were 3.4 times more likely to have an infant die with sudden infant death syndrome.

There is a much higher incidence in the north-west of England: 0.53 deaths per 1000 live births.

Measures in place to reduce the risk

In 1991, a campaign was launched to reduce the risk in England and Wales and this has contributed to a reduction by around 71%.

In 1992, the American Academy of Pediatrics launched its Back to Sleep campaign which has led to a drop of 50% in deaths.

Both of these campaigns widely advertised the risk that parents and carers were taking by placing their infants to sleep on their stomachs. Historically, this is how infants had always been put to sleep, and would be the advice of grandparents and health care professionals.

Advice to parents to help reduce the risks

There are a number of risk factors that can contribute to sudden infant death syndrome. The education of parents is paramount in helping to reduce the numbers of infant deaths that still occur:

- Always put the infant to sleep on his/her back
- Keep the cot in the adults' room for the first 6 months of age
- Recommend the baby is placed with his/her feet near to the bottom of the cot to prevent getting underneath bedding
- Do not smoke during pregnancy or after the birth of the infant
- Do not allow anyone to smoke in the same room as the infant
- Do not share a bed with an infant
- Do not sleep with an infant in an armchair or on a sofa
- Be more vigilant if taking drugs or alcohol
- Do not allow the infant to become too hot – keep bedding and clothing to a minimum and keep the room they are sleeping in cool rather than over-heated
- If the infant was born prematurely, was born with a low birth weight or born to a mother under the age of 20 years, the infant will have an increased risk. These infants should be observed more frequently.

Smoking

There is evidence to support that smoking can significantly increase the risk of sudden infant death syndrome. This applies to mothers who smoke during pregnancy, after pregnancy and any other adults who smoke around an infant. The environment an infant should be in is completely smoke-free as an infant in a smoky environment is eight times more likely to die from sudden infant death syndrome.

Key points

- Sudden infant death syndrome remains the biggest killer for infants less than 1 year old.
- Placing infants on their backs in a smoke-free environment can significantly reduce the risk of death.
- A health care professional has a huge responsibility in educating parents and carers.

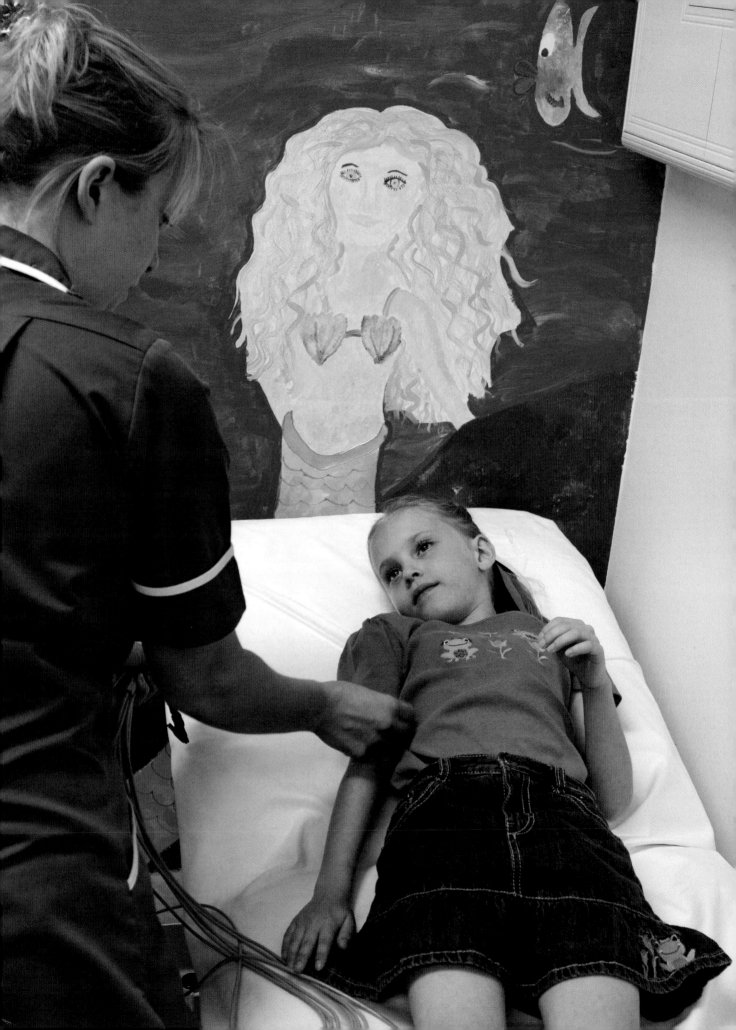

The developing child

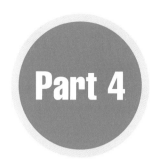

Part 4

Don't forget to visit the companion website for this book at www.ataglanceseries.com/nursing/children where you will find over 500 interactive multiple-choice questions to supplement your learning.

54 Nutrition in childhood

Figure 54.1 Nutritional assessment

Questions are directed here for the child in terms of a subjective and objective assessment but could be directed to parents or legal guardians

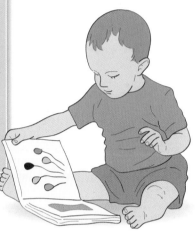

Subjective data

Practical questions for assessment of children's nutritional status

- What foods do you like? Include preferences including snacks, patterns and times of meals
- What foods don't you like? Include any allergies or diet restrictions
- What do you use to eat? Include any equipment
- When do you prefer to eat and drink? Include times and preference
- Does the child need any help? Include anyone who helps and following any observations of chewing and swallowing
- Does the child get tired? Note any fatigue or longer time taken over feeding

Objective data

Practical questions for assessment of children's nutritional status

- Weight is the most sound indicator of current nutritional status. It should be measured at regular intervals
- Usual approximate body weight is helpful. Use medical notes. Assess any change such as dry skin or tongue
- Height and length is a useful growth parameter and should be plotted on a percentile chart
- As head circumference growth during the first 2 years is very rapid, head circumference is a good indicator of nutritional intake and growth
- Fat distribution or musculoskeletal changes. Triceps skin-folds (TSF) measurements should be performed only by those trained in this method (e.g. dietitian, nutritional care specialist or medical staff)
- If problems are identified, the physical assessment might include some more in-depth assessments such as mid-arm circumference (MAC). This is made with a tape measure with the arm down in a fully relaxed position, and indicates muscle and fat stores

Figure 54.2 The importance of good nutrition

Good nutrition gives a child the best start in life and begins at an early stage. Childhood nutrition should be a balance between the vitamins, protein, carbohydrates and minerals required for healthy growth and development:

- **Bread, cereals, grains, potatoes, pasta and rice** provide energy, fibre, vitamins and minerals
- **Fruit and vegetables** provide fibre, vitamins and minerals, and are a source of antioxidants
- **Meat, fish, poultry and alternatives**, which include eggs and pulses, provide protein and vitamins and minerals, especially iron. Pulses also contain fibre
- **Milk and dairy foods** such as yoghurt and cheese provide calcium for healthy bones, growth and teeth, plus vitamins and minerals

Any healthy diet needs to be in association with regular physical exercise. Worryingly, research has found that many children and young people have inadequate intakes of many nutrients, including vitamin A, riboflavin (vitamin B2), zinc, potassium, magnesium, calcium and iron, particularly once they reach age 12+ and have more control over what they eat

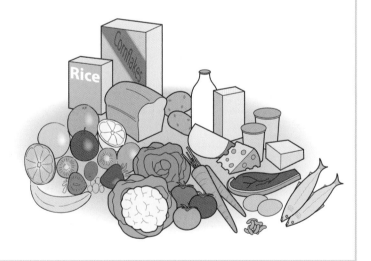

Importance of good nutritional assessment

This chapter focuses on the nursing assessment of children's and young people's nutrition, both when healthy and when ill. Assessment of children's and young people's nutritional status is important in order to plan and evaluate care. Poor nutrition complicates many diseases of childhood and affects both the physical and psychological well-being of children and young people.

In order to facilitate a good understanding of nutrition, Figure 54.1 contains a list of questions nurses could use when assessing children and young people. It is crucial that the nurse has a sound grasp of 'normal' development (see Chapters 59 and 60).

Nutrition in the under-fives

Healthy young children have a high energy requirement because of their rapid growth and increasing activity. As the young child

Children and Young People's Nursing at a Glance, First Edition. Edited by Alan Glasper, Jane Coad, and Jim Richardson.
© 2015 John Wiley & Sons, Ltd. Published 2015 by John Wiley & Sons, Ltd. Companion website: www.ataglanceseries.com/nursing/children

Table 54.1 Calorie intake for children

Age (years)	Calories per day	
	Boys	Girls
1–3	1230	1165
4–6	1715	1545
7–10	1970	1740
11–14	2220	1845
15–18	2755–3000	2110

Although obesity is a major problem, children and teenagers still need enough calories to grow and develop into healthy adults.

This chart gives a rough guideline to the daily calorie needs of boys and girls at different ages.

Children and young people who are very physically active may need more; those who are inactive may need less.

becomes more independent and adept at holding a spoon or drinking from a beaker, this is the time to introduce variety. As they have small stomachs, it is advisable to offer small frequent meals. To help prevent dental caries there should be restriction of sugary snacks such as fizzy drinks and sweets.

As the child develops, milk is no longer the main source of nutrients, although the under-fives should still drink a pint a day (440 mL). Whole-fat milk is recommended for those over 12 months and can be used until age 5 years to provide plenty of calories, unless the child is overweight or under medical care. Some evidence suggests semi-skimmed milk (but not skimmed) can be introduced after 2 years of age, but the overall diet must provide enough energy.

The diet must also be high in vitamins and minerals. In particular, a good supply of protein, calcium, iron and vitamins A and D is required. It is recommended that the pre-school child should progress from the very high energy diet of infancy (with about 50% of total energy coming from fat) to the diet for a 5-year-old which should have much greater emphasis on a lower fat content (but still about 35% of energy from fat).

Diet-related problems

Obesity is less likely in under-fives but is increasing in some countries. In a healthy diet, young children should not be put on weight reduction diets, but a healthy family approach to food and regular physical activity are important in avoiding excessive weight gain and obesity.

Worryingly, iron deficiency anaemia is common at this age, resulting from high requirements for growth and poor dietary intake, especially in the 'faddy or fussy eater'. It is associated with frequent infections, delayed development and poor weight gain. Vitamin C present in orange juice can enhance iron absorption from the gut.

Constipation is common in the under-fives and can be prevented by gradually increasing the amount of fibre in the child's diet. Foods high in fibre include vegetables, wholemeal bread, baked beans and high fibre white bread. A high fluid intake, not fizzy drinks, is also important.

Toddler diarrhoea is also common and may be linked with too many sugary drinks and fruit juice, especially between meals.

Nutrition in school aged children

The same principles apply for school aged children as for the under-fives. The younger school aged child, 4- to 6-year-olds, still need smaller and more frequent meals as they do not have large enough stomachs to cope with large adult-sized meals. The requirement for energy remains due to growth and activity, but gradually an 'adult style' healthy diet should be introduced, reducing high fat content foods and increasing fibre-rich foods.

Diet-related problems

An increasing number of school aged children are overweight or are being diagnosed as obese. Dr Mary Rudolf (2006), a community paediatrician from Leeds, UK, discovered that 14% of the children studied of primary school age were obese. In these situations, medical or dietetic referral is required. Nurses can also support any weight loss in encouraging a child to lose weight gradually and increase activity while their height also increases. This may require a healthy lifestyle for the whole family.

Nutrition in young people aged 12+

It is particularly important that young people over 12 years eat a healthy diet rich in vitamins and minerals. Growth in girls occurs prior to puberty and slows down thereafter while boys grow following puberty. Young people often have higher requirements for nutrients than adults in order to support growth. For example, 15- to 18-year-old boys need more thiamin (vitamin B1), niacin (vitamin B3), vitamin B6, calcium, phosphorus and iron than adult men. Similarly, 15- to 18-year-old girls need more niacin, calcium, phosphorus and magnesium than adult women.

The Food Standards Agency has provided guidance on the safe maximum consumption levels for oily fish: boys aged under 16 can have up to four portions of oily fish a week and girls up to two portions. The lower recommendation in girls is because substances found in oily fish can accumulate in the body and high levels may be detrimental to the developing fetus if they become pregnant later in life.

Diet-related problems

As young people become more independent, have new interests away from family life such as relationships, have concerns such as career choices and body image, their energy needs are paramount. At the same time, they may tend to develop health-compromising eating behaviours such as skipping meals, fad dieting, over-eating, or develop an eating disorder such as binge eating or anorexia. They need a diet that provides the high energy needed for this stage of life while delivering nutritious and convenient foods that promote long-term health. Medical help should be sought in eating disorders.

55 Breastfeeding

Figure 55.1 Choosing to breastfeed

The Baby Friendly Initiative in the United Kingdom and Ireland encourages health care professionals to promote and support breastfeeding. Children's nurses have a pivotal role in the promotion, protection and support of breastfeeding.

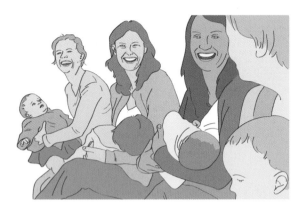

Breastfeeding is a normal way to feed and care for a baby. Breast milk is uniquely designed to provide the best nutrition and protection to meet the baby's needs and its properties can never be reproduced in formula milks. Colostrum is produced in the few first days. It is high in protein, immunoglobulins, vitamins, anti-infective agents, living cells and minerals – and helps babies to resist infection.

Breast milk is then produced. It is a constantly changing food that adjusts to the age and needs of the baby or child. Protection from infection is provided by iron binding in the baby's gut and maternally derived antibodies.

Children's nurses should actively promote breastfeeding as it offers many health benefits for both baby and mother. These health benefits extend beyond the breastfeeding period and into later life.

Children who do not receive breast milk

- Are more likely to develop ear, nose and throat infections
- Are more likely to develop gastroenteritis, kidney and chest infections
- Have a greater risk of obesity and of developing diabetes
- Have a higher risk of allergies and eczema
- Have an increased risk of sudden infant death syndrome
- Have a higher risk of necrotizing entercolitis (in the preterm baby)

Breastfeeding babies gain comfort, warmth and security close to the mother. For the mother, breastfeeding helps protect against breast and ovarian cancer, as well as help achieve and maintain a healthy post-pregnancy weight

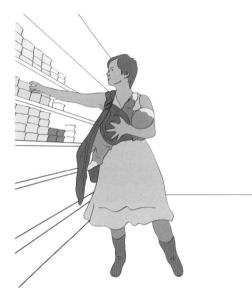

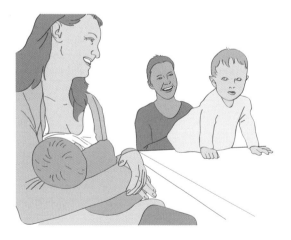

The World Health Organization recommends 6 months exclusive breastfeeding continued with complementary foods to 2 years of age or older. In the United Kingdom 74% of mothers, and 55% of mothers in Ireland, initially choose to breastfeed their baby. However, by 6 months these numbers are greatly reduced. Children's nurses can help the mother plan achievable goals in relation to breastfeeding and support her in sustaining breastfeeding.

Figure 55.2 Advice on breastfeeding

Breastfeeding support

A children's nurse can offer breastfeeding support by:
- Providing consistent and accurate information to families
- Providing reassurance and encouragement to families
- Providing the opportunity for families to discuss issues
- Proving the mother with evidence-based information on how to address any problems that may occur
- Assisting in getting timely assistance from trained peer support, relevant heath professionals, and mother to mother support

Initiating breastfeeding

Breastfeeding or expressing milk as soon after delivery as possible will aid breastmilk production. The breastfeeds should be frequent, effective, exclusive and on demand. It is advised to avoid giving a breastfed baby formula or use bottles initially, as this may lead to a reduction in milk production.

The baby may be unable to feed at the breast due to illness or abnormalities, or if the mother is away from the baby, she may choose to express her breastmilk by hand, hand pump or electric pump and it can be delivered by another method. The children's nurse should provide information on how to obtain, clean and use equipment and on the safe storage and delivery of the expressed milk.

Protecting breastfeeding

The children's nurse should be aware of and adhere to the International Code of Marketing of Breastmilk Substitutes (WHO/UNICEF)

Further information for both mothers and health professionals can be found at www.breastfeeding.nhs.uk (UK) and www.breastfeeding.ie (Ireland)

Attachment

It is important that the baby latches on to the breast with a widely open mouth, so that not just the nipple is in the baby's mouth but also the areola and underlying breast tissue. On attaching, the chin should touch the breast first and the baby's head allowed to tip back slightly so the tongue can reach as much of the breast as possible.

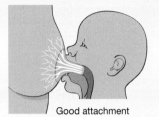 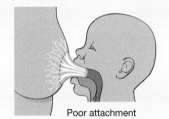

Good attachment   Poor attachment

Positioning

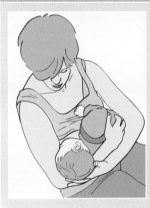

There are many different breastfeeding positions: the cradle hold, underarm hold, laid back and lying down.

There is no best way, and each mother and baby should try different positions in different circumstances. To facilitate the baby to self-attach and feed well, the principles are always the same: the mother should feel comfortable; the baby needs to be in a position that is close, facing the breast, straight and supported.

Signs that a baby is breastfeeding well

- Gaining weight after the first 2 weeks
- 2–3 wet nappies in the first 48 hours, then 5–6 every 24 hours
- Passing meconium by day 2, by day 3 a changing stool that is lighter and easier to clean. From day 4 and for the first few weeks at least two soft or runny yellow stools every day
- At least 8 feeds in a 24-hour period and feeds for 5–30 minutes at most feeds
- Breast and nipples should not be sore
- Baby is content and satisfied after most feeds

56 Bottle feeding

Figure 56.1 Examples of specialized milks

Pre-term hospital formula milk
– Aptamil Preterm, Cow & Gate Nutriprem 1 and SMA Gold Prem 1

Pre-term post hospitalization formula milk
– Cow & Gate Nutriprem 2, SMA Gold Prem 2

Colic and/or constipation
– Cow & Gate Comfort

Lactose intolerant
– SMA LF

Figure 56.2 Safe preparation of powdered infant formula

Here are four things to remember

1. Use equipment that has been cleaned and sterilised

2. Boil one litre (1L) of cold tap water and leave to cool for 30 minutes before using it to prepare feeds

3. Cool prepared feeds quickly

Source: How to prepare your baby's bottle (www.safefood.eu)
Reproduced with permission of Safefood

4. Either
• Use the feed immediately and throw away any left over within two hours; or
• Store made-up bottles in the back of the fridge at 5°C or less and use within 24 hours

Balanced nutrition is critical for the normal growth and development of the infant. Breastfeeding is the recommended method of infant feeding. However, by choice or necessity, some mothers may formula feed their infant. Formula companies must comply with legislation that governs the production, composition, marketing and distribution of formula milk. In particular, the composition of formula milk is adjusted to increase its similarity to breast milk. Protein, carbohydrate and fat content is modified, and important vitamins, minerals and trace elements are added. Despite such modifications formula milk continues to differ in the source and amounts of its constituents and does not contain the biologically active ingredients contained in breast milk. The nutritional composition of both breast and formula milk should satisfy the complete nutritional requirements of an infant until the introduction of complementary foods, around 6 months of age, and continue to contribute to nutritional intake for the first year.

Types of infant formula

Infant formula milk is commonly made from modified cow's milk which is either dominant in whey or casein protein. Choosing an infant formula milk is based on the infant's age and nutritional requirements, and in some circumstances an infant's medical condition.

Standard infant formula

First infant formulas should be based on the whey protein in cow's milk as whey is similar, although not identical, to the protein in breast milk. Whey-dominant formulas are suitable from birth to 1 year. Casein-dominant formula is marketed for hungrier infants. Casein is a more difficult protein to digest and it is thought, although not scientifically proven, that casein provides feelings of increased fullness and satiety. Casein-dominant formula has the same calorie and nutritional content as whey-dominant formula but the casein protein is less similar to the protein found in breast milk. A range of whey and casein-based formula milks are available for term infants (Table 56.1).

Follow-on formula is suitable for infants from 6 months of age. It contains additional iron and protein for growth and development. Infants do not have to switch from a first infant milk to a follow-on formula as the introduction of complementary foods will generally provide an adequate source of extra nutrients.

Daily fluid or feed requirements differ depending on the infant's age and weight (Food Safety Authority of Ireland 2011) (Table 56.2).

Specialized infant formula

A range of specialized infant formula milks are available for infants with specific nutritional requirements that cannot be met by standard formula. These specialized formulas should only be used on the advice of a health care professional. Examples are shown in Figure 56.1.

Partial or completely hydrolysed formula is recommended for infants with cow's milk allergy rather than using sheep, goat or soya-based formula.

Preparing infant formula

Infant formula is available as ready to feed (RTF) or powdered. RTF is a sterile formula that does not require refrigeration and is stored at room temperature. It is ready to feed to the infant and warming the feed is dependent on infant preference. Powdered infant formula is non-sterile and can be contaminated with a number of harmful bacteria including the *Cronobacter* species and *Salmonella*. It is therefore imperative that strict safety guidelines are followed in the preparation of powdered infant formula to ensure that the prepared feed is not contaminated by harmful bacteria. Key safety statements in relation to the safe preparation of formula feeds are presented in Figure 56.2 and the following guidelines.

Children and Young People's Nursing at a Glance, First Fedition. Edited by Alan Glasper, Jane Coad, and Jim Richardson.
© 2015 John Wiley & Sons, Ltd. Published 2015 by John Wiley & Sons, Ltd. Companion website: www.ataglanceseries.com/nursing/children

Table 56.1 Whey and casein-based formulas

	Examples	Protein/ g/100 mL	Energy/ 100mL
Whey-dominant	**Aptamil** – First Milk **Cow & Gate** – First Infant Milk **SMA** – First Infant Milk	1.3 (whey : casein = 0.8–0.9 : 0.4–0.5)	66–67
Casein-dominant	**Aptamil** – Hungry Infant Milk **Cow & Gate** – Infant Milk for Hungrier Babies **SMA** – Extra Hungry Infant Milk	1.6 (whey : casein = 0.3 : 1.3)	66–67

Table 56.2 Daily fluid or feed requirements

Age (months)	Approximate number of feeds in 24 hours	Daily fluid intake (mL/kg)
0–3	6–8, every 3–4 hours	150
4–6	4–6, every 4–6 hours	150
7–9	4	120
10–12	3	110

Guidelines: formula feeding an infant

1 Involve parents if present
2 Ensure that all nursing care is completed before the feed
3 Cleanse hands and work surface
4 Check that the formula is the correct type and volume, in date, the bottle is properly sealed and the cap is covering the teat
5 Place the bottle in bottle warmer with a small amount of water. Do not heat the feed in a microwave
6 Warm the bottle for less than 15 minutes
7 Check feed temperature by placing two drops of feed on the inner wrist. Milk should feel lukewarm, not hot
8 When warm, remove from the bottle warmer and use immediately
9 Place a bib on the infant
10 Carer or parent should be seated and comfortable
11 Place the infant in a semi-reclining position in the crook of the arm
12 Place the teat gently on the infant's lip and when the infant opens his/her mouth place the teat centrally on the tongue
13 Keep the bottle at an angle to ensure that the teat is always full of milk
14 Wind the infant regularly by placing the infant in an upright position and gently tapping or rubbing his/her back
15 Remember to communicate with the infant during the feed and monitor how the feed is being tolerated
16 When the feed is complete, wind the infant and place in a safe position in the cot
17 Discard any unfinished feed
18 Do not reuse or reheat feeds
19 Document the volume and type of feed and how the feed was tolerated by the infant
20 Empty the bottle warmer and clean and resterilize equipment

Guidelines: safe preparation of powdered infant formula

1 Wash hands
2 Cleanse the work surface with warm soapy water, rinse and dry
3 Wash and sterilize all equipment
4 Check that the powdered infant formula is in date
5 Check the required volume of water and the number of scoops of formula
6 Boil 1 L fresh cold tap water and allow it to cool for 25–30 minutes. This will ensure that the temperature remains greater than 70°C (to kill any bacteria that might be present in the powdered infant formula)
7 Do not use water from the hot tap, bottled or fizzy mineral water, spring or filtered water, or artificially softened water or water that has been boiled more than once
8 If boiled tap water is not suitable for drinking then boiled bottled water with a sodium content of less than 20mg can be used
9 Use the measurements on the bottle and pour in the required amount of boiled water
10 Use the leveller in the pack to level each scoop and add the required number of scoops of formula to the bottle of boiled water. Do not pack the powder into the scoop
11 Reseal the pack to protect against moisture and bacteria
12 If the bottle is not for immediate use, place the disc on the neck of the bottle, screw on the collar and shake until all powder is dissolved. Then cool and store in the back of the fridge at 5°C or less
13 If the feed is for immediate use, replace the disc with the sterile teat and cover the teat with the bottle cap and shake until all of the powder is dissolved
14 Cool the feed to the desired temperature by holding and swirling the bottle under running cold water or standing it in a large container of cold water. Ensure that the water does not reach the neck of the bottle. Use immediately

57 Feed calculations

Figure 57.1 Feed calculations

This chapter aims to show how to calculate the correct amount of feed required by an infant during a 24-hour period

The feed requirement should be calculated by using the equation:

Total mL/kg × weight of the infant (kg) = total feed requirement in 24-hour period (mL)

Once the volume required in a 24-hour period has been calculated, this figure can be used to calculate an hourly rate for if the infant is on a continuous feed:

Total feed requirement in 24-hour period / 24 = hourly rate for continuous feed (mL/hr)

The volume can also be used to calculate the total feed required every 3 hours (or whatever frequency necessary for bolus or oral feeds)

Total feed requirement in 24-hour period/8 (for every 3 hours), or / 6 (for every 4 hours) = feed required

Calculating the amount of feed required for bolus feeds can be slightly more difficult than calculating for continuous feeds as there is more maths involved. For example, if you wish to feed the infant every 3 hours, you need to be aware that the infant will require 8 feeds in a day as 8 × 3 = 24 hours. Similarly, if you wish to feed the infant every 4 hours, the infant will require 6 feeds in a day as 4 × 6 = 24 hours.

Example: A term baby has been admitted to a children's ward. The baby weighs 3 kg and should have 150 mL/kg/day of feed

How much feed does the baby require in a 24-hour period?

mL × kg – 150 × 3 = 450 mL (total feed requirement in 24-hour period)

The baby is to be fed continuously via a nasogastric pump. What should the hourly rate for continuous feed be?

450 mL (total feed requirement in 24-hour period) / 24 = 18.75 mL/hr

A couple of days later the baby is improving and requires feeding every 3 hours. How much feed will the baby require every 3 hours?

450 mL (total feed requirement in 24-hour period) / 24 (hours in a day) × 3 (hours) = 56.25 mL

The baby's parents request that the baby is fed every 4 hours. How much feed will the baby require every 4 hours?

450 mL (total feed requirement in 24-hour period) / 24 (hours in a day) × 4 (hours) = 75 mL

Children and Young People's Nursing at a Glance, First Edition. Edited by Alan Glasper, Jane Coad, and Jim Richardson.
© 2015 John Wiley & Sons, Ltd. Published 2015 by John Wiley & Sons, Ltd. Companion website: www.ataglanceseries.com/nursing/children

While it is well documented that breast feeding is the optimum form of nutrition for infants, sometimes it is not possible for breastfeeding to occur. The reasons for this could be maternal choice, problems with the technique required to breastfeed, the baby not taking enough feed to thrive or the baby being ill and therefore unable to breastfeed. Some babies are unable to feed orally and will require nutrition via a nasogastric or gastrostomy tube.

The amount of fluid that is required for a term baby who is receiving all of its nutrition from feed varies. If the baby is ill then the requirement may be restricted. Infants can be fed orally or via a nasogastric or gastrostomy route.

The premature infant should receive up to 220 mL/kg, which is dependent upon their gut tolerance and the fluid balance. To achieve an adequate level of nutrition the feed volume of the premature infant should be at least 150 mL/kg and they should be fed every 3–4 hours and not on demand to ensure that they are receiving the required nutrients.

The term baby should be fed on demand with 150–200 mL/kg until they have been established on a weaning programme.

The amount of feed that a baby requires will depend on their gut tolerance, if they have an acute illness and their current weight. It is normal practice that when a baby is acutely unwell the feed requirement that they receive is reduced to allow their gut to be rested and to allow the baby some recuperation time. If the baby is finding it difficult to feed orally then a nasogastric tube may be passed in the short term to ensure that they receive the required nutritional intake.

It is important that children's nurses understand how to calculate the feed requirement, volume for each feed and rate of each feed to ensure that the baby receives the optimum amount of nutrition and at an appropriate pace.

58 Percentile charts

Figure 58.1 Measuring head circumferences

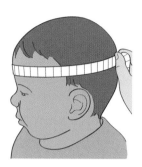

Why. Head circumferences provide information on head anomalies such as hydrocephalus or craniosynostosis, which may require treatment

When and Where. Neonates should have their first head circumference measurement taken after 36 hours, this allows moulding and oedema from birth to settle (Lindley et al. 1999; Sutter 1997). After this, children up to 2 years should have their measurement taken on each visit to clinic, doctor or hospital admission (May 2011)

How. Follow universal precautions at all times. Ensure the child is comfortable and settled to provide accurate measurement. The measuring tape should be placed above the ears and midway between eyebrows and hairline then around the occipital prominence of the back of the head (May 2011). This ensures the largest head circumference has been taken

Document. Always document on the correct gender centile chart, the child's health care records and local documentation paperwork

Figure 58.2 Measuring weight

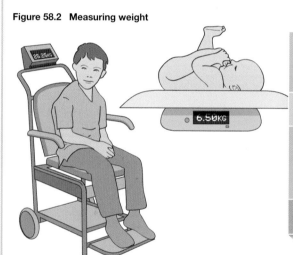

Why. Measuring weight is a useful tool in combination with height to determine the child's BMI. It indicates if the child is under or overweight for that child's age and gender. Additionally, it provides accurate medication and fluid requirements (RCN 2010)

When and Where. Weight should be taken in the morning for accuracy and should be taken on each visit to clinic, doctor or hospital admission

How. Follow universal precautions at all times. For neonates and infants remove all clothing and nappy. Children should wear minimal clothing and remove shoes. Use either baby scales or chair. Ensure scales are zeroed and place or ask the child to sit in the chair with feet on the ledge provided to ensure all weight is evenly spread

Document. Always document on the correct gender centile chart, the child's health care records and local documentation paperwork

Figure 58.3 Measuring height

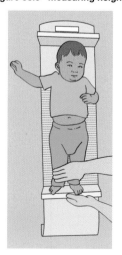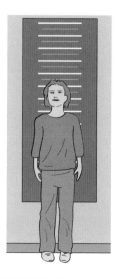

Why. In order to determine if a child is growing at a healthy rate. Measuring height is also useful tool in combination with height to determine a child's BMI

When and Where. Height should be taken in the morning for accuracy and should be taken on each visit to clinic, doctor or hospital admission

How. <2 years: the child should lie supine and measurement be taken on a roller mat. >2 years: or a standing height recorder. Feet should remain together and flat on the floor. The body should be straight with the head at 90° and the bottom to be against the backboard

Document. Always document on the correct gender centile chart, the child's health care records and local documentation paperwork

Children and Young People's Nursing at a Glance, First Edition. Edited by Alan Glasper, Jane Coad, and Jim Richardson.
© 2015 John Wiley & Sons, Ltd. Published 2015 by John Wiley & Sons, Ltd. Companion website: www.ataglanceseries.com/nursing/children

Definition

Percentile chats, now more commonly referred to as centile charts or growth charts, are used to show 'how common characteristics are' (Weller 2002), the 50th centile line thus showing the median or average of the population.

Background

The UK World Health Organization (WHO) growth charts are now used throughout the United Kingdom for the documentation on children's weight, height/length, head circumference and body mass index (BMI). The centile measurements are based upon statistics from breastfed children from non-smoking parents. Furthermore, the charts are suitable for all ethnicities (NHS Choices 2011). The charts represent the normal growth that a healthy child should follow, providing professionals with a surveillance tool to monitor whether a child is growing (or developing through puberty) as expected. The newer charts (Childhood and Puberty Close Monitoring Charts), published in June 2013, allow for the closer monitoring of children who may be of concern due to growth, nutritional or puberty problems (RCPCH 2013).

Potential triggers

There are a multitude of reasons that a child may not be growing as anticipated. For instance, a greater than expected increase in head circumference may indicate hydrocephalus. There may also be safeguarding reasons why a child may not follow a centile, for instance in cases of neglect the child may not gain weight as expected. These triggers should not be ignored and a full assessment should be carried out by a qualified health care professional.

The following charts are available:
- Early years chart 0–4 years
- Neonatal and Infant Close Monitoring (NICM) chart
- Personal Child Health Record (PCHR) charts – otherwise known as the 'Red Book'
- UK Down's Syndrome chart (DS) 0–18 years
- School age charts 2–18
- Childhood and Puberty Close Monitoring (CPCM) Chart
- Body Mass Index (BMI) chart (RCPCH 2013)

Key points
- The correct chart must be selected for the correct monitoring purpose and the child's age.
- The instructions on the chart must be followed exactly to ensure accurate records.
- Health care professionals must remember to date, time and sign their entries in the documentation.
- Any deviation from expected growth (e.g. sudden increase in head circumference) should be investigated by an appropriate professional.

59 Child development: 0–5 years

Figure 59.1 Gross motor development

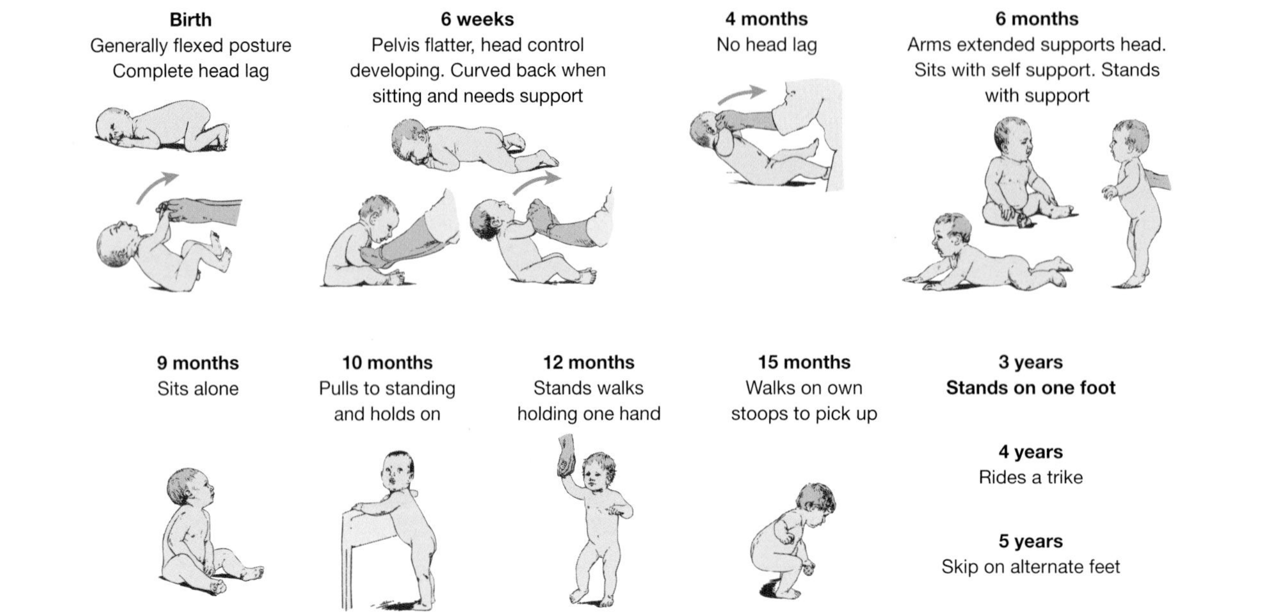

Birth
Generally flexed posture
Complete head lag

6 weeks
Pelvis flatter, head control
developing. Curved back when
sitting and needs support

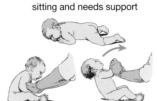

4 months
No head lag

6 months
Arms extended supports head.
Sits with self support. Stands
with support

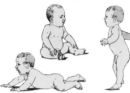

9 months
Sits alone

10 months
Pulls to standing
and holds on

12 months
Stands walks
holding one hand

15 months
Walks on own
stoops to pick up

3 years
Stands on one foot

4 years
Rides a trike

5 years
Skip on alternate feet

Figure 59.2 Fine motor development

(a) Manipulation

    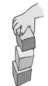

10 months
Points

12 months
Pincer grip

12 months

15 months

18 months

Pencil skills

  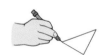

3 years
Draws circle

4 years
Draws a cross

5 years
Draws a triangle

(b) Grasping and reaching

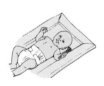   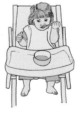 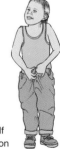

4 months
Holds and shakes
rattle

5 months
Reaches
for object

6 months
Moves object from
hand to hand

7 months
finger feeds

18 months
Spoon feeds

3 years
Dresses self
except button

Figure 59.3 Speech and language

3 months
Vocalizes

18 months
10 words

8 months
Dada mama

24 months
2 linked words

12 months
2 words with meaning

3 years
Full sentences

Figure 59.4 Social development

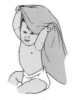 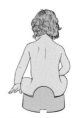

6 weeks
Smiles

4 months
Laughs

9 months
Plays peek a boo

About 2.5 years
Toilet trained by day

Children and Young People's Nursing at a Glance, First Edition. Edited by Alan Glasper, Jane Coad, and Jim Richardson.
© 2015 John Wiley & Sons, Ltd. Published 2015 by John Wiley & Sons, Ltd. Companion website: www.ataglanceseries.com/nursing/children

Growth and development occurs throughout the lifespan. Growth is an increase in the size of and the number of cells, resulting in an increase in size and weight of the whole, or any of its parts. It occurs in a continuous pattern, pace varies and the most rapid growth takes place *in utero*, in the first 2 years of life and in adolescence. Growth of the infant is measured by estimating the weight, length, head circumference and, in some instances, skinfold thickness.

Development is the increase in complexity of the individual, involving structure and function; the emerging of an individual's capacities through learning, growth and maturation. Development is measured using developmental scales and follows patterns of development (Table 59.1).

Development is divided into four major areas:

1 *Gross motor:* gross motor skills, primitive reflexes and postural responses
2 *Fine motor:* fine motor skills and vision
3 *Psychological:* emotional, behavioural, social
4 *Communication:* non-verbal communication, speech and language and hearing.

Factors influencing growth and development include prenatal and birth factors, genetic and chromosomal factors, health status, psychosocial factors including socioeconomic status, intrauterine and postnatal nutrition, and hormonal milieu.

Growth is rapid in the first year of life. Length is increased length by 50%, most of it occurring in the trunk. Weight doubles by the age of 5–6 months and triples by the end of the first year. The posterior fontanelle is usually closed by 2 months. Growth slows during the second year, with toddlers growing approximately 9–12.5 cm/year and gaining 220 g/month, head circumference increases 2.5 cm/year. The anterior fontanelle closes between 12 and 18 months. By the age of 2 years, birth weight has quadrupled to an average of 12.3 kg and the child is about half their adult height and has 20 teeth (Figure 59.1). At 2–3 years, toddlers grow 5–6.5 cm, gain 1.5–2.5 kg and head circumference has slowed to an increase of approximately 1.3 cm/year. Preschool children grow about 6.5–7.5 cm/year and gain 1.5–2.5 kg, weighing on average 14.5 kg. Not all body systems grow at the same rate. Full maturation is not complete until the end of the second decade.

Development is checked by assessing developmental milestones that children should reach by a certain age, some are essential to remember (Table 59.3).

Normal infant reflexes: neonatal behaviour is controlled by reflex. These reach a peak at 4–8 weeks of age and then begin to diminish from about 3 months old, except for the protective reflexes which include blink, parachute, cough, swallow and gag.

Table 59.1 Patterns of development

Pattern	Path of progression	Examples
Cephalocaudal	From head to toe	Head control precedes the ability to walk
Proximodistal	From the trunk to the tips of the extremities	The neonate can move arms and legs but cannot pick up objects with fingers
General to specific	From simple tasks to more complex	Progression from crawling to walking to skipping

Source: Devitt and Thain (2011).

Table 59.2 Dental development

Baby teeth	Erupt (months)	Lost (years)
Central incisor	8–12	6–7
Lateral incisor	9–13	7–8
Canine	16–22	10–12
First molar	13–19	9–11
Second molar	25–33	10–12

Table 59.3 Essential developmental milestones

Age	Milestone
4–6 weeks	Fixes to faces with eyes Smiles in response
6–7 months	Sits up unsupported
9 months	Gets to a sitting position
10 months	Pincer grasp Waves goodbye
12 months	Walks unsupported Two or three words with meaning
18 months	Feeds self with spoon Points to things Tower of 3–4 cubes Throws a ball without falling
24 months	Sentences of 2–3 words Runs Kicks a ball

Source: Miall et al. (2012).

60 Child development: 5–16 years

Figure 60.1 Child development 5–16 years

Physical changes are less obvious than at 0–5 years

Children grow taller, change shape and acquire new skills.
- By 5 years, the child's height and weight are increasing steadily at the rate of 5 cm and 2–3 kg/year
- Boys are on average 2.5 cm taller and 1 kg heavier than girls during early school years; however, by 12 years girls are both taller and heavier than boys

Age 6
Swings by arms, and skips with rope

Age 7
'Walks the plank', uses a bat and ball

Age 8–10
Hopscotch, skipping games

5–7 years
Reorganization of the brain occurs and ability to memorize and reason improves

By 7 years
Growth is nearly complete at 90% of final size. The volume of grey matter increases continuing to the second decade

Shape of the child's face changes from infancy to adulthood

- Eruption of permanent teeth erupt forces the shape of the jaw to change
- The jaw grows forward and the forehead becomes more prominent
- The head and eyes are extra large in children, by the age of 8 years the child's head is 90% of its adult size

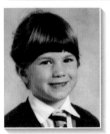
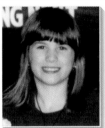
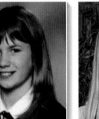
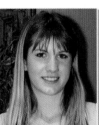

Pubertal growth spurt

- The rate of growth can double
- The final 20–25% of linear growth is achieved; this can be as much as 12.5 cm in a peak year
- Girls gain an average of 5–20 cm in height and 7–25 kg in weight
- Boys gain 10–30 cm in height and 7–30 kg in weight

Raging hormones

Testosterone production in boys rockets to 18x that of childhood and oestrogen 8x in girls

The normal age of **menarche** varies between 9 and 18 years

Developmental tasks of adolescence

- Leaving biological family
- Achieving a new relationship with parents
- Developing intimate, nurturing and caring relationships outside family
- Finding a career based on interest and capacity
- Becoming at ease with sexuality
- From dependence to independence…and to interdependence
- Change from concrete to abstract cognitive thinking
- Thinking about thinking
- Making more and more complicated decisions, analysing and hypothesizing

Figure 60.2 Growth rates for girls and boys

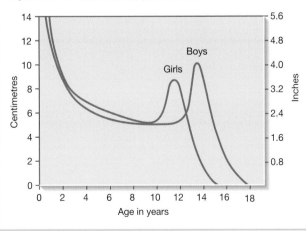

Figure 60.3 Chain of hormonal events in puberty

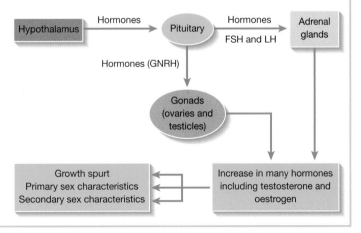

Children and Young People's Nursing at a Glance, First Edition. Edited by Alan Glasper, Jane Coad, and Jim Richardson.
© 2015 John Wiley & Sons, Ltd. Published 2015 by John Wiley & Sons, Ltd. Companion website: www.ataglanceseries.com/nursing/children

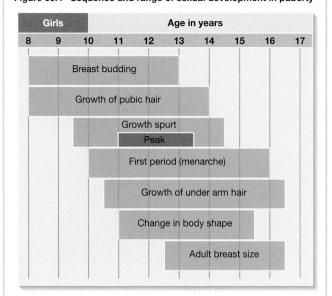

Figure 60.4 Sequence and range of sexual development in puberty

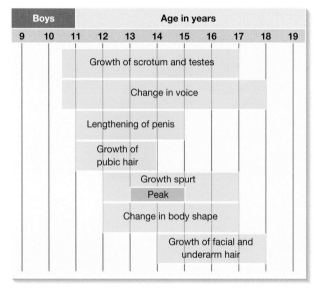

Between 5 years and puberty the physical changes in children are less obvious than at 0–5 years. However, as expected, children grow taller, change shape and acquire new skills. The 5-year-old draws a recognizable person or house, and writes their own name. They can hop, skip, swing, jump, balance, climb, dance and throw a ball. They also ride a two-wheel bicycle and begin to choose their own friends. They can undress and dress except for laces and ties and perform domestic and dramatic play, alone or with friends. Language in middle childhood continues to develop, both in vocabulary and complexity, with the child now able to correct their own mistakes and understand double meanings. There is an acceptance of rules but not necessarily an understanding of them and the child has a much better understanding of cause and effect.

Physically, the growth of the trunk and extremities now exceeds that of the head, the centre of gravity lowers and body proportions become slimmer. Growth hormone stimulates longitudinal growth in a dose-dependant manner and is reflected in

limb length. Girls stop growing sooner than boys as a result of epiphyseal unity under the effect of oestrogen secretion. Boys' longer growth is reflected in their greater height and longer arms and legs. The extremities grow first followed by neck, hip, chest, shoulder, trunk and depth of chest. Muscle growth follows that of bone and is therefore greater in boys. More fat is deposited in girls on the thighs, hips and buttocks, giving a smoother, more rounded body contour. In the cardiovascular system the systolic BP rises at an accelerated rate during puberty, pulse rate decreases, blood volume, haemoglobin, and red blood cells rise more in boys than girls, and by adulthood women have 1 million fewer red cells per mL than men. The size and capacity of the respiratory system increases, rate decreases and boys are able to take in more air at one breath because of their larger chest and shoulder size. This growth is reflected in peak flow rate, with normal ranges increasing from 150 L/min at 5 years to 240 L/min at 10 years and 400 L/min at 15 years. Oestrogen causes the skin of the female to develop a soft smooth thicker texture. The sebaceous glands are particularly active and the eccrine and apocrine sweat glands become fully functional. Body hair takes on the characteristic distribution patterns and the texture changes. The lymphoid system including the tonsils and adenoids decrease in size, improving asthma in some teens, and children start to lose their deciduous teeth. Permanent teeth appear at about the rate of 4 per year between the ages of 7 and 14 years.

Adolescence is a time of continued brain growth. There is no actual increase in number of neurons but growth of the myelin sheath continues until at least puberty, thus enabling faster neural processing which corresponds with the development of cognitive abilities. The more mature the brain, the more the prefrontal cortex works as a mechanism that enables a serious 'second thought' as decisions are made. This ability expresses itself in self-control and judgement. Younger teens may respond with less maturity because their brains are less mature. In early childhood and again at the onset of puberty, the prefrontal cortex fires up with new growth and millions of new neuro-connections are made, yet, after each growth spurt, the brain prunes away unused or unneeded connections. The connections that remain are more efficient, more powerful, and stronger. Research suggests that growth and changes in the prefrontal cortex continues well into the teen years.

During the pubertal growth spurt the rate of growth may double. The final 20–25% of linear growth is achieved; this can be as much as 12.5 cm in a peak year. Girls gain an average of 5–20 cm in height and 7–25 kg in weight. Boys gain 10–30 cm in height and 7–30 kg in weight (Figure 60.2).

The biological changes of puberty, which are considered to begin in adolescence, are universal but their expression, timing and extent show enormous variety depending on gender genes and nutrition. Puberty is triggered by a chain of hormonal effects controlled by the anterior pituitary in response to a stimulus from the hypothalamus (Figure 60.3).

During puberty, sexual development can be seen to occur in a set sequence, with variations in timing between individuals (Figure 60.4).

There are features of adolescent development that occur universally; the onset of puberty causes biological changes, the emergence of more advanced cognitive abilities are seen in cognitive changes, developing self-image, intimacy and relations with others (adults and peers) demonstrate emotional changes and finally the transition into new roles in society exemplify social changes.

61 Age-appropriate behaviours

Figure 61.1 Age appropriate behaviour

Determinants of behaviour

- Chronological age
- Parenting
- Developmental progress
- Prematurity
- Overall health and well-being
- Social and cultural environment
- Socialization
- Family structure and functioning
- Presence of illnesses or conditions in the child
- The child's global development
- Social functioning
- Impact of school and peers

Observation and record keeping

- Always consider the need to record growth, development, events and behaviours
- Be open and honest about issues when the need arises
- Adhere to the NMC Code principles on record keeping and referral

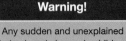

Warning!

Any sudden and unexplained behavioural change in children could be due to the presence of a brain tumour and so needs urgent assessment

Issues to consider

- Child's social and cultural circumstances
- Parenting behaviours and competence
- Parental reports of behaviour
- Where the child has a specific illness or condition impacting upon growth and development
- Children with learning disabilities
- Children with mental health problems
- Any history of abuse
- Bullying
- Substance misuse
- Influence of peer groups and antisocial behaviours

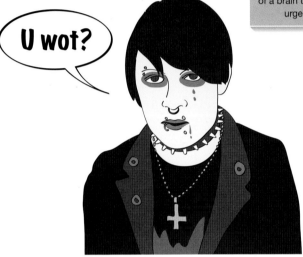

Children and Young People's Nursing at a Glance, First Edition. Edited by Alan Glasper, Jane Coad, and Jim Richardson.
© 2015 John Wiley & Sons, Ltd. Published 2015 by John Wiley & Sons, Ltd. Companion website: www.ataglanceseries.com/nursing/children

Assessing the development and behaviours of children encompasses a wide range of approaches measuring growth, cognitive ability, educational performance and social maturation, and also in specific circumstances such as behaviours in children with disorders. These methods help us to understand whether children are developing, evidenced through their behaviours, as well as identifying when they are not and the possible reasons for this. It is only through knowledge of what is appropriate at a certain age or level of development that nurses, and others, are able to identify delays. While it is possible to assess, measure and monitor development, children are individual in terms of their growth, self, health and well-being, all of which are impacted upon by their circumstances, culture, family and socialization. Changes in technology, availability of information and education also impact upon development and are issues to consider. Ultimately, children follow similar patterns of growth and development, some variance being deemed acceptable. However, absent, delayed or inappropriate behaviours are issues of concern and need to be identified, assessed and addressed appropriately.

Growth

Growth of children generally follows a similar pattern which is reflective of bone and neuromuscular development; this is the same on both sides of the body. Such growth and development can be assessed using growth (centile) charts which plot weight, height, head circumference and body mass index. These are based on averages for children of similar ages and stages of development and so allow the practitioner to ascertain any abnormalities or deviations, particularly in behaviour.

Development

Biological growth is the foundation for the child's overall development. However, as they age so do their abilities, skills and communication. These can be understood with reference to assessing the following factors.

Physical development

While growth continues, the child develops the psycho-motor skills necessary to function, which in turns supports their physical and non-verbal behaviour.

Cognitive development

Cognitive development includes aspects of personality, reasoning, concepts of self. The way in which the child behaves clearly reflects all of the above and these are particularly influenced by the relationships they have with carers.

Language development

Language acquisition is a crucial aspect of children's functioning and behaviour. Not only does it reflect their development, but is a part of how others perceive a child's behaviour.

Social development

Children learn social behaviours through observing others (predominately parents and peers) and by conditioning (e.g. rewards).

Role models are critically important for social learning and it is with reference to these that the child develops their own behaviours. Poor or dysfunctional role models may thus lead to the child developing and displaying inappropriate behaviours.

Age-inappropriate behaviours

There are a wide range of circumstances, conditions and illnesses that can result in age-inappropriate behaviour, impede appropriate behaviour or influence overall development.

Peer influence

Peers are a powerful influence on behaviour and can be valuable in developing a sense of esteem, group ownership and appropriate social behaviour. Equally, the shared behaviours of the group may be perceived as inappropriate and potentially antisocial.

Drug and alcohol-mediated behaviour

There is an increasing concern about young people's access to and use of alcohol and illegal drugs. Consumption of these may be linked to intra-familiar issues such as parental use, co-presence of family/parental discord and dysfunction as well as child abuse. Peer groups are also a powerful influence on children to participate in taking alcohol or drugs. Both substances impact on behaviour, often leading to disruption, antisocial incidents, criminal acts, self-harming and suicide in addition to the impact on their physiology.

Hospitalization

Children with chronic illness often attend hospital and are exposed to adult behaviour, medical language and environments that may impact on their development. As children develop, they may be perceived as being manipulative, 'knowing too much' and adult-like in their behaviours.

Sexualized behaviour

Sexual behaviour and relationships are often difficult issues for young people and their parents to contend with. Nonetheless, some children display behaviours such as displaying body parts, inappropriate touching, kissing and use of sexual language. When these occur, particularly at younger ages, it can be suggestive of child sexual abuse, access to pornography or mental health problems.

Learning disabilities

The many conditions that lead to learning disabilities means that children may display a wide range of behaviours which could be considered age inappropriate. These can be linked.

Mental health conditions

While mental health conditions will not cause age-inappropriate behaviour, they may impact on the child's overall development. In such cases they may 'act out' or display behaviours that are considered not to be consistent with the norm.

62 Common behavioural problems of childhood

Figure 62.1 Behaviour problems and strategies

The crying baby

- Wet or dirty nappy
- Too hot or too cold
- Hungry
- Wind
- Colic
- Environmental stress
- Reflux oesophagitis
- Teething

If sudden severe crying, consider:
- Any acute illness
- Otitis media
- Intussusception
- Strangulated inguinal hernia

Temper tantrums

- Normal, peak at 18–36 months
- Screaming
- Hitting
- Biting
- Breath-holding attacks

Strategies that may help
- Avoid precipitants such as hunger and tiredness
- Divert the tantrum by distraction
- Stay calm to teach control
- Reward good behaviour
- Try to ignore bad behaviour until calm
- Use time-out

Sleeping problems

- Difficulty getting to sleep
- Waking during the night
- Sleeping in parents' bed
- Nightmares and night terrors

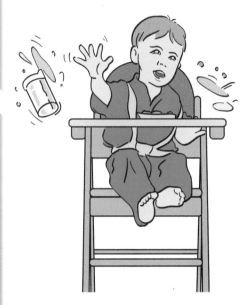

Eating problems in toddlers

- Food refusal
- Fussy eating – only eating a limited variety of foods
- Overeating
- Battles over eating and mealtimes
- Snacking
- Excessive drinking of juice

Unwanted habits

- Thumb sucking
- Nail biting
- Masturbation
- Head banging
- Hair pulling
- Bedwetting
- Encopresis (passing faeces in inappropriate places)

Aggressive behaviour

- Temper tantrums
- Hitting and biting other children
- Destroying toys
- Destroying furniture
- Commoner in boys and in larger families
- May reflect aggression within family
- Requires calm, consistent approach
- Avoid countering with aggression
- Use time-out and star charts

Figure 62.2 What you need from your evaluation

History

- Ask what is troubling the parents most – is it the child or other stresses in their lives, such as tiredness, problems at work or marital problems?
- What are the triggers for difficult or unwanted behaviour? Does it occur when the child is hungry or tired, or at any particular time of day?
- Colic tends to occur in the evenings; tantrums may be more common if the child is tired
- Does the behaviour happen consistently in all settings or is it specific to one place, e.g. the toddler may behave well at nursery but show difficult behaviour at home?
- Does the behaviour differ with each parent?
- How do the parents deal with the behaviour – do they get angry or aggressive, are they consistent, do they use bribery or do they give in to the toddler eventually?
- What strategies have the parents already tried to deal with the situation?
- Is there any serious risk of harm? Some behaviour, such as encopresis or deliberate self-harm, may reflect serious emotional upset. Most toddlers who are faddy eaters are growing well and do not suffer any long-term nutritional problems
- Babies with colic are usually less than 3 months old, go red in the face with a tense abdomen and draw up their legs. The episodes start abruptly and end with the passage of flatus or faeces

Examination

- The history usually contributes more than a physical examination
- If the parents are concerned about sudden-onset or severe crying in a baby, it is important to exclude serious infection such as meningitis or urinary tract infection, intussusception, hernias and otitis media

Management

- In most cases the parents can be reassured that the behaviour is very common, often normal and that with time and common sense it can be controlled
- With tantrums it can be helpful to use the **ABC** approach:

  A What antecedents were there? What happened to trigger the episode?

  B What was the behaviour? Could it be modified, diverted or stopped?

  C What were the consequences of the behaviour? Was the child told off, shouted at or given a cuddle?

- Generally, it is best to reward good behaviour (catch the child being good) and ignore bad behaviour. Star charts can be very useful: the child gets a star for good behaviour (staying in bed, etc.) and then a reward after several stars
- Parents should try hard not to be angry or aggressive as this may reinforce attention seeking behaviour

Children and Young People's Nursing at a Glance, First Edition. Edited by Alan Glasper, Jane Coad, and Jim Richardson.
© 2015 John Wiley & Sons, Ltd. Published 2015 by John Wiley & Sons, Ltd. Companion website: www.ataglanceseries.com/nursing/children

Common emotional and behavioural problems

These problems are seen so often that many would regard them as normal, although in a small minority the behaviour is so disruptive that it causes major family upset. GPs and paediatricians should be comfortable giving basic guidance on behaviour management to help parents through what can be a stressful, exasperating and exhausting phase of their child's development.

Crying babies and colic

Crying is usually periodic and related to discomfort, stress or temperament. However, it may indicate a serious problem, particularly if the onset is sudden. In most instances it is just a case of ensuring that the baby is well fed, warm but not too hot, has a clean nappy, comfortable clothes and a calm and peaceful environment. A persistently crying baby can be very stressful for inexperienced parents. It is important that they recognize when they are no longer coping and are offered support.

Infantile colic is a term used to describe periodic crying affecting infants in the first 3 months of life. The crying is paroxysmal, and may be associated with hunger, swallowed air or discomfort from overfeeding. It often occurs in the evenings. Crying can last for several hours, with a flushed face, distended and tense abdomen and drawn-up legs. In between attacks the child is happy and well.

It is important to consider more serious pathology such as intussusception or infection. Colic is managed by giving advice on feeding, winding after feeds and carrying the baby. It is not a reason to stop breastfeeding, but discontinuing cow's milk in the mother's diet can be helpful. Various remedies are available but there is little evidence for their effectiveness. Infantile colic usually resolves spontaneously by 3 months.

Feeding problems

Once weaned, infants need to gradually move from being fed with a spoon to finger feeding and feeding themselves. This is a messy time, but the infant needs to be allowed to explore his/her food and not be made to eat or reprimanded for making a mess.

Toddler eating habits can be unpredictable – eating large amounts at one meal and sometimes hardly anything at the next. At this age, mealtimes can easily become a battle and it is important that they are kept relaxed and the child is not pressurized into eating. Small helpings that the child can finish work best, and second helpings can be given if wanted. Eating together as a family encourages the child to eat in a social context. Feeding at mealtimes should not become a long protracted battle!

Sleeping problems

Babies and children differ in the amount of sleep they need and parents vary in how they tolerate their child waking at night. In most cases sleeping 'difficulties' are really just habits that have developed through lack of clear bedtime routine. Difficulty sleeping may also reflect conflict in the family or anxieties, for example about starting school or fear of dying. Successfully tackling sleeping problems requires determination, support and reassurance.

• *Refusal to settle at night.* Difficulty settling may develop if babies are only put to bed once they are asleep. A clear bedtime routine is important for older children; for example, a bath, a story and a drink.

• *Waking during the night.* This often causes a lot of stress as the parents become exhausted. It is important to reassure the child, then put them back to bed quietly. Sometimes a technique of 'controlled crying' can be helpful – the child is left to cry for a few minutes, then reassured and left again, this time for longer. Taking the child into the parents' bed is understandable, but usually stores up problems for later when it is difficult to break the habit.

• *Nightmares.* The child wakes as the result of a bad dream, quickly becomes lucid and can usually remember the content. The child should be reassured and returned to sleep. If particularly severe or persistent, nightmares may reflect stresses and may need psychological help.

• *Night terrors.* Night terrors occur in the preschool years. The child wakes up confused, disorientated and frightened and may not recognize their parent. He/she takes several minutes to become orientated and the dream content cannot be recalled. These episodes should not be confused with epilepsy. They are short-lived and just require reassurance, especially for the parents.

Temper tantrums

Tantrums are very common in the third year of life (the 'terrible twos') and are part of the child learning the boundaries of acceptable behaviour and parental control. They can be extremely challenging, especially when they occur in public.

The key to dealing with toddler tantrums is to try to avoid getting into the situation in the first place. This does not mean giving in to the child's every demand, but ensuring the child does not get overtired or hungry, and setting clear boundaries in a calm consistent way. It is generally best to ignore the tantrum until the child calms down. If this fails then 'time out' can be a useful technique.

The child is taken to a safe quiet environment, such as a bedroom, and left for a few minutes (1 minute for each year of age is a good guide) until calm. This is usually very effective as it removes the attention the child desires, and allows the parents time to control their own anger.

Unwanted or aggressive behaviour

Young children often have aggressive outbursts which may involve biting, hitting or scratching other children. These require consistent firm management, with use of time out and star charts for good behaviour. It is important not to respond with more aggression, as this sends conflicting messages. If aggressive behaviour is persistent, it is important to explore other tensions or disturbances within the family. In older children, the school may need to be involved.

Unwanted behaviours such as thumb-sucking, hair-pulling, nail-biting and masturbation are also common in young children. Most can be ignored and resolve with time. Masturbation can usually be prevented by distracting the child or dressing them in clothes that make it more difficult. Older children should not be reprimanded but informed that it is not acceptable in public.

Key points
• Emotional and behavioural problems are extremely common, to the point of being part of normal child development.
• Parents need to be encouraged that they can manage most behaviour with a clear strategy.
• A calm confident consistent approach to the child's behaviour is recommended.
• Parents should reward good behaviour and try to minimize attention given to undesirable behaviour.

63 Adolescent development

Figure 63.1 Who am I and how am I ?

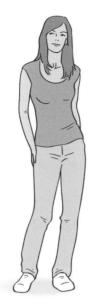

I need services that …

- Treat me with respect and make me feel welcome
- Have staff who are professional, knowledgeable, trustworthy, value me and know how to help me
- Listen, understand me, appreciate and my concerns and enable me to make informed choices
- Will not be shocked by my behaviour or lifestyle and can signpost me to other services if I need them
- Are accessible at times and locations that are suitable to me
- I can trust to treat what I say in confidence unless I am at risk of harm
- Develop and improve in response to my feedback

Adolescence is a period of development that presents the individual with numerous challenges as they progress through the transition from childhood to young adulthood. Growth and maturation make new behaviours possible, provide opportunities for intellectual development and learning but also presents hurdles and challenges to be overcome as new relationships develop and new experiences are encountered. These changes are important to the young person because they determine experience, impact on how others view and respond to them and influence the ways in which the young person sees him/herself. They also determine the path from education to the world of work and financial independence.

Physical development

The teenage years mean rapid physical change for both boys and girls. They experience a growth spurt of several inches a years for several years. Individual differences will be widespread because of factors such as sex and genetic inheritance. Physical changes involve the skeletal and nervous systems, leading to changes in shape and proportion, for example significant changes to hands and feet, arms and legs, and trunk. Strengthening of bones continues and is associated with thickening muscle fibres in boys and increased fat deposits in the breasts and hips in girls. Puberty also results in the development of sex characteristics which further differentiate the sexes. Hormonal upheaval may also affect teenage time keeping and sleep patterns; the sleep hormone melatonin, for example, is released at about 10pm in adults, but not until 1am in teenagers.

Brain development and changes in cognition (thinking)

The cerebral cortex of the brain governs learning and is concerned with increasingly complex thought, perception, language and memory, reflexivity and empathy as connections between neural pathways are made in response to repeated experiences. These form the 'hard wiring' of the brain and nervous system, a process that will be most successful with repeated positive learning experiences and less effective during periods of stress or inconsistency. Significant periods in the hard wiring of the brain have recently been shown to occur at around the age of 2 years and during the early teens when the synaptic connections are pruned and reorganized. During early and mid adolescence, young people may rely on more primitive areas of the brain leading to increased impulsivity and risk-taking. Gradually, increased myelinization of the new connections in the frontal cortex leads to an ability to transmit messages more effectively, hold in mind more multidimensional concepts and to think in a more strategic manner. These science-based understandings based on modern imaging techniques are consistent with the ideas of the cognitive developmental psychologist, Jean Piaget (1951), who saw early adolescence as a period characterized by new ways of thinking as the young person moves from thought processes based on concrete reasoning to more abstract thinking. This means that teenagers are likely to be more reflective in their thinking, and more concerned with ethical and philosophical dilemmas such as their place in society, moral dilemmas, altruism, politics and the meaning of life.

Identity

Erik Erikson (1950) saw acceptance of both self and society as a task that is especially important between onset of puberty and young adulthood. He saw this period of development to be characterized by an 'identity crisis' as young people struggle to resolve a sense of confusion to establish a consistent sense of themselves; trying out numerous roles to gain a sense of personal integrity and bringing together experiences, values and aspirations to answer the question 'Who am I?' The young person may discover their place in society or feel they stand outside society. An important aspect of this is maintaining a sense of being true to oneself while at the same time balancing this with the need to conform to the expectations of peers, culture and wider society. Later, this will lead to the young person becoming less self-absorbed and being able to overcome a sense of isolation to be able to develop an intimate relationship with another person. Erikson's 'storm and stress' view of adolescence has been challenged by other researchers who argue that the majority of teenagers will go through a relatively smooth transition from childhood to young adulthood.

Changing social relationships

Urie Bronfenbrenner (1979) developed an Ecological Systems Theory to demonstrate that no child or young person will develop in isolation. All young people will be influenced the sociocultural context within which they live and develop; their family, community, social institutions; culture and media, generation and political environment. Most important for young people will be their decreasing dependence on parents and the increasing influence of peers, who may provide a source of friendship, mutual support and positive learning experiences, but also may encourage negative health behaviours in more vulnerable young people such as smoking; experimentation with drugs and alcohol; pressure to engage in sexual experimentation; offending and violent gang culture.

Young people as service users

Young people may access health services from numerous agencies for a variety of reasons: access to health information, treatment for health problems or access to specific services such as stopping smoking, help with drug and alcohol misuse or contraception, and sexual health services. Most young people will treat services with respect, but some may initially present challenging behaviour in order to test out whether they can confidently trust the service provider not to be judgmental or shocked by their concerns. All young people have the right to be treated with dignity and respect and receive services that are accessible, welcoming and responsive to their needs and concerns as well as safeguard their well-being. Professionals and practitioners working in these services will need to demonstrate appropriate attitudes and values. They will also need to know about other services that could be additional sources of support for young people in challenging social circumstances.

64 Child health promotion

Figure 64.1 What is health promotion?

The World Health Organization (1984: 4) suggests that:
'Health promotion is the process of enabling people to increase control over, and to improve, their health.'

Health promotion embraces the concept of empowerment, both at an individual and collective level, thus enabling others to make their own decisions and equipping them with resources to determine their health circumstances.

Scenario

Each year a number of children visit their local accident and emergency departments following falls from their bikes. Many sustain head injuries as a direct consequence of not wearing a cycle helmet.

There are five key health promotion approaches that can be drawn on to try to remedy this situation (Ewles and Simnett 2003):
• Medical
• Behavioural
• Educational
• Client-centred
• Societal change

Figure 64.2 Approaches to health promotion

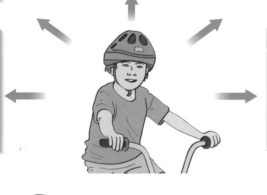

Medical

This approach requires the target population to comply with preventative medical measures. There may be an expectation that medical advice is followed in terms of cycle helmet wearing as this has the potential to reduce head injuries. There could also be an expectation that parents will have ensured that their children have had their immunizations, thus reducing the likelihood of a tetanus infection in the advent of a cycle fall.

Behavioural

This approach aims to promote behaviour that reduces the risk of ill-health. The type of healthy behaviours that are expected are normally identified by the professional. Therefore, cycle helmet wearing may be promoted within a school environment; alternatively, a children's nurse may choose to opportunistically promote this to children and their families when they are in the accident and emergency department.

Educational

This approach provides people with information, enabling them to make informed decisions. Ideally, children, young people and families should be given information about the wearing of cycle helmets as well as the opportunity to ask questions. Developmentally appropriate resources should be used to enhance the child's understanding. Individuals are encouraged to make their own decisions based on the knowledge that they have gained.

Societal change

This approach modifies the environment, both physically and socially, to make healthier choices the easier ones. Therefore, if it became usual practice, and socially accepted, that everyone wore a cycle helmet, it may make it easier for children and young people to comply.

Client-centred

This approach enables children, young people and families to identify their own health needs. Therefore, unless concerns about cycle helmet wearing are expressed, this would not automatically be addressed by the children's nurse.

Figure 64.3 Promoting health to children

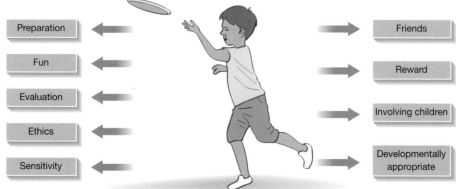

Preparation

Fun

Evaluation

Ethics

Sensitivity

Friends

Reward

Involving children

Developmentally appropriate

Children and Young People's Nursing at a Glance, First Edition. Edited by Alan Glasper, Jane Coad, and Jim Richardson.
© 2015 John Wiley & Sons, Ltd. Published 2015 by John Wiley & Sons, Ltd. Companion website: www.ataglanceseries.com/nursing/children

What is child health promotion?

'Health in childhood determines health throughout life and into the next generation...Ill health or harmful lifestyle choices in childhood can lead to ill health throughout life, which creates health, financial and social burdens for countries today and tomorrow'. (World Health Organization 2005: ix)

The above quote illustrates just how important the promotion of children's health is. Child health promotion focuses upon the enhancement of children and young people's overall health and well-being.

Do children's nurses need to promote health?

The Nursing and Midwifery Council (NMC) (2010) standards for pre-registration nursing education clearly indicate that nurses should be able to recognize unhealthy activities and promote the health and well-being of the people they work with. In addition, the Department of Health (2012) launched an initiative entitled Making Every Contact Count (MECC). This programme advocates that every health professional supports patients to facilitate healthier choices; there is a clear emphasis placed upon the role of nurses and it is suggested that all nurses, in any context, can make every contact count in order to positively influence the health of their client group. In terms of children's nursing, it may be advising a parent about areas such as children's immunization, sleep requirements, diet or dental hygiene; alternatively, it may be referring an adolescent who smokes to a Stop Smoking Service.

Involving children

The 'emergence of children's voice' (Prout and Hallett 2003: 1), and the need to involve children in a range of issues, has grown in acceptance and it is now widely established that the views and experiences of children should be taken into account wherever possible. Health promotion is no different and it is essential that children and young people be fully engaged in the promotion of their health from an early age.

Engaging with children requires tremendous skill and expertise and there are a range of factors that should be taken into account:
• *Planning.* The child and the nurse need to be clear about the aim of the health promotion initiative. Planning and organization are fundamental if success is to be achieved.
• *Developmental stage.* Taking the child or young person's cognitive developmental stage into account is crucial. If someone does not understand the approach taken, or if the strategy is perceived to be too 'babyish', there will be a lack of engagement. Similarly, physical capability and ability needs to be assessed to ensure that appropriate strategies are utilized.
• *Fun.* We all enjoy having fun so being able to portray a serious health message in a fun and creative manner can be a good way to engage children (particularly those at the primary school age) and enable them to remember the key issues. For example, a strategy to enhance handwashing may involve educating children about 'germs' and how they are spread. Children could be asked to dip their hands into bright paint, representative of germs, and then be asked to use soap and water to remove it. The remains of the paint on the children's hands after washing serves as a demonstration of how germs can then be spread to other areas, such as food.

• *Rewards.* Young children in particular enjoy a reward system (e.g. a certificate or sticker) if they, for example, successfully complete a game. However, the older age range are also responsive as long as the 'prize' is age appropriate – wrist bands and pens that reinforce the health message are frequently well received.
• *Friends.* It is widely recognized that children and young people of all ages enjoy spending time with their friends so health promotion activities that enable this are more likely to be engaging.
• *Sensitivity.* The time and context of any health promotion activity needs to be considered. For example, while a child is recovering from an acute illness and family members may well be experiencing increased stress levels, it may not be appropriate to discuss sensitive issues such as a child's excess weight. Perhaps discussion or referral to other health professionals may be more appropriate.

Ethics

Health promotion also presents some ethical challenges. The aim of health promotion is to do good, but sometimes there can be negative outcomes – for example, a children's nurse could advise a teenage girl to reduce her weight as she has a high body mass index, this would be perceived as being in the girl's best interests. However, if the girl started smoking because she had heard that this is a good appetite suppressant, there could be negative consequences. This is one reason why the evaluation of any health promoting activity is so important.

Evaluation

Evaluation is a key aspect of health promotion, in other words, has it worked? Does anything need to be changed for the future? This can be difficult to assess, but it is still important that evaluation is objectively considered. It can include simple strategies such as:
• The children's nurse's reflection on the activity
• Feedback from whoever the activity was aimed at.

Where is health promoted to children?

In summary, everywhere. All health professionals have a responsibility to be involved in the promotion of children's health, whether this is in an acute or primary care setting. Schools have been recognized as a key environment in which health can be promoted. However, emphasis has traditionally been placed upon the promotion of specific health needs such as diet, sexual health, drug and alcohol abuse, rather than fostering a more holistic and engaging health promotion approach. There is now a recognized need to develop strategies to redress this balance. One way could be the organization of a health promotion 'market', facilitated by health professionals, which exposes children and young people to a range of health promotion initiatives.

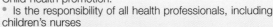

Key points

Child health promotion:
• Is the responsibility of all health professionals, including children's nurses
• Should involve families – in particular parents – as well as the children and young people themselves
• Must be carefully planned and be appropriate for the development stage and needs of the children or young people
• Should be evaluated
• Is complex, but everyone needs to rise to the challenge.

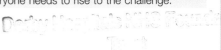

65 Immunity and immunization

Figure 65.1 Immunization

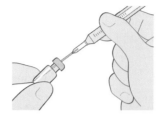

Aims of immunization

- Prevention of infectious diseases and their associated complications
- Prevention of outbreaks of disease
- Eradication of infectious diseases worldwide

Role of the nurse

Nurses are major contributors to immunization programmes. They regularly administer vaccines for childhood immunization programmes (see Chapter 66), annual influenza vaccination campaigns and travel vaccine schedules.

NMC Code of Conduct

Nurses have professional accountability when they undertake immunizations. This means that in order to administer immunizations safely and effectively they have a responsibility to work within their competence and keep their knowledge and skills up to date.

When working within the boundaries of their competence nurses ensure that no action or omission is detrimental to patients.

Figure 65.2 Safe administration of vaccinations

Patient Group Direction (PGD)

PGDs are legal written instructions for the supply and administration of vaccines to patients for whom no individual prescription exists.
They are used for groups of patients whose requirements and characteristics are consistent.

- Patients must meet specific inclusion and exclusion criteria stated in the PGD
- Nurses must be individually named and have signed the PGD to be eligible to use it

Consent

- Consent must be obtained before giving any vaccine to a patient
- There is no legal requirement that this must be in writing but a consent form can be a record of the information provided about the process, benefits and risks of immunization as well as the decision
- It is good practice to check the person still consents at each immunization episode

Contraindications

Vaccines should not be given when a patient has had an anaphylactic reaction to a preceding dose.
Live vaccines may be temporarily contraindicated in patients who are pregnant or immunosuppressed.
Vaccines may be postponed when a patient is acutely unwell or has a febrile illness. This is to prevent wrongly attributing new or worsening symptoms to the vaccine.

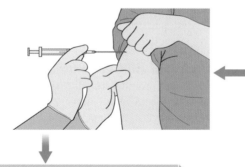

Adverse events following immunization

Common adverse events include:
- Pain, swelling or redness at the injection site
- Fever, malaise, headache
- Fainting and panic attacks

Anaphylactic reactions are extremely rare. Typically, onset is rapid and unpredictable with cardiovascular collapse, bronchospasm and angioedema. Anaphylaxis is treated using intramuscular adrenaline.

Documentation and record keeping

Accurate documentation is essential in order to monitor an individual's vaccine status as well as record what action or care was taken.
It is best practice to document the vaccine name, dose, batch number and expiry date as well as the site of administration.

Dealing with anxious people

Some people can be anxious about injections. Maternal anxiety can make children nervous. Teenagers can be nervous due to peer influence. To alleviate anxiety nurses should:

- Use a calm reassuring approach
- Use distraction techniques to divert attention from the procedure
- Prepare the vaccine out of sight of the patient
- Explain the procedure fully

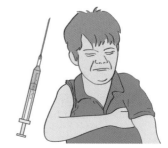

Children and Young People's Nursing at a Glance, First Edition. Edited by Alan Glasper, Jane Coad, and Jim Richardson.
© 2015 John Wiley & Sons, Ltd. Published 2015 by John Wiley & Sons, Ltd. Companion website: www.ataglanceseries.com/nursing/children

Immunity

Immunity is the ability of the body to protect itself from infectious disease. There are two types of immunity: innate and acquired.

Innate immunity

Innate immunity is present from birth and is a non-specific first line of defence. Innate immunity includes:
- Physical barriers such as intact skin and mucous membranes
- Chemical barriers such as saliva and gastric acid
- Phagocytic cells such as macrophages in the mucosa.

Acquired immunity

Acquired immunity is specific to a single organism or group of closely related organisms and is acquired through an active or a passive mechanism. Acquired immunity can be active or passive.

Active immunity is usually long-lasting and can be acquired through exposure to the natural disease or by vaccination. The body responds by producing antibodies and T lymphocytes to act against the infection. Vaccination provides immunity without the risk from the disease and its complications.

Passive immunity provides temporary protection to an individual by the transfer of antibodies. For example:
- Across the placenta from mother to child
- Transfusion of blood or blood products containing immunoglobulins.

How immunizations work

Immunization is a safe and effective way of preventing infectious disease. Vaccines are administered to an individual to provide protection by triggering active immunity and providing immunological memory. This prepares the immune system to respond quickly when exposed to natural infection in the future therefore preventing or reducing the severity of the disease. Vaccines are generally made from inactivated (killed) or attenuated (weakened) live organisms, or from their component parts or the toxins they produce.

Inactivated vaccines

Inactivated vaccines may require two or more injections to produce sufficient primary antibody response. Reinforcing doses are often given to provide longer term protection. Inactivated vaccines cannot cause the infectious disease they are intended to prevent.

Attenuated vaccines

Live attenuated vaccines induce the same immune response as natural infection and usually provide long-lasting antibody response after one or two doses. It does not usually cause the disease itself in healthy individuals.

Population immunity

The main aim of immunization is to protect the individual. People who have been vaccinated are less likely to be a source of infection to others, so reducing the risk of exposure to unvaccinated individuals. This means vaccination programmes can also benefit those who cannot be immunized. This is called population or herd immunity.

Safe immunization

Nurses must have received additional training to be authorized to administer immunizations. They must be competent in all aspects of immunization including contraindications and the recognition and treatment of anaphylaxis. In order to maintain patient safety and remain current on immunization policy and practice, NHS Trusts require nurses to receive regular update courses in immunization and resuscitation.

Safe storage of vaccines

The success of immunization programmes depends on vaccine potency. Vaccines are sensitive to heat, cold and light. Exposure to these conditions irreversibly reduces the effectiveness of vaccines and put patients at risk. This can lead to litigation issues if ineffective vaccines are administered. The Cold Chain is the system used for storing and transporting vaccines within the safe temperature range of 2–8°C and protected from light. Dedicated fridges are used, temperature is monitored daily and stockpiling is avoided to enable air to circulate and maintain a constant temperature.

Reporting adverse events

Vaccines are tested for quality, safety and efficacy before being licensed for routine use. Although adverse effects are identified prior to licensing, careful monitoring is required. The Yellow Card Scheme is a voluntary process for reporting suspected adverse reactions. The scheme is important in early identification of safety concerns. Vaccine safety is kept under constant review by a committee of experts who carefully review new evidence and make recommendations.

Immunization controversies

Immunization has caused controversy since first discovered by Edward Jenner over 200 years ago. False beliefs tend to flourish where there is limited understanding of the evidence. Dissemination of misleading and contradictory information has been facilitated in recent times by the internet and social media. Reporting in the media may give equal weight to both sides of an argument without giving due emphasis to a robust research base. This can result in a reduction in vaccine uptake and a resurgence of the disease.

One such controversy was that surrounding measles, mumps and rubella (MMR) vaccination following a study published by Wakefield et al. (1998). The findings of this research linked MMR to autism and gastrointestinal problems. The research was seriously flawed and the findings have since been withdrawn. Because of the research many parents opted not to vaccinate their children and as a result there has since been an increase in the number of cases of measles, predominantly in those who were unvaccinated. Measles is associated with serious complications including meningitis, pneumonia and hepatitis. By 2011, MMR coverage for population immunity had still not been achieved.

In order to inform practice and be able to respond to patients' concerns, nurses need to know where to find reliable information about current issues and have the skills to critically appraise research.

66 Childhood immunizations

Figure 66.1 Immunization schedule for children 2 months to 18 years

2 months:	diphtheria, tetanus, pertussis, polio, haemophilus influenza type B, pneumococcal
3 months:	diphtheria, tetanus, pertussis, polio, haemophilus influenza type B, meningitis C
4 months:	diphtheria, tetanus, pertussis, polio, haemophilus influenza type B, pneumococcal, meningitis C
12–13 months:	pneumococcal, haemophilus influenza booster, measles, mumps and rubella
3 years 4 months to 5 years:	measles, mumps and rubella, diphtheria, tetanus, percussis and polio
Girls 12–13 years:	three single doses over a year of human papillomavirus
13–18 years:	diphtheria, tetanus and polio

Immunizations should not be delayed because of:

- Minor infections (coughs and colds) without pyrexia
- Family history of bad reactions to immunizations
- The infant or child having had the illness (e.g. mumps)
- Prematurity
- Cerebral palsy
- Contact with an infectious disease
- Has asthma, hay fever or eczema
- The infant or child is on antibiotics, an inhaler or using steroid creams
- Breastfeeding
- Jaundice
- Underweight
- Being above the recommended age of immunization
- History of febrile convulsions or allergies

Immunizations are:

- Safe
- Free
- Very unlikely to cause allergic reactions
- Protection against some life-threatening illnesses

Health care professionals have a responsibility to:

- Promote immunization
- Reassure parents and carers
- Support parents and carers in their decision making
- Offer advice on pain control

Immunization saves lives
Be wise – immunize

Children and Young People's Nursing at a Glance, First Edition. Edited by Alan Glasper, Jane Coad, and Jim Richardson.
© 2015 John Wiley & Sons, Ltd. Published 2015 by John Wiley & Sons, Ltd. Companion website: www.ataglanceseries.com/nursing/children

There are many decisions parents and carers have to make about their infants and children, and immunizations are often an area that parents worry about, particularly with media hype and the misguided research on the adverse affects of immunizations on some children.

The benefits of immunizations outweigh the risks to the infant or child. Sharing information and reassuring parents and carers by health care professionals is paramount if we are to continue to ensure that some diseases do not return.

Smallpox was officially declared wiped out in 1980, and polio is heading towards eradication. Immunizations have saved more lives and prevented more serious diseases than any advance in recent medical history. There will be more potentially life-saving immunizations in the coming years as there are more than 150 new immunizations currently being tested.

Immunizations given at 2, 3 and 4 months

By about 2 months of age, the baby's natural immunity gained from his/her mother begins to diminish and so that is why the program starts at aged 2 months.

A 5-in-1 vaccine (DTaP/IPV/Hib) protects the infant against diphtheria, tetanus, pertussis, polio and haemophilus influenza type B.

The infant is also given PCV (pneumococcal) at 2 months and 4 months and meningitis C at 3 months and 4 months.

Immunizations given at 12–13 months

A booster of meningitis C and haemophilus influenza type B is given and a third dose of PCV (pneumococcal) along with MMR (measles, mumps and rubella).

Immunizations given at 3 years 4 months or soon after

A booster of MMR is given, along with a pre-school booster for diphtheria, tetanus, pertussis and polio (DTaP/IPV).

Immunizations given to girls at 12–13 years

Human papillomavirus immunization was commenced in 2008 to try to reduce the numbers of cervical cancer. The immunization program is given via three single injections over a period of a year. The girl will have protection for 6 years after the last dose, but it is still unknown how long protection will last.

Immunizations given to teenagers aged 13–18 years

A booster of diphtheria, tetanus and polio is given before the child leaves senior school.

Other immunzations available

Immunosuppressed children may be offered varicella immunization between the ages of 1 and 12 in one single dose. A child over 13 years will be given two doses given 4–8 weeks apart.

Tuberculosis immunization is given to infants and children who have a high chance of coming into contact with the disease and is given from birth to 16 years of age.

Influenza immunization is offered to children who have certain medical conditions or who are immunosuppressed once a year from 6 months of age.

Common problems

The 5-in-1 injection may cause redness and swelling at the site for a few days, and mild fever may last up to 10 days after the immunization.

The pneumococcal immunization causes redness and inflammation in 1 in 7 infants. Mild symptoms of irritability, raised temperature and digestive disturbances can occur.

The meningitis C vaccine can cause swelling and redness to the site. In toddlers, disturbed sleep and mild fever can occur, whereas older children may complain of headaches.

MMR can cause cold symptoms, fever, swollen salivary glands, for a few days up to 3 weeks after the immunization. Rash and loss of appetite can also occur.

Treatment

All the common problems are manageable and minor. Paracetamol for pain and discomfort according to prescription advice is recommended along with frequent fluids and rest.

When not to immunize

Immunization should be postponed if a child has a pyrexia (above 38°C).

If a child has had a bad reaction to a previous immunization, they may require assessment first, and future doses may be given in a hospital setting.

Only children who have had a confirmed anaphylactic reaction to an immunization will be advised not to have further doses.

Key points

- Immunizations are safe.
- Allergic responses are very rare.
- The benefits outweigh the risks.
- Immunization across the globe has saved millions of lives.

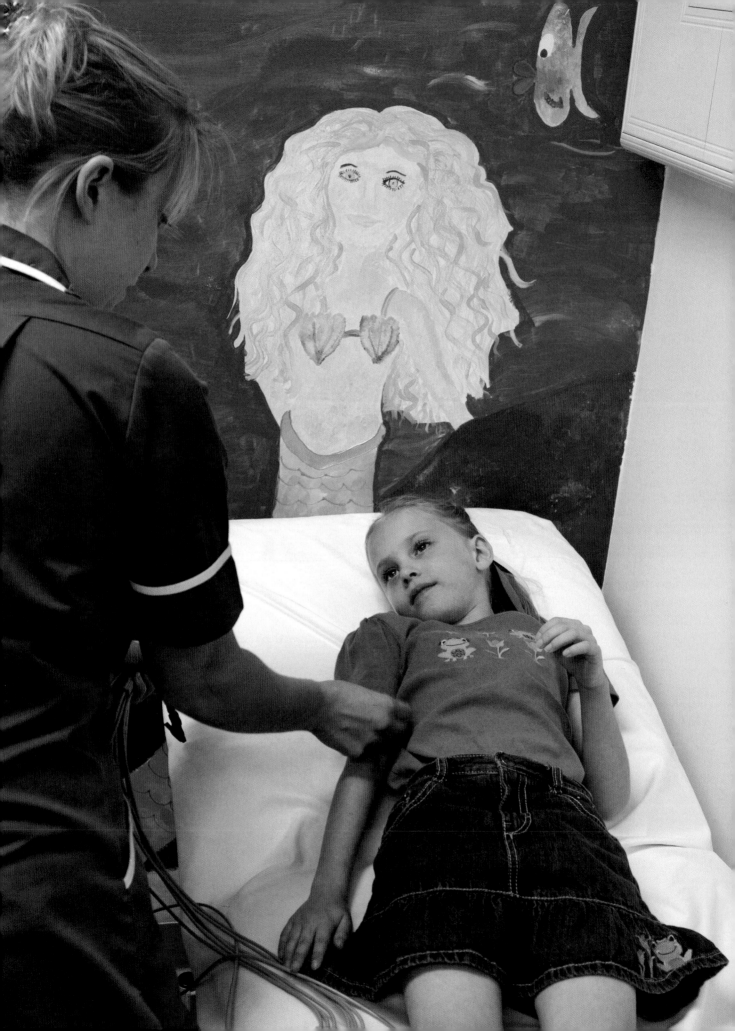

Child heath policy

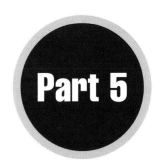

Part 5

Chapters

Don't forget to visit the companion website for this book at **www.ataglanceseries.com/nursing/children** where you will find over 500 interactive multiple-choice questions to supplement your learning.

67 Child health policy

Figure 67.1 Current UK Child health policies for health and social care

Policy

The English National Service Framework (NSF) for Children, Young People and Maternity Services (DOH 2004)

10 year visionary benchmarking document to optimize the health and safety opportunities for:

• Well children and young people
• Sick children and young people in hospital and community settings (and those with mental health problems, disabilities and complex health needs)
• Maternity services

Inequalities across these three areas impact upon child health, morbidity and lifespan opportunities

The Right Start:
The NSF for Children, Young People and Maternity Services (DOH 2004) was the first part of the English NSF to be published. Set rigorous standards for hospitalized children addressing three domains:

• Child-centred services
• Quality and safety of care provision
• Quality of settings and environment

The NHS and local authorities must evolve services to meet the standards

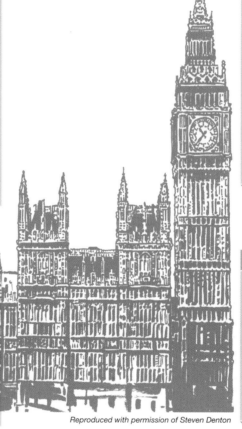

Reproduced with permission of Steven Denton

Regulation

• Established in 2008, the Care Quality Commission (CQC) is the principal regulator for health and social care in England, with powers to ensure safe quality care provision.
The CQC has 28 quality standards.

• The CQC and Ofsted ensure compliance with and progression towards NSF benchmarks via inspections. The CQC standards and NSF benchmarks, alongside similar policies across the four countries that make up the United Kingdom, form the backbone of UK child health standards

Recommendations

• The Children and Young People's Health Outcomes Forum recommend that, by 2013–2014, the DOH incorporate children and young people's views into patient surveys, in all care settings, to inform decisions about delivery of health care
• The 15 Steps Challenge: Quality Toolkit (for children and young people's inpatient services). Aims to evaluate and develop services from perspectives and experiences of children and their families

Child health policies aim to maintain or improve the health of children and young people. Within the United Kingdom, health inequalities remain prevalent, impacting upon the life experiences and opportunities for every child. Investment in these, alongside other measures to challenge child poverty, will influence the opportunities and safety for future generations. The current standards for children and young people, in the coalition government, are the National Service Framework for Children, Young People and Maternity Services (DOH 2004). This policy is far reaching in terms of its remit across health and social care boundaries. The standards recognize the need to invest in preconception care, because this influences the health of the developing child though to adulthood, the need to promote health for the well child (e.g. in terms of healthy eating to prevent obesity and promotion of exercise in home and school settings) and ensuring children who experience ill health receive exemplary care to enable them to achieve their potential.

Historically, landmark policies recognized the impact of hospitalization upon child development, as well as measures to promote the health and ensure the safety and protection of children in a range of settings. The policies promoted the need to have paediatric health and social care facilities and staff specifically trained in caring for children, young people and their families:

- Platt Report (HMSO 1959)
- Court Report (HMSO 1976)
- Children's Act (HMSO 1989)
- Welfare of Children and Young People in Hospital (HMSO 1991)
- Allitt Inquiry/Clothier Report (DOH 1994)
- Kennedy Report into Bristol Children's Heart Surgery (DOH 2001)
- Redfern Report into Liverpool Children's Hospital (DOH 2001)
- Seeking Consent: Working with Children (DOH 2001)
- Laming Report into the death of Victoria Climbié (DOH 2003)
- Children's Bill (DOH 2004).

This chapter provides a glimpse into government policy in the United Kingdon, which is vast and evolving. Health policy has been proactive in championing the specific needs of children and young people within society but embedding the recommendations is challenging. Regulation and coordination of the range of services and agencies that children and young people come into contact with are complex. The children's nurse has a key role in disseminating, promoting and collaborating interprofessional working with children and their families to ensure the best health outcomes for children and young people.

It is imperative that children's nurses keep up to date with evolving policies through professional updating (as part of professional regulation and through employers, e.g. local health organizations and trusts will have clinical governance procedures for implementing and developing national and local policy). Children's nurses have a responsibility to keep abreast of evolving evidence-based guidelines specifically for children, such as NICE Guidance. Keeping abreast of policies locally can be achieved by accessing managers and local intranet sites, as well as clinical governance teams. However, government policy relating to health care more often relates to the NHS as a whole and seeks to address changes to service provision for the entire population. Children's nurses therefore also have a key role in advocating for the specific rights of children and young people in relation to generic policy recommendations. The children's nurse is a gatekeeper who can influence and contribute to policy development, since there is still much work to be done to ensure equality of opportunities. The Report of the Children and Young People's Health Outcomes Forum (2012) recommended that the DOH and NHS Commissioning Boards should incorporate the views of children and young people into existing national patient surveys in all care settings by 2013–2014. This could ensure that the views of children form the starting point for policies to protect them. Furthermore, it is important to understand that there are implications in adhering to and following policy when working in any one of the four countries that make up the United Kingdom. Government policy, which was instigated from the Department of Health, may be adopted for use within Wales, Scotland or Ireland, or each country may choose to adapt their own policy (e.g. child safeguarding).

68 The rights of children in hospital

Figure 68.1 Ensuring the rights of children in hospital

The **Convention on the Rights of the Child** was adopted by the General Assembly of the United Nations in November 1989. It came into force in the United Kingdom in January 1992. Its primary aim is to provide a comprehensive set of principles and standards to guide and inform planning and practice for children and young people up to 18 years of age.

The **Children's Charter** was launched as part of the UK government's commitment to accountability in public services in 1996. It made a number of innovative pledges to children and their families. These pledges were based on good practice generated through years of published child health policy.

Action for Sick Children Millennium Charter

1. All children shall have equal access to the best clinical care within a network of services that collaborate with each other.
2. Health services for children and young people should be provided in a child-centred environment separately from adults so that they are made to feel welcome, safe and secure at all times.
3. Parents should be empowered to participate in decisions regarding the treatment an care of their child through a process of clear communication and adequate support.
4. Children should be informed and involved to an extent appropriate to their development and understanding.
5. Children should be cared for at home with the support and practical assistance of community children's nursing services, unless the care that they require can only be provided in hospital.
6. All staff caring for children shall be specifically trained to understand and respond to their clinical, emotional, developmental and cultural needs.
7. Every hospital admitting children should provide overnight accommodation for parents, free of charge.
8. Parents should be encouraged and supported to participate in the care of their child when they are sick.
9. Every child in hospital shall have full opportunity for play, recreation and education.
10. Adolescents will be recognized as having different needs from those of younger children and adults. Health services should therefore be readily available to meet their particular needs.

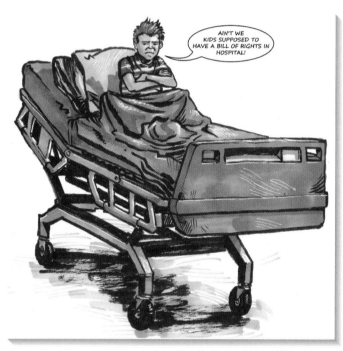

Reproduced with permission of Steven Denton

The **Welfare of Children in Hospital** (Committee of the Central Health Services Council 1959) **Platt Report** was a wake-up call for nurses involved in the care of sick children in hospital

National Service Framework for Children

This sets new standards for children and young people across health and social care boundaries in England

There are many barriers to the implementation of policy recommsendations in contemporary health care settings for children and young people. The welfare of children in hospital (Committee of the Central Health Services Council 1959) was the first of many reports specifically aimed at alleviating the psychological traumas perpetrated on children during a hospital stay. The Platt Report had profound and lasting effects on the welfare of children in hospital, not only in the UK, but also much further afield in countries such as Australia, New Zealand, Canada and the United States. In particular, Platt highlighted the necessity of nurses to appreciate the emotional needs of children in hospital in order to percive the child as a whole, and as a continuous developing person.

In 1995, the British Association for Community Child Health published *Child health rights: Implementing the UN Convention on the rights of the child within the NHS. A practitioners' guide.* This publication brought to the attention of all who work with children the mechanisms for the implementation of the UN Convention. This convention on the rights of the child was adopted by the General Assembly of the United Nations in November 1989. It came into force in the United Kingdom in January 1992. Its primary aim is to provide a comprehensive set of principles and standards to guide and inform planning and practice for children and young people up to 18 years of age. The 1990s was an era of public charters and The Patient's Charter: Services for Children and Young People (the Children's Charter) was launched in 1996 as part of the UK government's commitment to accountability in public services. It made a number of innovative pledges to children and their families. These pledges were based on good practice generated through years of published child health policy. For the first time, children and their families were given copies of this 'bill of rights' on admission to hospital. The charter was clear in highlighting the role and commitment of the NHS in protecting the mental health and well-being of every child admitted to hospital. Much of this charter was eventually enshrined within Action for Sick Children's Millennium Charter for children's health services which has stood the test of time and remains good practice (http://www.ascscotland.org.uk/default.asp?page=37)

Action for Sick Children Millennium Charter for Children's Health Services

- All children shall have equal access to the best clinical care within a network of services that collaborate with each other.
- Health services for children and young people should be provided in a child-centred environment separately from adults so that they are made to feel welcome, safe and secure at all times.
- Parents should be empowered to participate in decisions regarding the treatment and care of their child through a process of clear communication and adequate support.
- Children should be informed and involved to an extent appropriate to their development and understanding.
- Children should be cared for at home with the support and practical assistance of community children's nursing services, unless the care that they require can only be provided in hospital.
- All staff caring for children shall be specifically trained to understand and respond to their clinical, emotional, developmental and cultural needs.
- Every hospital admitting children should provide overnight accommodation for parents, free of charge.
- Parents should be encouraged and supported to participate in the care of their child when they are sick.
- Every child in hospital shall have full opportunity for play, recreation and education.
- Adolescents will be recognized as having different needs from those of younger children and adults. Health services should therefore be readily available to meet their particular needs.

Children and young people have rights when receiving health care, but especially the right to have someone they love with them wherever and whenever possible, and to be told what is actually happening or going to happen to them. They should be encouraged to ask questions and be given honest answers that they can understand. Importantly, they have the right to receive safe care and be protected from harm, from people who understand the needs of children and young people.

69 The NHS Change Model

Figure 69.1 The NHS Change Model

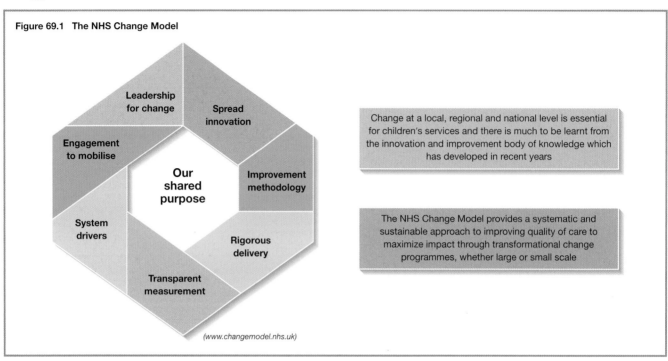

Change at a local, regional and national level is essential for children's services and there is much to be learnt from the innovation and improvement body of knowledge which has developed in recent years

The NHS Change Model provides a systematic and sustainable approach to improving quality of care to maximize impact through transformational change programmes, whether large or small scale

(www.changemodel.nhs.uk)

Application of the NHS Change Model to innovation in children's services

The National Service Framework for Children, Young People and Maternity Services (Department of Health 2003), stated 'Children and young people deserve the best care because they are the life-blood of the nation and are vital for our future economic survival and prosperity.' Yet while there are 12.4 million under-19-year-olds in England, 24% of the total population only 5% of the NHS budget is allocated to children's health care, indicating that children and young people do not have the priority required to make a difference to the future health of the population (Office for National Statistics 2010).

A confidential inquiry into child deaths found identifiable failure in the child's direct care in 26% of deaths, with potentially avoidable factors in a further 43% (Pearson et al. 2009). Death rates from illnesses that rely heavily on first access service, for example, meningococcal disease, pneumonia, and asthma, are higher in the United Kingdom than in Sweden, France, Italy, Germany and the Netherlands, and if the UK health system performed as well as that of Sweden, as many as 1500 children might not die each year (Wolfe et al. 2011). The Children and Young People's Health Outcomes Forum report (Department of Health 2012) states 'it is becoming increasingly evident that health outcomes for children and young people in our country are poor'. This is not what most people to believe. The system and country appears to be both 'sentimental and complacent'. Yet 'there is a deep wish within the system to try and get it right and improve many of the longstanding shortcomings for children and young people.'

Change at a local, regional and national level is therefore essential for children's services and there is much we can learn from the innovation and improvement body of knowledge which has developed in recent years. The NHS Change Model (2013) provides a systematic and sustainable approach to improving quality of care to maximize impact through transformational change programmes whether large or small scale.

The model brings together collective improvement knowledge and experience from across the NHS into eight key components. Through applying all eight components effective change can be achieved, the approach can fit each unique context as a way of making sense at every level of the 'how and why' for delivering improvement, to consistently make a bigger difference, whether it be reducing emergency admissions, transforming services as a result of user engagement or introducing new processes such a SBAR (Situation, Background, Assessment and Recommendation) to enhance communication.

Central to successful change is the agreement of a **shared purpose**, clarity of focus is essential so that the intent of the change programme is clear to all.

Evidence suggests that the **leadership** style and philosophy that is most likely to deliver change is one that generates a commitment to a shared purpose through collaboration. Role modelling of leadership behaviours, skills and attributes and setting of a high ambition for performance ensures connection to values and empowers others to commit to action. By doing these things, the scale and pace of improvement is maximized.

Change cannot be achieved in isolation. **Engagement** of the multidisciplinary team complemented by engagement of children, young people and families, education and voluntary organizations is essential if we are to collaboratively make services better. True co-production in improvement of services must be the ultimate aim. Mobilization enables all stakeholders to build relationships quickly focusing on creating 'urgency' for change from which to organize resources through developing 'commitments' to each other and to the common goal.

When we want to change something, even if it is just something small, conditions need to be right if the change is going to both work as we wanted it to, and also stay changed for the future. Key to both of these is whether the broad conditions for change, the **system drivers**, can be lined up to support what we are trying to do. These drivers might take the form of incentives for change such as commissioning for quality and innovation payments (CQUINs) or specific standards to be achieved if penalties are to be avoided. Aligning these drivers with the quality improvement intent and thereby making the best use of them is crucial.

Using an evidence-based **improvement methodology** ensures that the change will be delivered in a planned proven way. There is a range of methodologies available to support different kinds of change, such as Plan, Do, Study, Act (PDSA) cycles. With the use of effective evidence-based improvement methodologies, the adoption and systematic spread of change is more effective and delivery of leadership goals and the overall success of a change effort are more likely to be assured.

Evidence suggests that an effective approach for the **rigorous delivery** of change and the monitoring of progress towards planned objectives are essential to making that change a reality. A project management approach will increase the likelihood that changes will deliver the planned benefits, because accountabilities are shared and clear, and the scale and pace of improvement are enhanced. A rigorous approach requires discipline and focus.

Transparent measurement of the outcomes of change is crucial to provide evidence that the change is happening and the desired results are being achieved. Using appropriate measurement techniques ensures remedial action can be taken to mitigate risk, unforeseen consequences can be dealt with promptly and, importantly, that success can be celebrated.

We need to accelerate the speed and extent of the **spread and adoption of innovation, locally, regionally and nationally** in order to improve the quality of care, use of the NHS Change Model provides a framework to ensure we consistently improve outcomes for children, young people and their families.

70 Young person policy

Figure 70.1 Child health policy is the cornerstone of improvements in child health

'You're Welcome – Quality criteria for young people friendly health services' (2011)

The 'You're Welcome' standards designed to make young people welcome in the NHS are not enforceable

National Service Framework for Children, Young People and Maternity services standard 8 (2004)

Practical implications for children, young people and families with enduring complex health needs

Aiming High for Disabled Children: better support for families (2007)

This is designed to help disabled children, young people and their families get the support they need to live ordinary lives

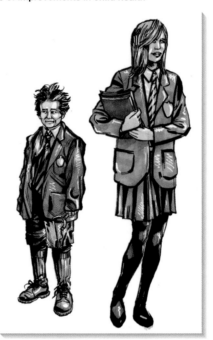

Reproduced with permission of Steven Denton

The 15 Steps Challenge for children and young people's inpatient services (2012)

'I can tell what kind of care my daughter is going to get within 15 steps of walking on to a ward'

Youth matters: evidence-based best practice for the care of young people in hospital (1998)

This document was designed to raise awareness of the plight of young people in hospital. The number of adolescent beds in UK children's hospitals and units is still low

Lost in transition: moving on well; moving young people between child and adult services (2008)

Bridging the gaps: health care for adolescents (2007)

Children and Young People's Nursing at a Glance, First Edition. Edited by Alan Glasper, Jane Coad, and Jim Richardson.
© 2015 John Wiley & Sons, Ltd. Published 2015 by John Wiley & Sons, Ltd. Companion website: www.ataglanceseries.com/nursing/children

The Department of Health's 'You're Welcome: Quality criteria for young people friendly health services' was first published in 2005 with the objective of helping commissioners and providers of health services to improve NHS and non-NHS health services. A new and enhanced version of this was published on 15 April 2011. 'You're Welcome' encompasses all contemporary health policy for young people (http://webarchive.nationalarchives.gov.uk/20130107105354/http://www.dh.gov.uk/en/Publicationsandstatistics/Publications/PublicationsPolicyAndGuidance/DH_073586).

The quality criteria provided in this good practice guidance should facilitate enhancements in local practice and help provide the evidence of what will improve the health care journeys and health outcomes for young people. To support the implementation of 'You're Welcome', the Department of Health has developed an easy to use self-review online tool (www.dh.gov.uk).

The prime message of 'You're Welcome' is that all young people are entitled to receive appropriate health care wherever they access it.

How can the 'You're Welcome' criteria help nurses improve health care for young people?

The quality criteria or standards developed by the Department of Health:

1 Involve young people in service improvement
2 Enhance young people's patient experiences
3 Increase young people's opportunities to share in decisions about their health.

The 'You're Welcome' criteria cover 10 themes, the first eight of which are relevant to all health care settings in both community and hospital. The final two are orientated towards improving specific services for young people.

1 Access. This indicator of quality is concerned with strategies that can be employed by nurses and others to ensure that services are accessible to young people.

2 Publicity. This indicator highlights the importance of effective publicity in raising awareness of the services available to young people, with significant emphasis on the importance of confidentiality.

3 Confidentiality and consent. This indicator concentrates on the topical theme confidentiality and consent and how this is operationalized by health care staff and significantly understood by the young people using the service.

4 Environment. This indicator addresses the environment of care and whether young people are welcomed by the health services.

5 Staff training, skills, attitudes and values. This indicator is dedicated to the importance of training and acquisition of young person caring skills, incorporating the attitudes and values that nurses and others need to deliver young people friendly services effectively.

6 Joined-up working. This indicator addresses some of the ways to ensure effective joined-up service delivery for young people.

7 Involvement in monitoring and evaluation of patient experience. This indicator is related to the full and unequivocal involvement of young people in all aspects of service design, configuration and delivery.

8 Health issues and transition for young people. This indicator has a number of components ranging from the identification of the health needs of young people as they emerge from transition into adult services through to the promotion of healthy lifestyles and the care and support of young people with complex health needs.

9 Sexual and reproductive health services. This indicator is orientated towards sexual and reproductive health of young people ranging from *Chlamydia* screening through to sexually transmitted disease testing and the use of high quality information packages.

10 Targeted and specialist Child and Adolescent Mental Health Services (CAMHS). This indicator is pertinent to targeted services ranging from counselling to specialist services (such as multidisciplinary teams or inpatient services).

How can nurses self-review their compliance to the 'You're Welcome' standards?

Accompanying the 'You're Welcome' policy is an easy to use self-assessment audit pack which can be loaded on to a laptop computer, notebook or tablet.

71 Child disability policy

Figure 71.1 Policies and guidance documents for disabled children and young people and those with complex health needs

Policy exemplars

Aiming High for Disabled Children (2009)

Designed to enhance service provision, better access to health care for disabled children and their families, and provide timely support

Together From the Start: Practical Guidance (2003)

Promoting the participation of parents with disabled children in the planning and delivery of service provision

Better Care: Better Lives (2008)

Providing better end-of-life care, improving outcomes and experiences for children, young people and their families who are living with life-threatening conditions

Valuing People: A New Strategy for Learning Disability for the 21st Century (2001)

Providing high-quality evidence-based multidisciplinary specialist services to meet the needs of disabled people

The main role of health policy is supporting or enhancing the care of patients and supporting children with disabilities and those with complex health needs to access mainstream health services. This is a key goal of government policy.

Children and Young People's Nursing at a Glance, First Edition. Edited by Alan Glasper, Jane Coad, and Jim Richardson.

Figure 71.2   Child health policy for improving standards of care for children with disabilities and those with complex health needs

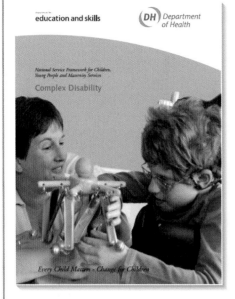

Key points when working with disabled children and their families (DfEs/DH 2003)

- Valuing the child
- A duty to see the child first and then their condition
- Using the child's name all the time
- Being positive during discussions
- Sharing the findings and diagnosis with both the child and parents
- Communicating in a respectful manner
- Awareness of safe guarding issues
- Improve the child's welfare

Pertinent policies

- Standard 8, National Service Framework for Children, Young People and Maternity Services: Disabled Children and Young People and Those with Complex Health Needs(NSF) (DH 2004)
- Aiming High for Disabled Children: Best Practice to Common Practice (DCSF and DH 2009)
- Aiming High for Disabled Children: Better Support for Families (DfES and DH 2007)
- Better Care: Better Lives (DH 2008)
- Nothing about us without us (DH 2001)
- Services for People with Learning Disabilities and Challenging Behaviour or Mental Health Needs (DH 2007)
- Together from the Start: Practical Guidance for Professionals Working with Disabled Children (birth to third birthday) and Their Families (DfES and DH 2003)
- Valuing People: a New Strategy for Learning Disability for the 21st Century (DfES and DH 2001)
- Valuing People Now: a New Three-Year Strategy for People with Learning Disabilities (DH 2009)

Promoting the 'whole child'. The interweaving of health, social care and education in the child's life

Children with complex health needs have traditionally been poorly served by society but does society value these children?

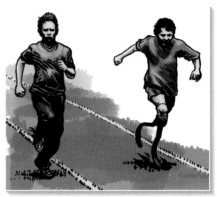

Reproduced with permission of Steven Denton

Other pertinent polices

- Better Care: Better Lives (DH 2008)
- Every Child Matters (DH 2003)
- Transition: getting it right for young people. Improving the transition of young people with long-term conditions from children's to adult health services (DH 2006)
- Report of the Children and Young People's Health Outcomes Forum (DH 2012

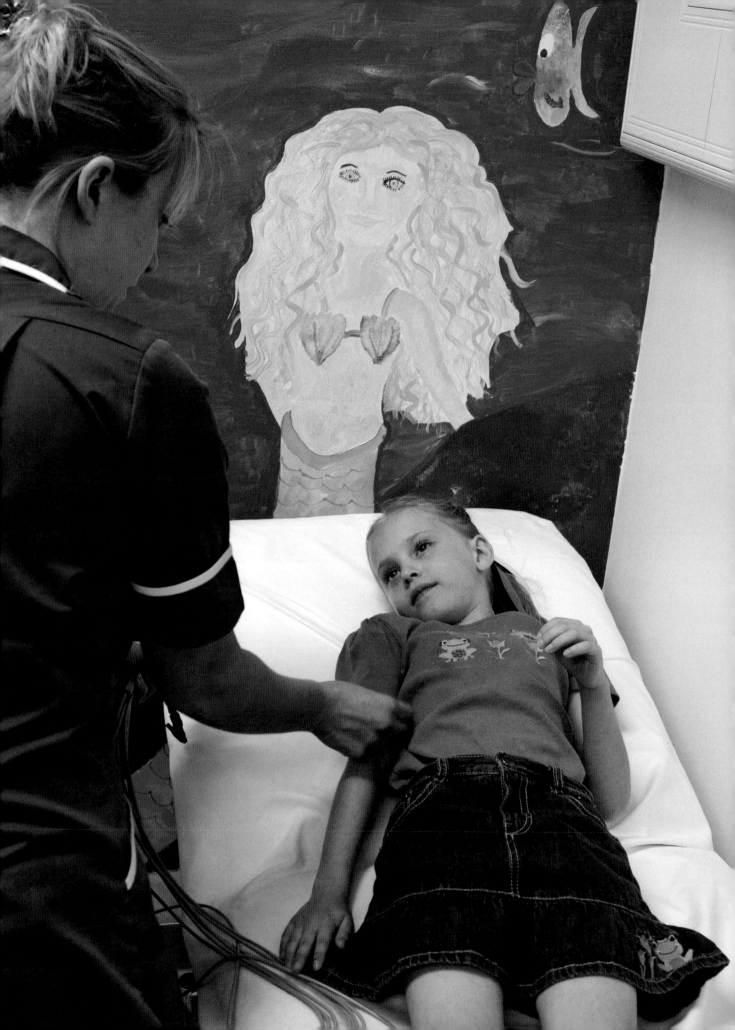

Nursing the sick child and young person

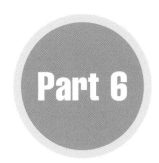

Part 6

Don't forget to visit the companion website for this book at www.ataglanceseries.com/nursing/children where you will find over 500 interactive multiple-choice questions to supplement your learning.

72 Pain assessment

Figure 72.1 Factors affecting a child's behaviour when in pain

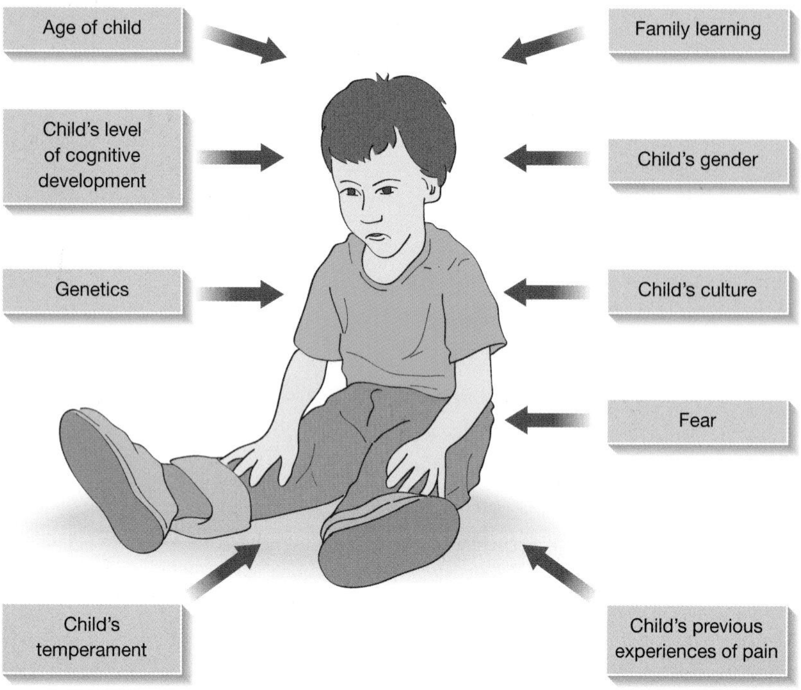

- Age of child
- Child's level of cognitive development
- Genetics
- Child's temperament
- Family learning
- Child's gender
- Child's culture
- Fear
- Child's previous experiences of pain

Figure 72.2 Key steps in pain assessment

- Record a pain history
- Assess the child's pain using a developmentally appropriate pain assessment tool
- Reassess pain having allowed time for pain-relieving interventions to work

Figure 72.3 Three approaches to assessing pain

- *Self-report:* what the child says
- *Behavioural:* how the child behaves
- *Physiological indicators:* how the child's body reacts

Figure 72.4 Self-report tools

These should be used with children who are:
- Old enough to understand and use self-report scale (e.g. 5 years and older)
- Not overtly distressed
- Not cognitively impaired

Figure 72.5 Some of the more commonly used and well-validated pain assessment tools

For non-verbal children
Revised FLACC
Children's Hospital of Eastern Ontario Pain Scale (CHEOPS)
COMFORT Scale – see http://bit.ly/YxQWOk

For verbal children
Faces Pain Scale-Revised (FPS-R) – see http://bit.ly/ve9FDW
Wong-Baker FACES Pain Scale – see http://painconsortium. nih.gov/pain_scales/Wong-Baker_Faces.pdf
Oucher – see http://www.oucher.org/the_scales.html
Numerical rating scale

Pain assessment is the first step in the management of pain. To treat pain effectively, ongoing assessment of the presence and severity of pain and the child's response to treatment is essential. However, pain assessment poses many challenges in children because of the subjective nature of pain, and developmental and language limitations. In addition, not all children behave in the same way when in pain and so the factors identified in Figure 72.1 need considering when carrying out a pain assessment.

Self-report tools

There are a plethora of pain assessment tools available. If you work on a general paediatric ward you are likely to have two or three tools available to cater for the ages of children cared for. Some of the most commonly used pain assessment tools are listed in Figure 72.5.

Faces pain scales

Faces pain scales are the most popular self-report tool. The design of faces scales is intended to enable a child to provide a representation of their pain intensity. Faces scales are popular with children but they need to be explained carefully to the child. It is important to note that faces pain scales are not designed to be used as observational scales; they should only be used as a self-report tool. Faces pain scales can be used by most children aged 5 years and over.

Numerical rating scale

When using a numerical scale, the child is asked to rate their pain from 0 to 10 (or 0 to 5). Very little research has explored the use of numerical pain rating scales in paediatrics but there is some evidence to support their use with children aged 8 years and older.

Behavioural cues

There are a number of behavioural cues that can be used to assess whether a child is in pain:
- Changed behaviour
- Irritability
- Flat affect
- Unusual posture
- Screaming
- Reluctance to move
- Aggressiveness
- Disturbed sleep pattern
- Increased clinging
- Unusual quietness
- Loss of appetite
- Restlessness
- Whimpering
- Sobbing
- Lying 'scared stiff'
- Lethargic

How these cues are displayed varies from child to child and so it is important to involve parents in assessing pain in order to ascertain the child's normal behaviour. A good rule of thumb is that a change in a child's normal behaviour should be considered an indication that they might be in pain.

Behavioural pain assessment tools should be used with infants, toddlers, pre-verbal, cognitively impaired and sedated children. If a child is overtly distressed (e.g. due to pain or anxiety), no mean-ingful self-report can be obtained at that point in time. In this situation the child's pain should be estimated using a behavioural pain assessment tool until the child is less distressed.

The revised-FLACC

The r-FLACC is a behavioural pain assessment tool that has good clinical utility. FLACC is an acronym for Facial expression, Leg movement, Activity, Cry and Consolability. The original version was revised in 2006. The FLACC has been validated for postoperative pain in children aged 2 months to 8 years, as well as procedural pain in children aged 5–16 years. The FLACC is also one of only three scales considered valid and reliable for the assessment of pain in children with cognitive impairment and has also been shown to be valid and reliable pain measure in the paediatric intensive care unit. Although the scale cannot be used in children who are intubated as 'cries' will not be audible, nor is it suitable for children who are paralysed or have impaired mobility as this will make it difficult to assess the 'leg movement' category.

Physiological cues

Physiological cues that can be used to assess pain are seen in Table 72.1. Other physiological indicators of pain include sweating and dilated pupils. On their own, physiological indicators do not constitute a valid clinical pain measure for children. A multidimensional tool that incorporates physiological and behavioural indicators, as well as self-report is therefore preferred whenever possible.

Reassessment of pain

A key component of caring for a child in pain is reassessing their pain at regular intervals. This enables the child's response to pain management interventions to be reviewed. Children should have their pain assessed:
- When they visit an emergency department or an ambulatory clinic
- On admission to hospital
- At least once per shift
- Before, during and after an invasive procedure.

Following surgery and/or if the patient has a known painful medical condition pain should be assessed hourly for the first 6 hours. After this, if the pain is well controlled, it can be assessed less frequently (e.g. every 4 hours). If the pain is not well controlled, regular assessment should continue.

Table 72.1 Physiological signs used to assess pain

Observation	Change indicating pain
Heart rate	Increases when in pain (after an initial decrease)
Respiratory rate and pattern	There is conflicting evidence about whether this increases or decreases, but there is a significant shift from baseline. Breathing may become rapid and/or shallow
Blood pressure	Increases when a child is in acute pain
Oxygen saturation	Decreases when a child is in acute pain

73 Pain management

Figure 73.1 The stages of pain management

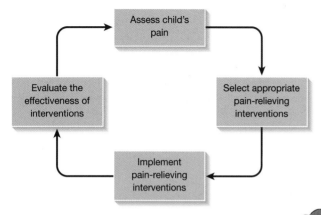

- Assess child's pain
- Select appropriate pain-relieving interventions
- Implement pain-relieving interventions
- Evaluate the effectiveness of interventions

Figure 73.2 The three P's of pain management

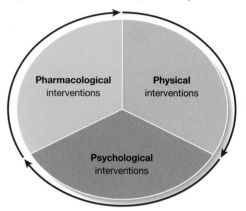

- Pharmacological interventions
- Physical interventions
- Psychological interventions

Figure 73.3 Interventions

Pharmacological interventions

- Administering prescribed analgesic drugs is the mainstay of acute pain management
- Should adhere to the World Health Organization's two-step ladder
- Multimodal analgesia should be used

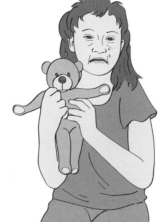

Physical and psychological interventions

Interventions that can be used include:

- Acupuncture
- Distraction
- Guided imagery
- Music therapy
- Relaxation

Figure 73.4 The WHO two-step approach to pain management

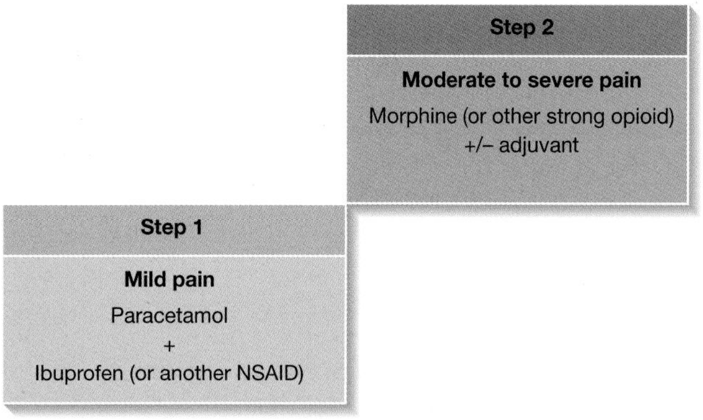

Step 2

Moderate to severe pain

Morphine (or other strong opioid) +/– adjuvant

Step 1

Mild pain

Paracetamol
+
Ibuprofen (or another NSAID)

Table 73.1 Consequences of unrelieved pain

Physical effects

- Rapid, shallow, splinted breathing, which can lead to hypoxaemia and alkalosis
- Inadequate expansion of lungs and poor cough, which can lead to secretion retention and atelectasis
- Increased heart rate, blood pressure and myocardial oxygen requirements, which can lead to cardiac morbidity and ischaemia
- Increased stress hormones which in turn increase the metabolic rate, impede healing and decrease immune function
- Slowing or stasis of gut and urinary systems, which leads to nausea, vomiting, ileus and urinary retention
- Muscle tension, spasm and fatigue, which leads to reluctance to move spontaneously and refusal to ambulate, further delaying recovery

Psychological effects

- Anxiety, fear, distress, feelings of helplessness or hopelessness
- Avoidance of activity, avoidance of future medical procedures
- Sleep disturbances
- Loss of appetite

Other effects

- Prolonged hospital stays
- Increased rates of readmission to hospital
- Increased outpatient visits

Children and Young People's Nursing at a Glance, First Edition. Edited by Alan Glasper, Jane Coad, and Jim Richardson.
© 2015 John Wiley & Sons, Ltd. Published 2015 by John Wiley & Sons, Ltd. Companion website: www.ataglanceseries.com/nursing/children

Why managing pain in children is important

Painful experiences are part of life for every child. Pain has an important purpose, serving as a warning or protective mechanism; people who are unable to feel pain often suffer extensive tissue damage. However, unrelieved pain has a number of undesirable physical and psychological consequences (Table 73.1). When these adverse effects are considered the need to manage children's pain effectively is clear.

Summary of current guidelines

A review of clinical guidelines relating to the management of pain in children and young people indicates that effective management of pain requires nurses to:
- Take a pain history on admission
- Assess pain using a validated pain assessment tool
- Reassess pain following the implementation of pain-relieving interventions
- Discuss the child's pain management with their parents or carers
- Involve the child in decisions about their pain management
- Ensure the child has appropriate analgesic drugs prescribed
- Administer analgesic drugs as prescribed
- Use appropriate physical and psychological interventions
- Prepare the child for painful procedures
- Use analgesic creams for planned painful procedures
- Ensure pain assessments are recorded on a flow chart
- Document the pain-relieving interventions used and their effectiveness in the child's notes.

What does pain management involve?

Pain is a biopsychosocial phenomenon. This means that when managing pain in children pharmacological, physical and psychological interventions need to be used.

Aims of pain management

The aims of managing acute pain in children are to:
- Rapidly identify pain
- Prevent pain if possible
- Control pain by administering analgesic drugs
- Use multimodal analgesia
- Monitor to prevent adverse events
- Address emotional components of pain
- Continue pain control after discharge from hospital.

Pharmacological interventions
Non-opioids
Paracetamol

Paracetamol is appropriate for mild pain. It is thought to act by inhibiting prostaglandin synthesis in the brain. Paracetamol has antipyretic activity but minimal anti-inflammatory effects. Paracetamol can be administered via oral, rectal or intravenous routes. Due to their immature liver function, newborn babies require reduced doses.

Non-steroidal anti-inflammatory drugs

Non-steroidal anti-inflammatory drugs (NSAIDs), such as ibuprofen and diclofenac, are used for mild to moderate pain. They act

by inhibiting the synthesis of prostaglandins by inhibiting the production of COX-1 and COX-2 enzymes. NSAIDs have antipyretic activity as well as anti-inflammatory and analgesic activity. Any easy way of remembering the adverse effects of NSAIDs is by using the acronym SKAB:

Stomach — NSAIDs can cause gastric irritation
Kidneys — NSAIDs should not be given to people with impaired kidney function
Asthma — NSAIDs can exacerbate symptoms in some people with asthma
Bleeding — NSAIDs should not be given to people with impaired platelet function.

Important point: these adverse effects can occur with *all* routes of administration, not just the oral route.

Opioids

Opioids, such as morphine, diamorphine and fentanyl, are used for treating moderate to severe pain. Adverse effects of opioids include:
- Vomiting
- Constipation
- Respiratory depression
- Bronchoconstriction
- Pruritus (itching)
- Urinary retention.

Multimodal analgesia

Multimodal analgesia is the combination of two or more analgesic drugs with different mechanisms of action. This improves children's pain scores and allows for lower drug doses of analgesic drugs, thus minimizing adverse effects.

WHO two-step approach to pain management

The 2012 World Health Organization (WHO) analgesic ladder offers a two-step strategy for treating pain and recommends analgesic drugs are given according to pain severity. Analgesic drugs should be given around the clock to start with and then as needed to keep the child pain free (Figure 73.4).

Addiction

Addiction is a psychological dependence on drugs. Many health care professionals worry that patients will become addicted to opioids. However, in reality this rarely happens. If children are on opioids for more than a few days they may become tolerant to the drug and need an increased dose to keep them pain free – this does not mean they are addicted. Likewise, if a child is on opioids for more than 3 days or so they are likely to experience withdrawal symptoms if the drug is stopped abruptly. Again, this does not mean the child is addicted to the drug but rather that a weaning protocol needs to be implemented.

Physical and psychological interventions

Several physical and psychological interventions can be used to enhance the effectiveness of the analgesic drugs administered. Some of the interventions used most often for the child in acute pain are outlined in the Figure 73.3. The clinician needs to choose an intervention that is appropriate for the age and development of the child.

74 Preoperative preparation

Figure 74.1 Preoperative preparation

- Preadmission clinic
- Fasting guidelines
- Hospital admission
- Patient safety and risk management
- Effects of hospitalization
- Informed consent

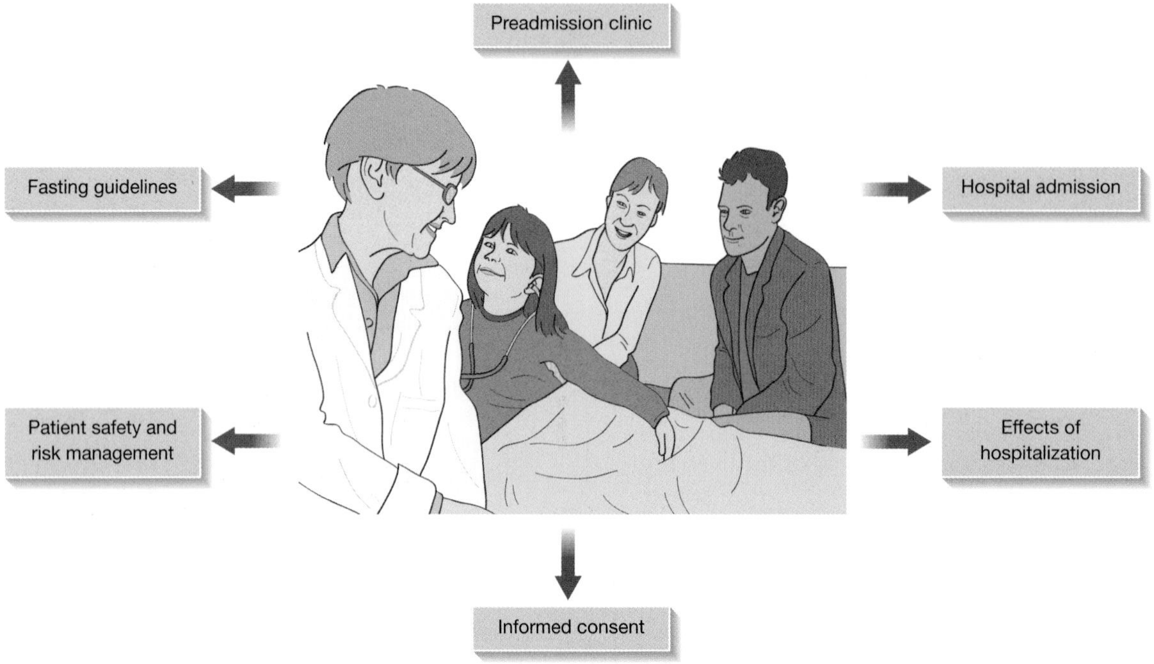

Figure 74.2 Preoperative checklist

	Yes	No	N/A	Theatre
Identity band present				
Clinical observations and weight recorded				
Loose teeth/fillings/caps/crowns/braces				
Fasting: time of last food, time of last fluids				
Bath/shower; passed urine				
Prosthetics: aids, jewellery, nail varnish removed, body piercings				
Local anaesthetic applied: Ametop Emla (please circle)				
Allergies				
Premedication given				
Consent form signed				
Medicine prescription record included				
Investigation records; blood results				
Discharge letter attached				
Seen by Dr Seen by anaesthetist				
Signed:	Ward nurse		Date	
Signed:	Theatre		Date	

Children and Young People's Nursing at a Glance, First Edition. Edited by Alan Glasper, Jane Coad, and Jim Richardson.
© 2015 John Wiley & Sons, Ltd. Published 2015 by John Wiley & Sons, Ltd. Companion website: www.ataglanceseries.com/nursing/children

Preadmission clinic

These services are nurse-led clinics that aim to prepare patients for admission to hospital for elective surgery. Patients are assessed in relation to medical fitness for the procedure. These clinics also offer patients and their families information about the planned surgery, deal with any concerns they may have and provide post-surgery and discharge information. Some tests or investigations may be carried out at this appointment. Following attendance at the preadmission clinic patients will receive confirmation of their date of admission.

Hospital admission

Patients and their families are usually admitted on the day of their surgery. Admission processes and associated documentation are completed including a comprehensive assessment of the child and family's needs and preoperative procedures such as patient identity, vital signs, weight and any relevant investigations indicated by the surgical team.

Effects of hospitalization

Hospitalization can be a daunting experience for children and their families. Children need to gain knowledge and understanding of why they are in hospital and what is likely to happen during their stay. A warm welcome and a friendly approach can do much to reduce anxiety, alongside developing a sound therapeutic relationship.

Informed consent

Informed written consent is a legal requirement and good practice both in elective and emergency procedures. Children should be involved in this process whether or not of an age to consent (16 years), alongside parents or carers. Information pertaining to the benefits, risks and complications of the procedure need to be discussed by the surgeon and family to ensure informed consent has been achieved.

Patient safety and risk management

Many factors contribute to the safety of the patient in the preoperative period, including patient identification, potential risks to safety (i.e. allergy status, prosthetics, loose teeth, laboratory reports or other investigation results). Indication of the site of surgery should also be observable, checking the child has voided, and skin and nail preparation has occurred. Premedications or local anaesthetics may be prescribed and administered prior to surgery.

Fasting guidelines

In order to ensure that the child's safety is maintained in the preoperative period, it is vital to ensure the required fasting times are adhered to: 6 hours for solid foods, 4 hours for breastfeeds and 2 hours for clear fluids. This minimizes the risk of the child aspirating stomach contents during the anaesthetic procedure. If the child has a prolonged period of fasting or an underlying medical disorder it may be necessary for the child to receive intravenous replacement fluids.

75 Postoperative care

Figure 75.1 Phases of postoperative care

Immediate phase (recovery unit)	Intermediate phase (children's ward)	Discharge phase
Airway – will require equipment (artificial airway) and positioning to maintain patency of airway; observe for vomitus/secretions in the airway; suctioning equipment	Nurse child beside oxygen and suction – aim to maintain airway independently	Child is able to maintain airway independently or airway patency is as prior to admission
Breathing – close observation of the child's breathing pattern and supportive care in the form of oxygen is administered	Observe effort, rate, depth and rhythm closely in the initial period after return to ward; be aware of the effects of opiods	Breathing pattern should have returned to within normal limits for the patient
Circulation – assessment of perfusion – centrally and peripherally, capillary refill time, manual heart rate/pulse to assess strength, rate and rhythm	Continue to monitor, as in the immediate phase – observe colour of child's lips and nail beds	Normal perfusion and circulatory performance is achieved
Clinical observations – monitored very closely in the recovery room, respiratory rate, heart rate/pulse, blood pressure, temperature, oxygen saturation levels, level of consciousness	As per ward policy or guideline; however, continues to be monitored closely (i.e. half-hourly to hourly), physiological data recorded as per early warning systems or ward policy	These should have returned to within normal limits for the individual, parents advised re observation of child's recovery from surgery (i.e. temperature checking)
Wound management – close observation of wound sites, dressings or drains for signs of primary haemorrhage	Wound assessed for any sign of oozing, swelling, bleeding and/or pain at sight – record findings. Ensure any dressings remain in situ. Ensure surgeon speaks to child and parents prior to discharge	Written and verbal advice given regarding care of wound in home, any dressings, suture removal and analgesia. Referral to local community children's nursing team may be necessary
Pain management – can be patient or nurse controlled, commenced in perioperative period, need to monitor effectiveness, need for additional analgesics	Accurate assessment of the degree and severity of child's pain using an age-appropriate pain scoring tool is vital, in order to measure and effectively control pain	Pain management strategies discussed with parents prior to discharge. Advice re safe storage of medications in the home
Fluid replacement – consider prolonged fasting times, theatre time, postoperative instructions, may be necessary for the child to have intravenous (IV) fluid therapy	Record the site of child's IV cannula, closely monitor for potential complications, reintroduction of oral fluid intake and discontinuation of IV replacement therapies	Ensure IV cannula is removed prior to discharge, noting condition of site and removal in the patient's notes
Nutrition – introduction of clear oral fluids, when child fully alert, as per surgeon's instructions, small amounts initially	Offer light diet – toast or ice cream – when child feels ready to eat	Child should be tolerant of a light diet prior to discharge
Mobilizing – recovery position initially until regains consciousness, change of position if this is restricted postoperatively, bed rest until return to ward area	Gentle mobilization as tolerated or as condition permits	Able to mobilize gently
Elimination – monitor postoperative elimination; observe for possible urinary retention, postoperative nausea and vomiting (PONV) – record frequency, amount and nature	Monitor and record intake and output chart, noting any signs of dehydration or urine retention. Manage any episodes of PONV	Ensure child has passed urine prior to discharge. Child is not experiencing any PONV
Complications – numerous potential problems, most common – hypoventilation, primary haemorrhage, nausea and vomiting	Raised body temperature, risk of shock, respiratory depression, intermediate haemorrhage, nausea and vomiting, signs of wound infection	Wound dehiscence, advice regarding how to manage any possible complications (e.g. secondary haemorrhage following discharge)
Psychological care – communicate with the child – what is happening, parental presence in recovery room	Parents and child kept fully informed and included in all aspects of postoperative care and decisions	Parents happy to take child home and have necessary information and support to continue care at home
Discharge planning – when fit for return to ward, child and family discharged in line with hospital criteria	Ongoing communication with child and family regarding potential discharge date and time and resources to support discharge	Health education and promotion opportunities – restricted activities, importance of nutrition in healing, supplies and letter for general practitioner. Contact numbers for ward to parents

Children and Young People's Nursing at a Glance, First Edition. Edited by Alan Glasper, Jane Coad, and Jim Richardson.
© 2015 John Wiley & Sons, Ltd. Published 2015 by John Wiley & Sons, Ltd. Companion website: www.ataglanceseries.com/nursing/children

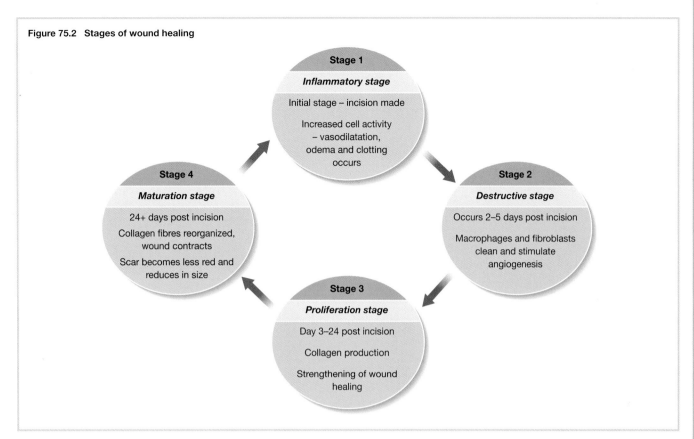

Figure 75.2 Stages of wound healing

Stage 1

Inflammatory stage

Initial stage – incision made

Increased cell activity – vasodilatation, odema and clotting occurs

Stage 2

Destructive stage

Occurs 2–5 days post incision

Macrophages and fibroblasts clean and stimulate angiogenesis

Stage 3

Proliferation stage

Day 3–24 post incision

Collagen production

Strengthening of wound healing

Stage 4

Maturation stage

24+ days post incision

Collagen fibres reorganized, wound contracts

Scar becomes less red and reduces in size

Community perspective

Transition from hospital to home can be a complex and lengthy process. It may require discharge planning from the point of admission, by making practical plans with the child and parent in relation to identifying needs post-surgery and resources required, aiming to avoid a failed discharge or readmission for the child and family. The early identification of needs and initiation of effective communication pathways between the hospital and the community children's nurse, health visitor and other appropriate members of the multidisciplinary team should achieve a timely and successful discharge. Additional resources or expertise such as the tissue viability nurse may become involved with patients and families who experience issues with wound healing or choice of dressings. The importance of adhering to and completing treatment regimes following discharge should be emphasized and supported by community nursing teams until the child and family no longer require the input of such services. Infection prevention and control is a key aspect of ongoing care for the child and family, ensuring that all personnel involved in care delivery, whether in the hospital or community, are aware of effective hand hygiene and maintain good standards of hygiene around wounds until effective wound healing is complete.

76 Pressure area care

Figure 76.1 Development of pressure ulcers

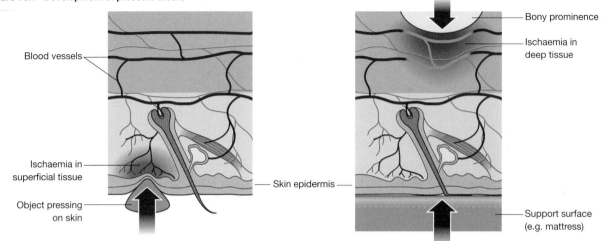

Blood vessels

Ischaemia in
superficial tissue

Object pressing
on skin

Skin epidermis

Bony prominence

Ischaemia in
deep tissue

Support surface
(e.g. mattress)

Figure 76.2 Some common sites for pressure ulcers

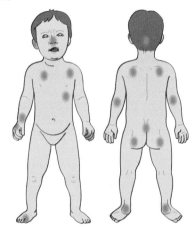

- **Ears** (nasogastric tube pressing)
- **Nose** (endotracheal tube, CPAP mask, nasogastric tube)
- **Chest** (ECG electrodes)
- **Wrist** (nameband in neonates)
- **Hand** (IV cannula)
- **Fingers** (oxygen saturation probes)
- **Iliac crest** (support surface)
- **Toes** (oxygen saturation probe)

- **Occiput** (support surface)
- **Shoulders/scapulae** (support surface)
- **Elbows** (support surface)
- **Sacrum and ischial tuberosities** (support surface)
- **Heels and maleoli** (support surface)

Pressure damage is caused by the external pressure of the support surface or objects pressing on the skin and underlying tissues, with enough pressure to reduce blood flow and for a long enough time to cause tissue ischaemia (Figure 76.1). In this case, pressure damage starts at the skin and may progress to deeper ulceration if pressure is not relieved. This can be seen initially as redness of the skin that does not blanch on light finger pressure (category 1 pressure ulcer). Pressure damage may also start in deep tissues at a bony prominence. If a child is lying in one position for a long period of time, tissues are compressed between the support surface and the bony prominence. The support surface may distribute skin pressure, but internal pressure will be concentrated at the bone. In this case, the ischaemia starts where the bone is pressing on muscle, and tissue damage progresses towards the skin. This may be first seen as swelling, heat and discoloration over the area of ischaemia. Both deep and superficial pressure ulcers can be very painful.

About half of pressure ulcers seen in children appear to be related to objects (such as medical devices) pressing or rubbing on the child's skin. All areas where devices may press or rub on the child's skin must be inspected frequently and, if possible, a cushioning layer should be placed between the device and the child's skin. Children with reduced mobility must have their position changed and skin inspected frequently.

Categories of pressure ulcers

The European Pressure Ulcer Advisory Panel and the National Pressure Ulcer Advisory Panel (2009) categorized pressure ulcers. This is useful when describing any lesions in patient records. Category I pressure ulcers usually heal without complications if the source of the localized pressure is removed. Moisture lesions (such as nappy rash) should not be confused with pressure ulcers.

Category/Stage I: intact skin with non-blanchable redness of a localized area usually over a bony prominence.

Category/Stage II: partial thickness. Loss of dermis presenting as a shallow open ulcer with a red pink wound bed, without slough. May also present as an intact, open or ruptured serum-filled blister.

Category/Stage III: full thickness tissue loss. Subcutaneous fat may be visible, but bone, tendon or muscles are not exposed. Slough may be present but does not obscure the depth of tissue loss. May include undermining and tunnelling.

Category/Stage IV: full thickness skin loss with exposed bone, tendon or muscle. Slough or eschar may be present on some parts of the wound bed. Often includes undermining and tunnelling.

The 2014 NICE Guideline CG179 recommends that all children who need nursing care or who have reduced mobility should have an initial pressure ulcer risk assessment documented. Children deemed to be at risk should have skin assessment and preventative action recorded in their care plan. Pressure ulcer risk assessment should be repeated whenever a child's condition changes.

77 Managing fluid balance

Figure 77.1 Common causes of fluid imbalance

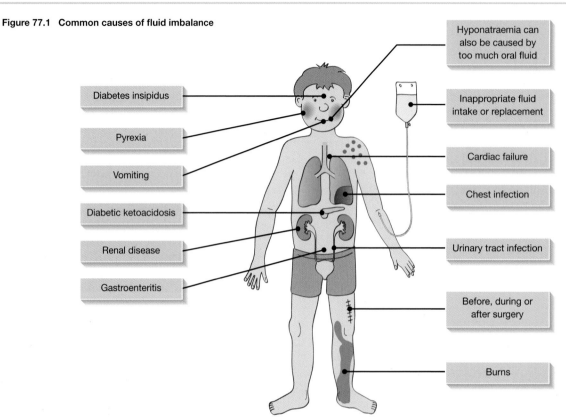

- Diabetes insipidus
- Pyrexia
- Vomiting
- Diabetic ketoacidosis
- Renal disease
- Gastroenteritis

- Hyponatraemia can also be caused by too much oral fluid
- Inappropriate fluid intake or replacement
- Cardiac failure
- Chest infection
- Urinary tract infection
- Before, during or after surgery
- Burns

Figure 77.2 What you need from your evaluation

History

- How long has the child been unwell?
- Any history of vomiting or diarrhoea or recent gastroenteritis in the family?
- Has the child been pyrexic?
- In an infant or young child: have the nappies been wet?
- In an older child: is the child passing urine?
- Is the child able to tolerate any oral fluids? How much and what type of fluids have been offered?

Key observations/investigations

- Temperature, pulse, respirations, blood pressure
- Capillary refill time
- Weight
- Urinalysis
- BM
- Glasgow coma scale
- Blood for urea and electrolytes
- Blood gas analysis in the ill child

Assessing the child: signs and symptoms of dehydration

- Pallor
- Sunken eyes
- Sunken fontanelle
- Dry skin/mucous membranes
- Presence of lethargy or irritability
- Reduced urinary output
- Weight loss
- Increased capillary refill time (>2 seconds)
- Cool, mottled extremities
- Decreased tissue turgor
- Increased pulse and reduced blood pressure
- Dehydration may be mild, moderate or severe

Assessing the child: signs and symptoms of over-hydration

- Altered urinary output
- Generalized or peripheral oedema
- Cerebral oedema: altered consciousness or seizure activity
- Weight gain

Children and Young People's Nursing at a Glance, First Edition. Edited by Alan Glasper, Jane Coad, and Jim Richardson.
© 2015 John Wiley & Sons, Ltd. Published 2015 by John Wiley & Sons, Ltd. Companion website: www.ataglanceseries.com/nursing/children

Distribution of body fluids

Fluids are contained within a number of compartments in the body. Intracellular fluid is contained within the cells. Extracellular fluid, contained outside the cells, is further subdivided into three types: interstitial fluid that surrounds the cell (e.g. that found in cartilage or connective tissue); intravascular fluid, found within the blood vessels; and transcellular fluid found in body cavities (e.g. cerebrospinal or intestinal fluid). Body fluids and associated electrolytes are in constant motion around the body by diffusion, osmosis and active transport in order to achieve a state of homeostasis. Thus, the body works continuously to achieve optimal fluid balance.

Mechanisms of fluid balance

The kidneys have a vital role in fluid balance by filtering plasma fluid during the formation of urine. There are three additional key mechanisms that control fluid balance in the body: thirst, antidiuretic hormone and the renin-angiotensin-aldosterone system.

Management of the child with fluid imbalance

As with any aspect of children's nursing, a family centred approach is essential. Careful and appropriate information sharing, involving the child and family, open communication and thorough preparation, including play and distraction techniques, will help to reduce anxiety. Ongoing monitoring and assessment of the child, together with the multidisciplinary team, and adherence to local policies are key aspects of ensuring safe and effective care. Appropriate measuring, recording and reporting of all intake and output in the fluid balance chart and documentation in the nursing notes are also vital. Some children (e.g. those with meningitis or electrolyte disturbance) may need fluid restriction, while those in specialist areas may have very individual requirements. Communication with the medical team is paramount.

Oral fluid requirements

Oral fluids are the preferred option for maintaining fluid balance in children where possible. If the child has a history of vomiting, an oral rehydration solution (ORS), such as Dioralyte, given orally or via a nasogastric tube, may be recommended. Parents have a key role in encouraging ORS intake (as opposed to water or other oral fluids) in small but frequent amounts. However, many children who are ill require intravenous therapy. Oral requirements for neonates vary according to hospital policies. However, as a general rule, by 5 days old onwards, 150 mL/kg/day body weight are required.

Intravenous fluid requirements

The choice of the intravenous fluid will be governed by local policy and the individual assessment of the child. If shock is present, a rapid bolus of 0.9% sodium chloride may initially be given. The fluid deficit, based on the estimated percentage of dehydration, may also be calculated and is normally replaced by sodium chloride 0.9% over the next 48 hours if the child is hypo- or hypernatraemic. This should take account of any boluses given. Large volumes of IV medication and ongoing losses should also be taken into consideration when calculating IV fluid requirements. Maintenance fluids are calculated by the formula below. For example;

- 6-kg infant would require $6 \times 100\,\text{mL} = 600\,\text{mL/day}$ or $6 \times 4 = 24\,\text{mL/hr}$.
- 25-kg child would need $1000 + 500 + 100 = 1600\,\text{mL/day}$ or $40 + 20 + 5 = 65\,\text{mL/hr}$.
- Maximum daily amounts should be specified in local policies.

Fluid requirements	Per day (mL/kg)	Per hour (mL/kg)
For the first 10 kg	100	4
For the second 10 kg	50	2
For each kg over 20 kg	20	1

Ongoing monitoring and assessment of the child, accurate recording, reporting and evaluation are key aspects of the children's nurse's role as a member of the multidisciplinary team.

Key points

- Assessing and managing fluid imbalance is an important part of the nurse's role.
- Optimal multidisciplinary working is essential.
- Accurate calculation of fluid requirements and knowledge of suitable fluid therapy is vital.
- Ongoing monitoring of the child and accurate documentation is key.

Acknowledgement. The authors would like to thank Dr Claire Anderson and Dr Jarlath McAloon for their assistance in the preparation of this chapter.

78 Administering medication

Figure 78.1 Medication procedure

1 Before you make a start

- Familiarize yourself with your local medicines policy and procedures
- Be aware of NMC Code of Conduct (2008), NMC Standards for Medicines Management (2010)
- Understand why your patient has been prescribed this medication, check the care plans as well as dose, possible adverse effects, contraindications and special precautions
- Check prescription charts regularly. Omission is the second most common reason for medication error (NPSA 2009)
- Gather together the prescription chart, keys and second RN to act as checker if required
- Wash your hands

2 Check prescription chart

- Has the correct patient identification. Full name, NHS number and/or hospital number if required by local policy
- Has a completed and signed confirmation of allergy status on the front of the chart
- Provides a clear legible prescription of medication to be administered. If this appears ambiguous it is safer to request that the prescription chart is rewritten. Prescriptions should include date of prescription, the generic drug name, route, dosage, date and time to be administered and the prescriber's printed name and signature
- Remember All checks should be completed independently

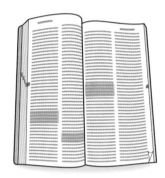

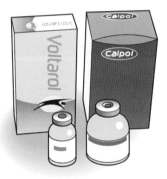

3 Preparing the medicine

- With the second checker, select the correct medication and check that it is within the expiry date. Consider formula/spoon/oral syringe preference for children
- Check that the dose prescribed is correct for the age and weight of the patient using a reference source (e.g. BNF for Children (BNFC))
- Independently calculate the volume of liquid or number of tablets required. Compare answers. Recalculate if you disagree
- Measure the dose required. Both practitioners should witness all stages of the process and confirm the amount prepared. Both nurses should undertake final bedside checks together

4 Administering the medicine

- Check that the patient's name, date of birth and NHS number on the name band correlate with these details on the prescription chart
- If possible, ask the patient/parent to tell you his/her name and date of birth
- Check the allergy section on the prescription chart for contraindications to administration
- Explain purpose of the medication to the patient/family and gain consent for administration
- The patient/family/non-registered nurse/play specialist may wish to be involved in the administration procedure. Remember This must always be performed under the supervision of an RN who remains accountable for any delegation of this task

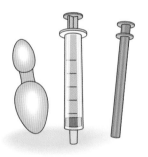

5 Closing the intervention

- After administering the medication both nurses should sign the prescription chart to evidence that the medication has been given
- Offer the patient a drink, particularly if the medicine has an unpleasant taste
- Record reasons for non-administration of the drug on the prescription chart and in the nursing documentation
- Make the patient comfortable. Offer bravery rewards if appropriate. Ask whether there are any further interventions required. Inform the patient and/or family when you will be returning
- Dispose of equipment safely with clean spacers as required. Wash your hands
- Observe patient for adverse effects

Children and Young People's Nursing at a Glance, First Edition. Edited by Alan Glasper, Jane Coad, and Jim Richardson.
© 2015 John Wiley & Sons, Ltd. Published 2015 by John Wiley & Sons, Ltd. Companion website: www.ataglanceseries.com/nursing/children

Contemporary issues

The administration of medicines to children and young people is a complex procedure, not least because of the intricate weight related calculations, frequent inability of the patient to identify or advocate for him/herself and the widespread use of unlicensed medications in this patient group. Therefore, the caution issued by the Nursing and Midwifery Council (NMC 2010) that medication administration is not purely a mechanistic act but one that demands thought and professional judgement, is particularly salutary in this patient group.

Although the use of medications that are not licensed for use in neonates, children and young people has traditionally been common, this practice has recently been deemed unacceptable (Department of Health 2012). Work is currently underway to work with the pharmaceutical industry to develop medicines that are safe and suitable for administration to neonates, children and young people.

Involving the child, young person and family

The admission process for children and young people should assess and record details of the child or young person's prescribed medication, together with their preferences for when this is usually taken and how all medications are usually given (e.g. tablet, syrup, spoon, syringe). Many children's hospitals operate parent administration procedures that maintain home routine, facilitate integrated family and health care partnership working and help to protect against medication errors (Crawford 2012). The role of the children's nurse in this process is to provide support to families but remain mindful of the NMC (2010) requirement to ascertain that medication has been administered as recorded.

Medications dispensed by hospital pharmacies for discharge frequently do not include guidance on usage. NICE (2009) estimate that 33–50% of all patients with long-term conditions do not take medication as directed, potentially at a cost of over £100 million per year. As children and young people are reliant upon parental understanding of medicine regimes for their well-being, they are particularly vulnerable. The children's nurse therefore has a key role in explaining rationale for dose, frequency, specific instructions and adverse effects of medication to children, young people and their parents and carers. Where hospital leaflets are unavailable, www.medicinesforchildren.org.uk is a valuable resource.

Medicines safety

Medication error was the most frequently reported adverse incident reported during an NPSA (2009) patient safety review. Ten per cent of errors affected the 0–4 year age group. The most common error was incorrect dose, followed by omitted doses and incorrect frequency. The Report of the Children and Young People's Health Outcomes Framework (2012) states that the actual number of incidents and the harm they cause is unknown as reporting is not yet mandatory. There are plans to change this position from April 2013. It is widely acknowledged that although these events are preventable, health care providers will never achieve a position of zero medication incidents (Chang and Mark 2011). What is important is that children's nursing learns from these events and as advocated by the Children and Young People's Health Outcomes Forum (2012), initiate bundles of interventions to reduce their frequency.

Calculation formula

$$\text{Dose} = \frac{\text{What you want}}{\text{What you have}} \times \text{Amount it is in}$$

For example: you need to administer 60 mg paracetamol which comes as a 120-mg in 5-mL preparation:

$$\text{Dose} = \frac{60}{120} \times 5 = \frac{1}{2} \times 5 = \frac{5}{2} = 2.5\,\text{mL}$$

Units of measurement

1 gram (g) = 1000 milligram (mg)
1 milligram (mg) = 1000 microgram (μg)
1 microgram (μg) = 1000 nanogram (ng)
1 litre (L) = 1000 millilitres (mL).

Calculating IV fluid rates

$$\text{Rate} = \frac{\text{Volume}}{\text{Time}}$$

Example 500 mL over 4 hours

$$\text{Rate} = \frac{500}{4} = 125\,\text{mL/hour}$$

79 Drug calculations

Figure 79.1 Principles of drug calculations

The metric system

To undertake drug calculations it is imperative to understand the units of measurement used in the prescribing and administration of drugs. The units are expressed using the Système Internationale within the standard metric system of weights and measures (Blair 2011).

Units	Abbreviations	Conversions
Kilogram	kg	1 kg = 1000 g
Gram	g	1 g = 1000 mg
Milligram	mg	1 mg = 1000 microgram
Microgram	Do not abbreviate	NA
Litre	L	1 L = 1000 mL
Millilitre	mL	NA

Fractions

A useful resource when undertaking drug calculations is to learn common fractions expressed as a decimal. This is helpful when calculating dosages from ampules.

$\frac{1}{2}$ = 0.5	$\frac{1}{4}$ = 0.25	$\frac{1}{5}$ = 0.2
	$\frac{2}{4}$ = 0.5	$\frac{2}{5}$ = 0.4
	$\frac{3}{4}$ = 0.75	$\frac{3}{5}$ = 0.6
		$\frac{4}{5}$ = 0.8

Worked example

If you require half of a 1-mL ampule you will require 0.5 mL

Proportions

Many calculations that are undertaken on a children's ward are based on weight and volume. This is because a dosage weight of drug has been dissolved in a volume of liquid. For example, an elixir that contains the dose strength of 125 mg in 5 mL means that in every 5 mL of liquid will be 125 mg of the drug.

Strength of the medicine	125 mg in 5 mL
If you halve the dose	62.5 mg in 2.5 mL
If you double the dose	250 mg in 10 mL

Dividing and multiplying by 10, 100 and 1000

Many drug doses and stock strengths are given in multiples of 10. A useful skill is to be able to recognize when a dose is a multiple of 10 or 100 and understand their relationship.

10 mg	= 10 × 1 mg
100 mg	= 10 × 10 mg
20 mg	= 10 × 2 mg
50 mg	= 10 × 5 mg
1000 mg	= 10 × 100 mg

Formula method

This method requires relevant numerical figures to be inserted into an equation, which once solved provides the necessary volume of liquid or number of tablets that need to be administered

- **What you want (presciption) ÷ What you have (stock strength) × What its in (volume) = Volume to be administered**

- **What you want (prescription) ÷ What you have (stock strength) = Number of tablets to be administered**

Worked examples

- You need to administer 120 mg paracetamol
  The dose strength available is 120 mg paracetamol in 5 mL
  = 120 ÷ 120 × 5 = 5 mL

- You need to administer 25 mg prednisolone
  This is available in 5 mg tablets
  = 25 ÷ 5 = 5 tablets

Children and Young People's Nursing at a Glance, First Edition. Edited by Alan Glasper, Jane Coad, and Jim Richardson.
© 2015 John Wiley & Sons, Ltd. Published 2015 by John Wiley & Sons, Ltd. Companion website: www.ataglanceseries.com/nursing/children

Numeracy

It is vital that paediatric nurses have sound numeracy skills to assist them within a range of health care activities. One such activity is drug calculation and administration. Poor numeracy skills may lead to medication errors. While recognizing that medication errors are multifactorial, lack of competence in basic calculation is often reported as a key area of concern for many trusts (Fry and Dacey 2007).

Nursing and Midwifery Council

To ensure that nurses are equipped with a high level of numeracy skills the Nursing and Midwifery Council (NMC) has established key competencies within the Essential Skills Clusters for pre-registration nursing students that must be met in order for students to be allowed to progress onto the professional register (NMC 2010a). It has also provided standards for some post-registration qualifications (NMC 2010b). However, many qualified nurses do not feel confident in their numerical competence and that they would benefit from regular revision of the common numeracy skills required for the calculations undertaken within their area of practice (Fry and Dacey 2007; Hutton 2009).

Skills

The NMC has determined that nurses must be proficient in long division, multiplication and fractions to undertake drug calculations successfully (NMC 2010b). There are several resources that could provide assistance to nurses in utilizing a multifaceted approach to drug calculations. These include being exposed to drug calculations within their area, having basic numeracy knowledge, possessing calculator skills and being proficient in the effective use of equipment, such as syringes (Wright 2009).

Estimation

Being able to estimate the answer sought is essential in drug calculations. Many medication errors occur as the practitioner has not thought through what a sensible answer or dose would be. A moment taken to approximate the calculation will prevent serious errors, such as a misplaced decimal point (Hutton 2009).

Using a calculator

Paediatric nurses should be able to undertake non-complex drug calculations without the use of a calculator. A calculator provides an answer to the equation that is keyed in; if the equation is incorrect it is easy to generate the wrong answer. However, it would be acceptable to calculate the dose needed and then check the answer using a calculator. For more complex drug calculations, it may be necessary to use a calculator, although the correct answer should be estimated to ensure the calculation is correct.

Checking the dose

Before administering a drug to a child the nurse must be sure that the prescribed dose is correct. While errors may be made by prescribers as well as those who administer the prescription, accountability sits with both. Double checking is recommended for complex drug calculations. Checking must involve each nurse independently undertaking the calculation and then both checking the answer together (NMC 2010b). There are some academics who believe that double checking may increase the risk of error as each become complacent and rely on the other to spot an error. This is why it is imperative that nurses undertake the calculation independently before doing it jointly.

Recommendations for practice

Medication administration incidents are most frequently due to the wrong dose, delayed or omitted medication or the wrong medication being administered (NPSA 2009; Nursing Times 2012), with the most frequently cited error being calculation error. Health care organizations must ensure that they implement routine and regular assessment of their clinical staff's numeracy skills. This should form part of their mandatory clinical update and continued professional development. It is hoped that the implementation of such strategies will lead to an increased awareness of the importance of numeracy and thus an improved quality of care of patients and a reduced risk of medication errors (Warburton 2010).

Key points
- Understand professional responsibility and accountability.
- Understand units of measurement.
- Possess sound knowledge of calculation formulas.
- Estimate the required volume and/or number of tablets.
- Double check when appropriate.
- Employers should demonstrate yearly assessment of practitioner's numeracy skills.

80 Enteral and nasogastric feeding

Figure 80.1 Troubleshooting nasogastric tube placement

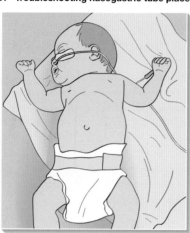

- The position of the tube should always be checked prior to administering any medication or feed
- Confirming tube position can sometimes be difficult
- Some medication such as H2 receptor blocking agents can alter the pH readings
- It can also be difficult to assess the pH of the stomach contents in children who are receiving continuous feeds
- Tips to try and check correct position:
  - ask the child to have a small drink if possible and safe to do so
  - reposition the tube to try to increase the amount of aspirate collected
  - reposition the child on their left side as this can increase the aspirate obtained
  - inject 10–20 mL air into the tube and then aspirate
- If no aspirate can be obtained then it may be necessary to confirm the position of the tube using X-ray. Local guidelines should always be followed in these cases

Figure 80.2 Administering a bolus feed

- Collect equipment and feed:
  - use correct personal protection equipment (PPE)
  - syringes
  - feed checked for correct child and expiry date
  - pH paper
  - water for flushing tube
- Wash hands and put on PPE
- Check tube position
- Check amount of feed to be delivered
- Attach syringe to nasogastric tube
- Administer feed slowly using gravity
- Flush nasogastric tube with water or air
- Dispose of all equipment following local policy
- Document actions

Figure 80.3 Administering a continuous feed

- Collect equipment and feed:
  - use correct PPE
  - syringes
  - feed checked for correct child and expiry date
  - pH paper
  - giving set
  - pump
- Wash hands and put on PPE
- Check tube position
- Check amount of feed to be delivered
- Prime giving set and place in pump
- Set hourly rate and volume to be administered on pump following local guidelines
- Dispose of all equipment following local policy
- Document actions

Figure 80.4 Administering medication

- Collect equipment and medication
- Check medication following local guidelines
- Wash hands and put on PPE
- Check tube position
- Administer each medication, flushing with water between each one
- Flush tube at finish
- Document actions

Children and Young People's Nursing at a Glance, First Edition. Edited by Alan Glasper, Jane Coad, and Jim Richardson.

Enteral feeding

Enteral feeding is used when a child cannot maintain their own nutritional intake. The main reasons for using enteral feeding are as follows:
• Children who are unable to feed orally because they have a swallowing problem
• Children who are unable to feed orally because they have breathing difficulties that are compromising their feeding
• Children who are unable to maintain an optimal nutritional intake because they need a high calorie diet or supplementation of their nutritional intake.

Enteral feeding can be short or long term and the chosen route for enteral feeding will be determined by its duration. It is important that children, young people and their carers are involved in the decision to start enteral feeding and all the options are explained to them. The child should also have a complete physical and nutritional assessment undertaken before commencing enteral feeding. The involvement of the multidisciplinary team is important in managing enteral feeding, particularly if the child is going to be discharged home with enteral feeding in place.

There are different routes by which children can be fed enterally:
• Orogastric
• Nasogastric
• Gastrostomy.

Nasogastric feeding

Nasogastric (NG) feeding is the most common form of enteral feeding. There are different types of NG tube available. Tubes for short-term use are made from polyvinylchloride (PVC) and can be left in place for 3–10 days. These types of tubes can also be used orally. Tubes for long-term use are made of polyurethane and usually have a guide wire to assist insertion. These tubes can remain in place for up to 6 weeks but the individual manufacturer's guidelines should be followed. Before insertion of the NG tube it is important to explain the procedure to the child and family and to gain informed consent for the procedure.

Inserting an NG tube

Before inserting an NG tube it is important to choose the correct size. This is usually decided by the size of the child's nostril. The NG tube should not obstruct the nostril and the child should be able to breathe around the tube. The most commonly used sizes are 6 fr and 8 fr. The appropriate length of tube should also be chosen, again dependent on the size of the child. The procedure for inserting the tube:
• Prepare child and family.
• Collect all the equipment required:
  ○ Correct size tube
  ○ pH paper
  ○ Appropriate size of syringe (usually 20 mL)
  ○ Tape to secure the tube
  ○ Sterile water to flush the tube once the position has been established
  ○ A drink with a straw or dummy for the child to suck on if appropriate.

• Wash hands and put on personal protective equipment.
• Open the tube and check it is intact and suitable to use.
• Measure the tube using the NEX measurement (nose, ear xiphisternum).
• If necessary lubricate the end of the tube with sterile water.
• Pass the tube gently into the child's nostril, advancing it along the nasopharynx into the oral pharynx. If any resistance is met or the child starts coughing or having difficulty breathing the tube should be withdrawn.
• Once the measured length has been reached the tube should be temporarily secured and tested using the pH paper.
• An aspirate of 5.5 or less indicates the tube is in the correct position.
• Once the correct position has been confirmed the tube should be secured ensuring the child's skin is protected if necessary. Size of tube and date of insertion should be recorded in the child's records.

Orogastric feeding

Orogastric (OG) feeding is not a common choice but it may be used for some groups of children where it is not possible to pass an NG tube. These may be children (usually infants) who are for example receiving continuous positive airway pressure (CPAP) non-invasive ventilation or who have a diagnosis of choanal atresia. Children admitted to the accident and emergency department with a suspected basal skull fracture should always have an OG tube passed. The procedure for passing an OG tube is very similar to that of passing an NG tube. The key differences:
• The tube is passed through the mouth
• The measurement is from the xiphisternum to the lips
• Care must be taken when securing the OG tube not to damage the lips or gums.

Gastrostomy feeding

Gastrostomy tubes provide a more long-term enteral feeding solution for children who are unable to maintain their nutritional status by oral feeding. A gastrostomy tube is inserted surgically by making an incision and placing the tube directly into the stomach through the abdominal wall. The tube is then held in place either by an internal flange or by a balloon. The type of fixation is dependent upon the type of tube.

All gastrostomy tubes will need the stoma site to be cared for. This involves cleaning around the site as part of normal washing once the child is 2 weeks post insertion. The stoma should also be observed for signs of infection such as redness, swelling or exudate. The tube should be rotated through 360° according to the manufacturer's instructions. This is to prevent the tube adhering.

The administration of feeds is similar to the procedure for NG feeding. The main differences are:
• There is no need to check the position of the tube
• The tube must be flushed with water before and after the feed
• If it is a button device then the extension set must be fixed on prior to the feed being administered.

81 The feverish child

Table 81.1 Thermoregulatory responses

Thermoregulatory responses to cold (body warming mechanisms)	Thermoregulatory responses to heat (body cooling mechanisms)
Vasoconstriction	Vasodilatation
Shivering	Sweating
Increase in basal metabolic rate (BMR) mediated by adrenal medullary and thyroid hormones	Decrease in BMR
Warmth seeking behaviour	Cold seeking behaviour

Figure 81.2 The fever cycle

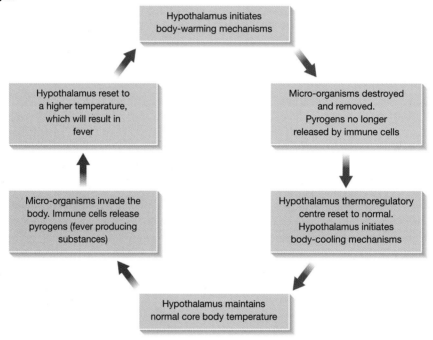

Figure 81.3 The tie course of a typical febrile episode

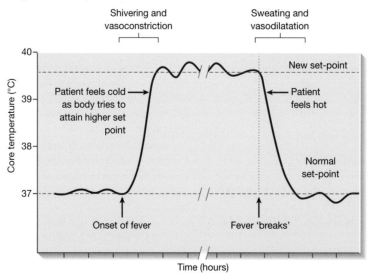

From Pocock G and Richards CD. (2004) Human Physiology:
The Basis of Medicine, 2nd edition. With permission of Oxford University Press

Children and Young People's Nursing at a Glance, First Edition. Edited by Alan Glasper, Jane Coad, and Jim Richardson.

Fever

Fever is defined as a rise in temperature above the normal range 'set-point' that is not associated with exercise or a high ambient temperature (Pocock and Richards 2004). It is one of the most common symptoms of illness in children (NICE 2007). To facilitate an understanding of fever it is necessary to review the key points associated with thermoregulation.

Thermoregulation

The maintenance of a constant core body temperature is vital for normal cell function, as the rates of all metabolic processes are highly temperature dependent (Pocock and Richards 2004).

Core temperature refers to the temperature around the internal organs. This is carefully controlled during health. A normal core temperature for an infant is between 36.5°C and 37.6°C, whereas in an older child it is between 36°C and 37.5°C (Glasper et al. 2010). Shell temperature refers to the surface or skin temperature and may vary considerably according to the ambient temperature. The skin can tolerate a wide range of temperature (Pocock and Richards 2004).

Thermoregulation is an example of a negative feedback homeostatic loop. The loop operates to regulate core temperature around a set-point. For a normal core temperature to be maintained, it is necessary that **heat loss from the body = heat gained by the body**. Mechanisms of heat loss include radiation, conduction and convection. Heat is generated by all the active cellular processes of the body (metabolism).

There are two populations of thermoreceptors: peripheral (located in the skin) and central (located within deeper structures including the central nervous system). Peripheral receptors monitor skin (shell) temperature. Central receptors monitor core temperature. The hypothalamus is the major integration centre for information from the thermoreceptors. It acts as the body's thermostat, set at around 37°C. When it is informed of a change in temperature, it organizes appropriate effector responses to restore normal temperature. Effector mechanisms are designed to restore normal core temperature and include autonomic, endocrine and somatic responses closely integrated with behavioural responses (McCance and Heuter 2010) (Table 81.1).

Physiology

Fever is usually associated with infectious disease and is caused by chemicals called exogenous **pyrogens** which are sometimes derived from bacteria (bacterial endotoxins) or viruses but more often are secreted by cells of the immune system (monocytes, phagocytes), endogenous pyrogens in response to infection. In fever, the control centre perceives normal temperature as being too low. Heat conservation and heat production then drive the temperature up to its new set level. The rise in the set point is due to the action of pyrogens that have the ability to readjust the hypothalamus. An example of a pyrogen is interleukin 1 (IL-1). It acts on the hypothalamus to stimulate the production of prostaglandins, which in turn act to reset the set point of the hypothalamus to a higher level. This is a rapid process, the temperature rising within 8–10 minutes of the release of IL-1. Pyrogens appear to induce fever by resetting the hypothalamic thermostat so that heat conservation mechanisms are initiated to raise the core body temperature to the new higher value (Figure 81.2).

Therefore, the child with a rising temperature will shiver, display signs of cutaneous vasoconstriction and will feel cold. Once the cause of infection has been removed from the body, the hypothalamic set point returns to normal and heat loss mechanism will be initiated. The child sweats, displays signs of vasodilatation and feels hot until the core temperature returns to normal (Pococks and Richards 2004) (Figure 81.3).

Clinical assessment

A mild temperature elevation (less than 38°C) in an otherwise healthy child should be left to run its course. A high temperature needs to be investigated and managed.

- Check for any immediately life-threatening features
- Use traffic light system to check for symptoms and signs that predict the risk of serious illness
- Look for a source of fever and check symptoms and signs associated with specific diseases
- Measure and record temperature, heart rate, respiratory rate, capillary refill time and assess for dehydration (NICE 2007).

Other points to consider:
- Is child shivering?
- Position of the child: fetal position or splayed out?
- Skin colour: pale or flushed?
- Are they sweating?
- Level of consciousness?
- Urine output (Glasper et al. 2010).

Note: The 'traffic light' system is a tool for prioritizing children with fever by assessing the presence of certain symptoms. Features associated with fever in children have been categorized by potential seriousness into three groups – 'green' (low risk), 'amber' (intermediate risk) and 'red' (high risk) – to help health care professionals identify the risk of serious illness (NICE 2007).

Management

Although fever may be regarded as part of the natural response to infection as it reduces the rate at which viruses and bacteria replicate, antipyretic drugs are often used to reduce temperature so that the child feels comfortable.

- Do not routinely give antipyretic drugs to a child with fever with the sole aim of reducing body temperature
- Antipyretics do not prevent febrile convulsions and should not be used specifically for this purpose
- Do not administer paracetamol and ibuprofen at the same time but consider using the alternative agent if the child does not respond to the first drug (NICE 2007).

82 Infectious childhood diseases

Children's nurses will come in contact with infectious diseases as part of their everyday practice. The ability to diagnose these quickly will result in the quick and safe isolation of the child, providing optimum care for the family while protecting public safety. This chapter outlines the main infectious diseases identified by the Health Protection Agency (2010). Readers should also consider the traffic light system contained within the NICE (2013) guidance. This traffic light system provides a framework to assess the severity of the illness encountered by the child.

Table 82.1 Childhood infections

Rashes and skin infections*	Infectious period	Symptoms	What to do
Chickenpox *1–3 weeks	1–2 days before the rash appears, but continues to be infectious until the blister crust over	• Mild flu-like symptoms: ○ general malaise ○ aching, painful muscles ○ moderate to high fever • Rash starts as red itchy spots that blister. Fluid in the blister turns cloudy and crusts over. The crusting naturally falls off after 1–2 weeks	There is no cure for chickenpox as it is a viral infection but care could include: • Analgesia and antipyretic treatment • Fluids • Strategies to reduce scratching • Cool light cotton clothing • Those who are newborn, pregnant or immunosuppressed may be administered antiviral treatment
Measles *7–18 days	Symptoms usually disappear 7–10 days after the onset of the illness	Symptoms start around 10–12 days with: • High fever • Coryza (runny nose) • Conjunctivitis (non-purulent) • Koplik spots • Rash appear around 4 days after the initial symptoms. Start small red spots behind the ears, moving to face and head before clustering and spreading over the body • Photophobia (light sensitivity)	There is no specific treatment for measles as it is a viral infection but care could include: • Analgesia and antipyretic treatment • Gentle cleaning of the eyes • Regular fluids • Darkened room
Rubella *2–3 weeks	1–5 days after the appearance of the rash	• Cold-like symptoms • Distinctive red–pink rash starting behind the ears before spreading around face, neck, trunk and the rest of the body. Rash last approximately 3–7 days • Swollen lymph nodes • Moderate to high temperature	There is no specific treatment for rubella as it is a viral illness but care could include: • Analgesia and antipyretic treatment • Fluids • Strategies to reduce scratching • Cool light cotton clothing
Impetigo *1–3 days for streptococcal infections and 4–10 days for staphylococcal infections	If untreated the sores will remain infectious as long as they persist	• Can occur anywhere on the body but general starts around the nose and mouth • Starts as a small itchy inflamed area that blisters releasing yellow fluid that forms honey-coloured crusts • This fluid is highly contagious	Impetigo is treated with antibiotics that may be administered orally or topically. Strict infection control measures should be implemented to reduce the risks of cross-infection within the home to include the child's own towel and washing equipment
Diarrhoea and vomiting infections			
Rotavirus *1–3 days	May remain infectious for up to 8 days after the loose stools subside	• Starts with a high fever and vomiting followed by 3–8 days of watery diarrhoea • Abdominal cramps • Signs of dehydration	• Fluid to prevent dehydration such as rehydration drinks • Analgesia and antipyretic treatment • Good hygiene and possibly barrier creams for anal area
Escherichia coli 0157 *1–10 days	Several weeks after the symptoms subside	• Severe abdominal cramps • Diarrhoea (often bloodstained) • Moderate fever • Most people recover within 5 days but there is a risk of kidney damage and severe illness	As above
Shigella *12 hours to 6 days	During the acute phase and up to 4 weeks after the symptoms have subsided	• Severe abdominal cramps • Diarrhoea (often bloodstained) • Moderate fever • Nausea and vomiting	As above
Cryptosporidiosis *3–12 days after contact	Should not return to school for 48 hours after the symptoms have subsided and should not attend public swimming pools for 14 days after symptoms	This is a parasitic infection that may have no symptoms. When ill the child presents with gastroenteritis like symptoms lasting around 12–14 days	As above

Table 82.1 (*Continued*)

Diarrhoea and vomiting infections

Salmonella *12–72 hours after infection	This can range from several days to several weeks	• Severe abdominal cramps • Diarrhoea (often severe) • Moderate fever • Nausea and vomiting	As above

Respiratory infections

Influenza *1–4 days	One day before and 5 days after the symptoms subside	• Headache • Fever (38–40°C) • Aching muscles and joints • Chest pains • Lack of appetite • Fatigue and weakness • A runny nose and sore throat • Dry cough • Chills and shivering • Vomiting or diarrhoea	There is no specific treatment for influenza as it is a viral illness but care could include: • Analgesia and antipyretic treatment • Fluids • Rest
Tuberculosis (TB) *2–12 weeks	A child is considered at the end of the infectious period when the frequency and intensity of the cough has improved or having received 2 weeks of adequate treatment	• A productive persistent cough that may contain blood • Progressive breathlessness • Lack of appetite and weight loss • Night sweats • Extreme tiredness and fatigue	Pulmonary TB is treated using a 6-month course of a combination of antibiotics. The usual course of treatment is: • Two antibiotics – isoniazid and rifampicin – every day for 6 months • Two additional antibiotics – pyrazinamide and ethambutol – every day for the first 2 months
Pertussis *Average 7–10 days (range 5–21 days)	21 days after the onset of symptoms	There are three stages to this illness: *Catarrhal stage:* usually 7–10 days with coryzal features, low grade temperature and a mild occasional cough progressively deteriorating *Paroxysmal stage:* usually 1–6 weeks but could last for up to 10 weeks. Presenting with numerous, rapid and productive cough with a high-pitched whoop in older children, cyanosis, vomiting and exhaustion *Convalescent stage:* usually 7–10 days presenting with a general recovery, less persistent cough which disappears over a 2–3 week period	Treatment is supportive and includes close attention to respiratory effort and exhaustion Small frequent meals help reduce the paroxysmal cough and fluid management helps with hydration Erythromycin may be prescribed to reduce the period of infectivity but has little influence on the disease progression

Others infections

Conjunctivitis *1–3 days for bacteria; 1–12 days for viruses	Usually while symptoms are present but some viruses could remain infective for 14 days after the start of symptoms	The eye appears red and may feel 'gritty', with a watery or yellow discharge One eye is usually involved at first but both eyes are usually affected within a few hours	Viral infections will resolve without treatment, topical antibiotic drops/ointments may be prescribed for a bacterial infection Eye toilet and strict hygiene helps to avoid the spread of infection
Meningitis *2–7 days following exposure	The child is not contagious 24–48 hours after administration of antibiotics	Initial clinical features include severe headache, fever, nausea and vomiting, feeling generally unwell. More specific symptoms include severe lethargy, joint and muscle pain, breathing difficulties. Symptoms related to meningitis include stiff neck, photophobia, confusion and possible seizures. Symptom relates to septicaemia include cold hands and feet, leg pain, abnormal skin colour, confusion and a non-blanching purpuric rash	Treatment includes assessment for raised intracranial pressures and deteriorating neurological status. Fluid management and intravenous antibiotics are the mainstay treatment while treating symptoms as they present
Mumps *Around 17 days	Just before the swelling of the parotid gland to 9 days after the onset of the symptoms	• Swelling of the parotid glands causing pain and difficulty swallowing • Headaches • General malaise • Moderate to high temperature • Loss of appetite and abdominal pain	There is no specific treatment for rubella as it is a viral illness but care includes: • Analgesia/antipyretic treatment • Fluids • Warm or cool compresses to the swollen glands may reduce discomfort • Soft, light diet

*Incubation period.

83 Assessing infectious diseases

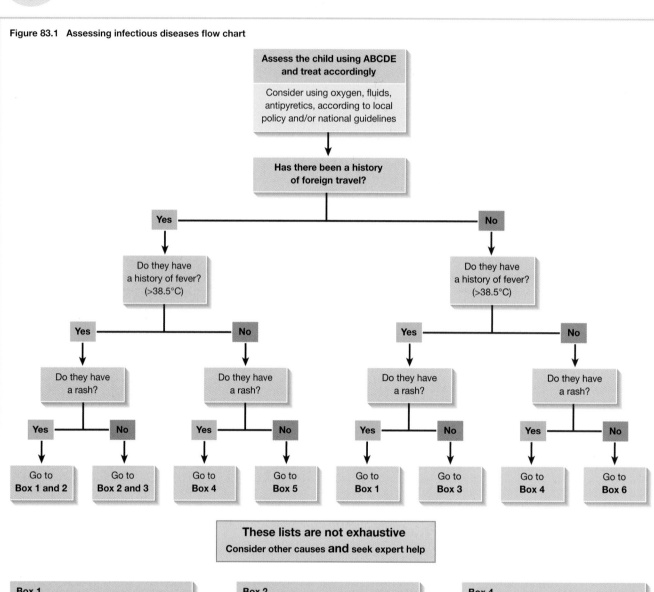

Figure 83.1 Assessing infectious diseases flow chart

Assess the child using ABCDE and treat accordingly

Consider using oxygen, fluids, antipyretics, according to local policy and/or national guidelines

Has there been a history of foreign travel?

Yes → **Do they have a history of fever? (>38.5°C)**

No → **Do they have a history of fever? (>38.5°C)**

Yes → **Do they have a rash?** → Yes: Go to Box 1 and 2 / No: Go to Box 2 and 3

No → **Do they have a rash?** → Yes: Go to Box 4 / No: Go to Box 5

Yes → **Do they have a rash?** → Yes: Go to Box 1 / No: Go to Box 3

No → **Do they have a rash?** → Yes: Go to Box 4 / No: Go to Box 6

These lists are not exhaustive
Consider other causes **and** seek expert help

Box 1

Consider

- **Macules/papules:** measles, rubella, human herpes virus 6 (roseola), enterovirus, infectious mononucleosis, Lyme disease
- **Purpura/petichiae:** meningococcal septicaemia, enterovirus, *Haemophilus influenzae*
- **Vesicles:** chickenpox, shingles, herpes simplex virus, hand-foot-and-mouth disease (slapped cheek)
- **Bullae/pustules:** staphylococcal/ streptococcal impetigo and scalded skin
- **Desquamation:** Kawasaki's disease and scarlet fever

Box 2

- Malaria
- Dengue fever
- Typhoid
- Cholera
- Helminth infections
- Worms
- Rheumatic fever

Box 3

- Meningitis
- Upper respiratory tract infection
- Pneumonia
- Urinary tract infection
- Viral infection
- Osteomylitis
- Bacterial gastroenteritis
- Mumps
- Post vaccination fever
- Tuberculosis
- Encephalitis

Box 4

- Consider incubation stage of infectious disease
- Consider boxes **1, 2** or **3**
- Treat the fever
- Observe and monitor **ABCDE**

Box 5

- Likely to be at convalescent stage
- Monitor rash and symptoms
- Further treatment not likely

Box 6

- Further action not required

Acknowledgement to Ellie Forbes, Matron for Child Health, and Dr Matt Halkes, Director of Clinical Education, South Devon Healthcare NHS Foundation Trust

Children and Young People's Nursing at a Glance, First Edition. Edited by Alan Glasper, Jane Coad, and Jim Richardson.
© 2015 John Wiley & Sons, Ltd. Published 2015 by John Wiley & Sons, Ltd. Companion website: www.ataglanceseries.com/nursing/children

What is infectious disease?

If the host (the human) sustains injury or pathologic changes in response to a parasitic infection, the process is called an infectious disease. The health of the host and the virulence of the micro-organism will determine the severity of an infectious disease, which can range from mild to life-threatening.

Infectious agents

In order to survive, an infectious agent must be able to multiply, emerge from the host, reach a new host and infect the new host. The agents of infectious disease include: viruses, bacteria, rickettsiae, chlamydiae, fungi, parasites and prions. Some of the key infectious agents are discussed here.

- **Viruses** can have an immediate effect on the host (e.g. influenza), or they could be latent (or dormant; e.g. herpesvirus and adenovirus, retrovirus (HIV), anthropod-borne virus, enterovirus).
- **Bacteria** are extremely adaptable: streptococcal, staphylococcal, Lyme's disease, Weil's disease, mycoplasmas.
- **Rickettsiae** combine the characteristics of viral and bacterial agents to produce disease in humans and depend on the host cell for essential vitamins and nutrients: arthropods – fleas, ticks, lice.
- **Fungi** are free-living and found in every habitat. They are separated into two groups: yeasts and moulds. Fungi include ringworm and athlete's foot.
- **A parasite** is a member of the animal kingdom that infects and causes disease in other animals and includes protozoa, helminths and arthropods. Protozoan infections include malaria, amoebic dysentery and giardiais. Helminths are a collection of wormlike parasites which include roundworms, tapeworms and flukes. The parasitic arthropods include ticks, mosquitoes, biting flies, mites, lice and fleas.
- **Prions**: Infective protein agents (e.g. Creutzfeldt–Jakob disease).

Epidemiology

Epidemiology means the study of factors, events and circumstances that influence the transmission of infectious disease in human populations. It is a science of rates; infectious diseases must be classified according to incidence, portal of entry, source, symptoms, disease course, site of infection and virulence factors. The purpose of epidemiology is then to predict, avert and appropriately treat potential outbreaks.

Incidence is the term used to describe the number of new cases of an infectious disease that occurs within a defined population (e.g. 1000 people) over a specified period of time (e.g. monthly).

Portal of entry

The portal of entry refers to the process by which the pathogen enters the body. **Penetration** is a disruption to the integrity of the skin by accident (burn or abrasion), medical procedure (catheterization), skin lesion (impetigo), inoculation or animal or arthropod bite. **Direct contact** with infected tissue or secretions such as sexually transmitted diseases (gonorrhoea, syphilis) or from mother to child during gestation or birth (rubella, cytomegalovirus, herpes simplex viruses, HIV). **Ingestion** is the entry of the pathogenic micro-organisms or toxins through the oral cavity and gastrointestinal tract. Contaminated water and food are a common source of entry for many bacterial, viral and parasitic infections (e.g. cholera, typhoid, traveller's diarrhoea and hepatitis A). **Inhalation** is responsible for the most deaths of children under 5 years because of the vast array of pathogens that invade through the respiratory tract: bacterial pneumonia, meningitis and sepsis, tuberculosis; viruses such as measles, mumps, chickenpox, influenza, respiratory syncytial virus and the common cold.

The portal of entry does not necessarily dictate the site of infection; ingested pathogens, for example, may cause liver disease.

Source

The source is essentially the who, what, where and when of disease transmission, and refers to the location, host, object or substance from which the infectious agent was acquired. The source could be the host's own microbial flora, external sources (such as soil, water and air), another human being, from an animal to human, or arthropod vectors. The source can also denote the place; for example, hospital-acquired infections or community acquired; and the likely vehicle for transmission, such as faeces, blood, body fluids, respiratory secretions and urine. Infected objects that are shared from person to person or complex combinations of sources can also spread infections.

Symptomatology

The symptoms of an infectious disease may be specific and reflect the site of infection (rash); conversely, there may be non-specific symptoms that are shared by a number of infectious diseases. Symptomatology is the collection of signs and symptoms (the clinical picture) expressed by the host during the course of the disease.

Accurate history taking and documentation is crucial to be able to aid in the diagnosis.

Disease course

There are five distinct stages that the infectious disease takes once entering the host:

1 **Incubation period**: the time taken to produce recognizable symptoms, which could be hours to days;
2 **Prodromal stage**: initial appearance of symptoms;
3 **Acute stage**: the maximum impact of infectious process;
4 **Convalescent stage**: the containment of the infection and repair of damaged tissue;
5 **Resolution stage**: the total elimination of the pathogen with no residual signs or symptoms.

Site of infection

The site of an infectious disease is determined by the type of pathogen, the portal of entry and the effectiveness of the host's immunological defence system. Infectious diseases affect one or more of the following systems: **respiratory, intestinal, blood and skin**.

Virulence factors

The substances or products that are generated by infectious agents to enhance their ability to cause disease are known as **virulence factors**.

Treatment and protection

The diagnosis of an infectious disease requires two criteria: (i) the recovery of the probable pathogen from the infected sites; and (ii) accurate documentation of clinical signs and symptoms.

Most infectious diseases are self-limiting and require little or no intervention. The choice of treatment for an infectious disease may be medicinal by using antimicrobials, immunological with antibody preparations or vaccines, or surgical. The goal of treatment is complete removal of the pathogen from the host and normal physiological function to damaged tissues. By far the best treatment of an infectious disease is **prevention**. Good handwashing techniques, clean water, a healthy diet and immunizations are fundamental in preventing the spread of infectious diseases.

84 Prevention of infection

Figure 84.1 Five moments for hand hygiene

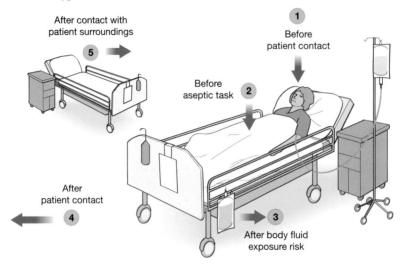

After contact with patient surroundings

5

Before patient contact

1

Before aseptic task

2

After patient contact

4

After body fluid exposure risk

3

Reproduced with permission of the World Health Organization

Figure 84.2 How to wash your hands

1. Wet hands with water
2. Apply enough soap to cover all hand surfaces
3. Rub hands palm to palm
4. Rub right palm over the back of the left hand with interlaced fingers and vice versa
5. Palm to palm with fingers interlaced
6. Backs of fingers to opposing palms with fingers interlocked
7. Rotational rubbing of left thumb clasped in right palm and vice versa
8. Rotational rubbing, backwards and forwards, with clasped fingers of right hand in left palm and vice versa
9. Rinse hands with water
10. Dry hands thoroughly with clean towel

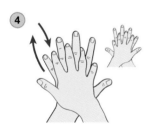

4

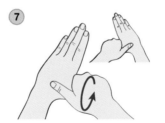

7

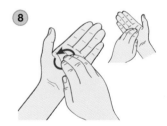

8

Context and definition

Florence Nightingale, in her *Notes on Nursing*, paraphrased the principle, 'First do the sick no harm'. Nowhere is this more important than in the prevention and control of infection in health care settings.

Approximately 10% of patients will acquire an infection during an episode of health care. This can result in:
- Increased suffering and distress
- Physical and psychological harm, lasting damage or even death
- The need for additional drug treatment with risk of adverse effects

- Extended hospital stays with additional exposure to risk
- Additional costs to the NHS.

Prevention and control of infection

Children are particularly vulnerable to health care associated infection. The younger the child, the more vulnerable he/she is as the immune system matures and becomes more efficient across childhood. Some groups of children are particularly at risk of acquiring infections:
- Children with intrinsic immunodeficiency (e.g. severe combined immunodeficiency (SCID))

- Children with acquired immunodeficiency (e.g. following chemotherapy, radiotherapy or corticosteroid use)
- Chronically unwell children
- The unimmunized.

Specific pathogens
- Staphylococci (e.g. methicillin-resistant *Staphyloccus aureus* (MRSA))
- Streptococci
- Enterococci (e.g. *Escherichia coli*)
- Respiratory syncytial virus (RSV)
- Rotavirus, etc.
- Hepatitis A, B and C
- HIV
- Fungi (e.g. *Candida*).

Actions to control transmission of infections
- Understanding the chain of infection and how this can be broken
- Hand hygiene
- Protective equipment
- Cleanliness
- Decontamination
- Patient accommodation (e.g. source isolation and protective isolation)
- Proper handling and disposal of waste
- Proper handling and disposal of sharps
- Proper handling of laundry.

Breaking the chain of infection
- Infectious agent
- Reservoirs
- Portal of exit
- Means of transmission
- Portal of entry
- Susceptible host.

Hand hygiene
Effective hand hygiene is the single most important thing the children's nurse can do to protect those in her care. It begins with:
- Bare below the elbow, short sleeves, no wristwatch or jewellery (except wedding ring which should be moved during cleansing to ensure that the area under it is cleansed)
- Care of skin and nails – nails kept short to allow proper cleansing and no nail varnish which could become a reservoir for contaminants
- A cleansing technique that covers the whole surface of the hands and wrists
- Use of sanitizing gel to decontaminate socially clean hands
- Use soap and water to decontaminate visibly soiled hands
- Not using hands to operate taps and bins
- Proper hand drying
- Appropriate skin care.

Proper use of sterile or non-sterile gloves does not remove the need for hand decontamination.

When is hand decontamination necessary?
(Figure 84.1)
- Before touching a patient
- Before a clean or aseptic procedure
- After body fluid exposure risk
- After touching a patient
- After touching patient's surroundings.

Hand decontamination technique – gel
1 Palmful of decontaminant into cupped hand.
2 Cover entire surface of hands and wrists.
3 Rub hands palm to palm.
4 Rub right palm over the back of the left hand and vice versa.
5 Rub palm to palm with fingers interlaced.
6 Rub backs of fingers to opposing palms with fingers interlocked.
7 Rotational rubbing of left thumb clasped in palm of right hand and vice versa.
8 Rotational rubbing backwards and forwards of clasped fingers of right hand in left palm and vice versa.
9 Once dry, hands are safe.

Hand decontamination technique – soap and water
(Figure 84.2)
1 Wet hands with water.
2 Palmful of liquid soap into cupped hand.
3 Cover entire surface of hands and wrists.
4 Rub hands palm to palm.
5 Rub right palm over the back of the left hand and vice versa.
6 Rub palm to palm with fingers interlaced.
7 Rub backs of fingers to opposing palms with fingers interlocked.
8 Rotational rubbing of left thumb clasped in palm of right hand and vice versa.
9 Rotational rubbing backwards and forwards of clasped fingers of right hand in left palm and vice versa.
10 Rinse hands with water.
11 Dry hand thoroughly with a single use towel.
12 Use towel to turn off tap.
13 Once dry, hands are safe.

Protective clothing
- Uniforms should be appropriately laundered and used.
- Protective clothing such as disposable aprons should be used in line with local policy.
- Appropriate use of gloves. NB These do not remove the need for hand decontamination.

Appropriate patient accommodation
- Single room use for infectious patients to prevent spread to others with source isolation techniques. On occasion, cohort isolation may be appropriate (e.g. RSV).
- Single room use for the particularly vulnerable to acquiring infections (e.g. infants under 1 year).

85 Hyponatraemia and its prevention

Figure 85.1   The effects of hyponatraemia and hypernatraemia on the cell

Normal	Hypernatraemia	Hyponatraemia
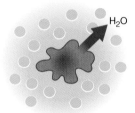		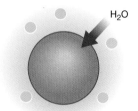
Normal cell size; normal serum Na concentration	Cell shrinks as H_2O is pulled **out** of cell	Cell swells as H_2O is pulled **into** cell

Causes of hyponatraemia include:

- Loss of sodium
- Excess water intake or retention
- Syndrome of inappropriate antidiuretic hormone (SIADH)
- Inappropriate fluid management (e.g. miscalculation, over-infusion of IV fluids or oral fluid overload)
- Inappropriate choice of IV fluid
- Incorrect reconstitution of formula milk

Assessing the child: signs and symptoms of hyponatraemia

May be asymptomatic but may include:

- Nausea and vomiting
- Headache
- Irritability
- Altered consciousness and lethargy
- Seizures
- Apnoea
- Respiratory arrest

Children and Young People's Nursing at a Glance, First Edition. Edited by Alan Glasper, Jane Coad, and Jim Richardson.
© 2015 John Wiley & Sons, Ltd. Published 2015 by John Wiley & Sons, Ltd. Companion website: www.ataglanceseries.com/nursing/children

Movement of body fluid and electrolytes

Body fluids and associated electrolytes are in constant motion around the body by diffusion, osmosis and active transport in order to achieve a state of homeostasis. Thus, the body works continuously to achieve optimal fluid and electrolyte balance. Electrolytes are substances that develop an electrical charge when dissolved in water and play an important part in controlling the osmosis of water between body compartments and its movement in and out of the cells. Sodium of one of the most important electrolytes in the ill child.

Sodium

Most sodium is kept outside the cells and potassium inside via the sodium–potassium pump mechanism. The movement of sodium and water are closely related; generally where one goes, the other follows. Thus, under normal circumstances, the sodium–potassium pump prevents too much water entering the cells. In hyponatraemia, a low serum sodium level means that the extracellular fluid is very dilute and water is drawn into the cells (Figure 85.1). This can result in cerebral oedema and brain herniation. A high serum sodium or hypernatraemia has the opposite effect but can also have serious neurological consequences (Figure 85.1), although further discussion of this is beyond the remit of this chapter.

What is hyponatraemia?

Normal sodium levels are 135–145 mmol/L. Hyponatraemia occurs when levels fall below these limits and is not uncommon in the child with fluid and electrolyte imbalance. Severe hyponatraemia occurs when plasma sodium levels fall below 130 mmol/L and severe acute hyponatraemia occurs when a normal plasma sodium falls below 130 mmol/L in less than 48 hours (Playfor 2013). This is a potentially life-threatening event that needs careful monitoring, care and treatment by the multidisciplinary team. Children are more at risk of detrimental effects of hyponatraemia because they cannot tolerate over-hydration, they have a higher brain : skull size ratio (meaning that there is little space for expansion as the brain cells fill with water) and hormonal changes render female adolescents, in particular, more prone to its development. Other children particularly at risk include those with central nervous system conditions, sepsis, gastroenteritis or those in the perioperative period. Stress, pain, nausea, certain anaesthetics or types of ventilation can cause what is known as the syndrome of inappropriate antidiuretic hormone (SIADH). This hormone normally conserves water in the body in times of dehydration; however, in SIADH it is produced unnecessarily and this can cause hyponatraemia resulting from the retention of water.

Management of the child with hyponatraemia

As with any aspect of children's nursing, a family centred approach is essential. Careful and appropriate information giving, involving the child and family and open communication will help to reduce anxiety. Good communication within the multidisciplinary team, and adherence to local policies are key aspects of the children's nurse's role in ensuring safe and effective care for the hyponatraemic child. Ongoing monitoring and assessment of the child for signs and symptoms of hyponatraemia and fluid imbalance (see Chapter 77) are key. Accurate recording and reporting of all intake and output in the fluid balance chart (including the child's daily weight) and documentation in the nursing notes are also of vital importance. In particular, the type, amount and rate of intravenous (IV) fluids should be recorded accurately together with any losses (e.g. gastric losses) that may need to be replaced. The child receiving IV fluids should be closely observed and their blood, urea and electrolytes (including BM) obtained on a regular basis and results evaluated by the multidisciplinary team. IV requirements should be adjusted accordingly if the child is also taking oral fluids. Hourly observation of the IV site, for the presence of inflammation and/or phlebitis (using an appropriate tool), is also an important part of the role of the nurse.

Treatment of hyponatraemia may involve the administration of sodium chloride solution (according to local policy) to raise serum sodium levels and/or fluid restriction. In general, correction of sodium levels should not be too rapid as this can result in neurological damage. Regular blood tests (urea and electrolytes) and urine collection for osmolality and electrolytes will be required as directed by the individual child's situation. The children's nurse has key role in supporting the family and ensuring that these tests are carried out and results reported back to appropriate medical staff in a timely manner.

Preventing hyponatraemia

Children's nurses, as members of the multidisciplinary team, may help prevent hyponatraemia by having a thorough working knowledge of suitable types and amounts of fluids for children in their care along with normal serum electrolyte levels. All professionals working with sick children should be familiar with local policies. They also need to be aware of the causes of hyponatraemia, the factors that put some children particularly at risk and an understanding of SIADH. Specific clinical guidelines have been developed throughout the United Kingdom for local use in response to the National Patient Safety Alert 22 'Reducing the risk of hyponatraemia when administering intravenous infusions to children'. It is imperative that children's nurses adhere to such guidance along with other members of the multidisciplinary team. Regular training, supervision and adequate reporting of incidents or near misses will help to ensure the safety of children at risk of hyponatraemia.

Key points
- The children's nurse should have a good knowledge of local fluid management policies.
- Multidisciplinary working and communication are key.
- Accurate assessment, reporting, good record keeping and ongoing monitoring of the child will help to reduce and manage the risk of hyponatraemia.

Acknowledgement. The authors would like to thank Dr Claire Anderson and Dr Jarlath McAloon for their assistance in the preparation of this chapter.

86 Thermal injuries

Figure 86.1 The SAFE approach

Shout for help

Assess the scene for danger

Free the area around the child for danger

Evaluate the casualty

Figure 86.2 Lund and Bowden assessment tool

	At birth	0–1 year	2–4 years	5–9 years	10–15 years
A. Half a head	9.5%	8.5%	6.5%	5.5%	4.5%
B. Half of thigh	2.75%	3.25%	4.0%	4.25%	4.5%
C. Half of leg	2.5%	2.5%	2.75%	3.0%	3.25%

Figure 86.3 Classification, assessment, management and complications

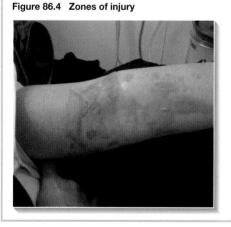

Classification

- Scalds
- Friction or contact burns
- Flame burns
- Flash burns
- Chemical burns
- Electrical burns
- Radiation burns
- Sunburn
- Extreme exposure to cold
- Child abuse

Complications

- Burn shock and hypovolaemic shock
- Fluid and electrolyte imbalance
- Hypermetabolism
- Hypothermia
- Infection
- Contractures
- Compartment syndrome
- Scarring, disfigurement and disability
- Multisystem organ failure

Assessment

Thermal injuries necessitate a structured approach as per Advanced Paediatric Life Support Guidelines (ABCDEFG), and a systematic response. Assessment and overall management of thermal injuries can be subdivided into the following phases of care:
- Rescue
- Resuscitate
- Review
- Resurface
- Rehabilitate
- Reconstruct
- Review

Management

- Pain assessment and management
- Fluid resuscitation
- Photographs
- Wound assessment using validated assessment tools
- Burns assessment tools
- Blister debridement
- Cleanse wounds according to evidence-based guideline and local policy

Figure 86.4 Zones of injury

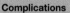

Thermal damage to tissue may be described in three zones:

1. **Zone of hyperaemia:** superficial damage when the damaged skin appears warm and red
2. **Zone of stasis:** the microcirculation is damaged resulting in changes to capillary permeability which allows fluids to leak from the vascular system into the interstitial space resulting in local oedema and resultant shock if extensive wounds are present
3. **Zone of coagulation:** the deepest area where damaged cells occlude blood vessels. The obstructed microcirculation prevents the humoral compartments of the immune response targeting the burned tissue

Severity of thermal injury

1. **Local:** oedema, fluid loss, significant circulatory alterations and development of thrombi
2. **Systematic:** may involve multiple system response including cardiovascular, gastrointestinal, renal and increased metabolism and body temperature

Thermal injuries have been described as some of the worst injuries for infants and children. Children experience physical and psychological trauma, which may leave disfigurement and disability. Approximately 50 000 children under the age of 5 years incur thermal injuries annually, the impact of which upon the child and the family cannot be quantified. Moreover, the evidence would suggest that accident prevention does not reduce the incidence of thermal injuries, particularly in the younger age group.

Incidence

The highest incidence occurs in children under 5 years. The most common thermal injury is scalds from hot water (66%), with a gender ratio higher in males than females. As young children become more mobile and curious their exposure to household thermal hazards increases. There may be seasonal and regional differences that affect the pattern of burn injuries. Cultural and

Children and Young People's Nursing at a Glance, First Edition. Edited by Alan Glasper, Jane Coad, and Jim Richardson.

socioeconomic factors may increase the risk patterns of thermal injuries in any community.

Priorities (Figure 86.1)

- Stop the burning and arrest any further damage.
- Assess if fluid resuscitation is required.
- Assess and mange pain.
- Communication with the child and family.

Total body surface area

The total body surface area (TBSA) affected can be estimated using a range of methods to assess whether a minor or major thermal injury is involved.

TBSA >10% is classified as major burns. Children whose burns make up 10% or more of TBSA are considered critical and require urgent hospitalization. Fluid resuscitation is calculated using the Parkland Formula which estimates the amount of fluid required over the 24-hour period following injury. Half the fluid is administered in the first 8 hours and the remainder is given over the subsequent 16 hours.

TBSA <10% is classified as minor burns unless there is associated smoke inhalation.

Assessment tools

It is important to remember that the burn itself is being assessed and surrounding areas of redness (erythema) should be excluded.

Wallace rule of nines. An acknowledged formula but based upon adults (estimates an adult head being 9% of total body area). It has the potential to be adapted for children but it does not take account of different surface area variations for children at different ages.

1 per cent rule or rule of palms. The surface area of a child's palm, including fingers, is considered to be 1%. It has been suggested that a more accurate figure for a child's palm is 0.5%.

Lund and Bowden assessment. Considered the most accurate tool for assessing percentage burns for children as it takes account of body surface changes with age (Table 86.1).

Burns

Fatal burns in children are often associated with house fires and are the second most common cause of accidents and deaths in childhood, with 50% of fatalities associated with smoke inhalation and the remaining 50% of deaths attributed to burn injuries. Death is attributed to massive fluid loss, hypovolaemic and neurogenic shock, and overwhelming infection.

Thermal injuries in children follow patterns related to both developmental level and socioeconomic status. Those children at greater risk are those who cannot protect themselves. An infant will rely totally upon another for protection, while an older child may be able to alert an adult (e.g. igniting a lighter or matches and 'STOP', 'DROP' and 'ROLL'). Children with disabilities and/or complex care needs have an increased risk because of their inability to protect themselves.

Depth of burns

First degree burns (superficial thermal injury)

- Only the epidermis is involved
- Potential for the formation of serous-filled blisters
- Pain
- Blanching of skin when pressure is applied
- Healing occurs within 5–7 days.

Treatment Initiate first aid and wounds should heal spontaneously with reasonable care.

Second degree burns (partial thickness thermal injuries)

- Loss of epidermis and partial loss of dermis
- Potential for blistering
- May blanch when pressure is applied
- Red in colour
- Potential for decrease in sensation
- Scarring may occur
- May require skin graft.

Treatment

- Remove burned clothing, clean with tepid water and leave blisters intact
- Pain relief
- Check immunization status.

Third degree burns (full thickness)

- Epidermis and dermis are destroyed
- Absence of serous-filled blisters
- White appearance of the skin
- No blanching on pressure
- Sensation is absent
- Grafting will facilitate healing.

Treatment

- Establish and maintain a patent airway. Initiate advanced life support if necessary
- Remove burned clothing but keep the child warm
- Cover burn to prevent contamination
- Pain management
- Nil by mouth until transported to specialist burns centre
- IV fluids and 100% oxygen.

Fourth degree burns

Fourth degree burns are rare. Damage extends through deeply charred subcutaneous tissue to muscle and bone. Fourth degree burns may be caused from prolonged exposure to flames or high-voltage electrical shock.

Treatment As per full thickness burns.

Compartment syndrome

This is a surgical emergency. It occurs when severe oedema causes a tourniquet-like effect that compromises the circulation and entraps nerves.

Scalds

A child becomes scalded far more quickly than an adult as it takes only 1 second for a child to sustain a scald when exposed to liquid at 60°C (the average setting point is 55°C in British homes). The features of any scald are defined by their causal factors such as agent, mechanism and intent (accidental or intentional), coupled with physical characteristics of the injury.

Accidental scalds in children. Accidental scalds in children are often described as **spill injures** where the child reaches out and accidentally pulls hot liquid over him/herself. This typically leads to a scalded area over the upper trunk face and/or arms. The scald usually has an irregular edge and is variable in depth, being deepest at the initial point of contact.

Intentional scald/thermal injuries. Severe burns are reported in an estimated 10–12% of children who have suffered physical abuse. Intentional injuries from hot boiling water usually affect the back or lower limbs with or without including the buttocks or perineum. They may also affect the arms and/or both legs in a **glove** or **stocking** manner. Forced immersion scald or burn injuries are consistently described as the most common mechanism of intentional thermal injuries. Local safeguarding policies and procedures should be initiated.

87 Childhood fractures

Figure 87.1 Common sites of childhood fractures

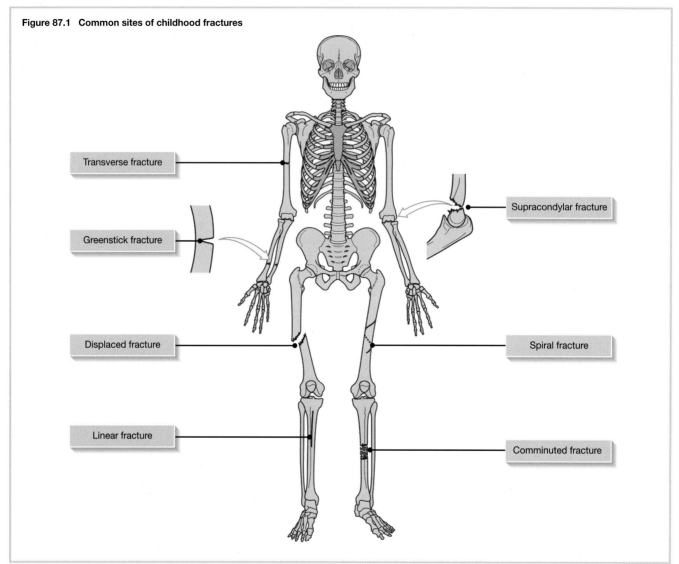

Children and Young People's Nursing at a Glance, First Edition. Edited by Alan Glasper, Jane Coad, and Jim Richardson.
© 2015 John Wiley & Sons, Ltd. Published 2015 by John Wiley & Sons, Ltd. Companion website: www.ataglanceseries.com/nursing/children

A fracture is defined as a break in the continuity of a bone (Hamblen and Simpson 2007). During play children undertake activities that can increase the risk of injury resulting in a fracture. The child with a fracture may present with pain, swelling, deformity, loss of function and movement; the diagnosis can be confirmed by X-ray.

There are two main classifications of fractures: closed and open (Dandy and Edwards 2009). For a closed fracture the skin remains intact whereas for an open fracture there is damage to the skin that communicates with the fracture site. This is also known as a compound fracture. Fractures can be displaced, where the bone fragments are not in alignment, or undisplaced.

Types of closed fractures

Transverse: the fracture is horizontal across the bone

Linear: the fracture is vertical.

Oblique: –the fracture is at an angle of <90°.

Spiral: the fracture runs in a spiral around the bone and is a result of a rotational force. Non-accidental injury should be suspected if this type of fracture is seen in an immobile infant.

Comminuted: a fracture that consists of more than two fragments.

Compression: this is where a bone has been crushed.

Avulsion: a fragment of bone has been pulled away from the site of ligament insertion.

Greenstick: this is an incomplete fracture where the bone remains intact on one side but breaks on the other. This is like trying to snap a new branch on a tree, hence its name.

Buckle: Compression of a long bone leading to a buckle.

The healing process

The fractured bone initially bleeds then forms a haematoma. The inflammatory process begins when necrotic bone and the haematoma are removed by macrophages and osteoclasts. Osteoid (bone) tissue develops, forming a callus at the fracture site. There are two types of bone cell: osteoblasts develop new bone and osteoclasts remove necrotic bone and are involved in bone resoption. After a few weeks the callus hardens and the bone develops mechanical strength. This area then consolidates with mature bone. After approximately 1 year, remodelling has occurred and the normal bone shape is restored. This can occur in children where there has been a significant malalignment of the fracture. This healing process is quicker in children than adults.

Management

Fracture of a bone is painful so any child who sustains a fracture should be assessed for pain and given analgesia accordingly. If the fracture is displaced, the bone ends need to be realigned to regain the position and length of the bone fragments and correct deformity. This is known as reduction. Methods of reduction are closed manipulation performed under general anaesthetic, traction (see Chapter 89) and by open operation. Not all fractures need reducing and can be treated with simple splintage such as neighbour strapping or use of a sling/collar and cuff. Following reduction, the fracture needs to be immobilized to maintain the position. This can be done by the application of a plaster of Paris cast (see Chapter 88), continued traction or by internal or external fixation. Internal fixation involves a surgical operation whereby the bone fragments are secured by using a metal plate and screws, screws/wires or an intramedullary nail. External fixation involves the insertion of pins into the fragments of bone which are then attached to a rigid bar or frame (the fixator) (Hamblen and Simpson 2007). Rehabilitation commences immediately after the initial treatment to promote healing and prevent joint stiffness in order to restore function.

Pin site care

The pins from skeletal traction or external fixator are a vehicle for hospital-acquired infection due to the nature of the pins penetrating the skin. There has been much debate as to the most effective methods of cleaning pin sites which led to the Royal College of Nursing (2010) developing guidelines based upon consensus:

• Clean pin sites weekly using alcoholic chlorhexidine and non-shedding gauze

• Cover with a wound dressing that keeps moisture and exudate away from the wound and secure with a bung that gives light compression

• Increase frequency of dressing changes if an infection is present or the dressing is excessively wet.

Complications

Injury to other structures/organs: injury to the brachial artery following supracondylar fracture of the humerus.

Compartment syndrome: increased pressure within the muscle compartments causing compression of the nerves, blood vessels and soft tissue by bleeding or tight dressings/cast (see Chapter 90).

Delayed union: normal healing does not occur as expected. This is less likely in children especially young children and infants.

Mal union: where the bone heals in an abnormal position.

Non-union: the bone fragments do not heal.

Fat embolism: release of fat from the fracture site of long bones into the circulation and lungs.

Osteomyleitis: an infection of the bone from a contaminated wound of a compound fracture or pin site. This is difficult to eradicate.

Avascular necrosis: death of bone due to loss of blood supply.

Growth restriction: caused by damage to the growth (epiphyseal) plate in children who have not reached growth maturity.

88 Plaster care

Figure 88.1 Removal of synthetic cast using an oscillating plaster saw

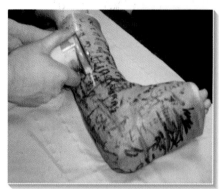

The blade rubs through the cast. Bony prominences should be avoided when removing the cast

Figure 88.2 Application of cast

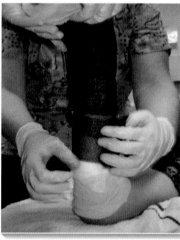

Following application of a layer of padding, the cast material is applied to the limb. The child needs to be in a comfortable position during this process

Figure 88.3 Completed cast

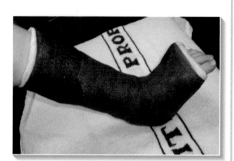

Children and Young People's Nursing at a Glance, First Edition. Edited by Alan Glasper, Jane Coad, and Jim Richardson.
© 2015 John Wiley & Sons, Ltd. Published 2015 by John Wiley & Sons, Ltd. Companion website: www.ataglanceseries.com/nursing/children

Plaster casts are applied for a variety of reasons. They can consist of plaster of Paris or synthetic materials such as fibreglass, depending on the reason. It is important for the nurse to know the reason why the cast is being applied, what type of material is required and how long it is to remain in place. It is also essential when applying lower limb casts to know whether the child is allowed to bear weight.

Reasons for application

- Treatment of fractures
- Following orthopaedic surgical procedures
- To improve function by stabilization of a joint
- To correct and prevent deformities
- To provide pain relief
- To permit early ambulation and weight bearing
- To make a mould of a limb for splints to be made.

Preparation of the child

Prior to application the child and the parent or carer should be provided with an explanation of the process of applying the cast and the reason. Consent should be obtained. Demonstrating the procedure on a doll is a useful method in younger children and can also be used as a method of distraction. It is important to make the child as comfortable as possible; small children may need to be seated on their parent's knee. Therapeutic holding may need to be considered (see Chapter 38).

Applying the cast

The aim is to apply a good cast that fits well, is not too tight, is smooth on the inside, using only enough materials to provide an effective cast without making it too heavy. The layers also need to be smoothed to ensure bonding (Miles et al. 2000). It is important to ensure the child has received adequate analgesia before attempting to apply the cast. If the cast is applied following surgery the child may still be anaesthetized during the procedure. It is important to position the limb correctly and ensure the child has their privacy and dignity maintained throughout as clothing may need to have been removed to expose the area requiring the cast. The procedure should be documented in the care records.

Indentation should be avoided when handling a wet cast as this can lead to pressure on the skin under the cast. The cast should be allowed to dry naturally to avoid separation of the layers. This can take 24–48 hours for plaster of Paris; synthetic materials take between 30 minutes and 1 hour. The newly plastered limb should be supported on a pillow to prevent pressure. It may be necessary to elevate the limb to assist in reducing swelling, especially following a fracture. Upper limbs can be placed in a sling whereas lower limbs should be elevated on a pillow. This elevation should be no more than 10 cm above the heart. It is important to check for swelling and neurovascular status of the limb which can occur due to the fracture or surgical procedure or if the cast is too tight (see Chapter 90).

Potential problems

As well as the neurovascular complications, it is important to observe for the following problems.

- **Cracking/softening/breakdown of the cast**. If areas of the cast are likely to come into contact with bodily fluids, such as a hip spica, waterproof or absorbent tape should be applied to the edges to keep the cast clean. Parents should be advised to use a smaller nappy that tucks under the edge of the cast and a larger one that goes over the spica. The child should be advised not to get the their cast wet or put weight on it until dry.
- **Indicators of pressure**. Pressure or cast sores can occur if the underlying padding is uneven or insufficient over bony areas or a poor application technique is used. The cast being too loose or too tight can also be a contributory factor. Damage to the skin can be caused by the insertion of objects being pushed down the plaster by younger children or to relieve itching by older children. Signs of a cast sore are an offensive smell, staining of the cast from an oozing wound, burning pain and pyrexia. Younger children may be irritable.
- Allergic reactions to the casting material.
- If following a surgical procedure the cast should be observed for signs of bleeding.
- Children in spica casts may develop bloating of the abdomen.

Caring for a child in a cast can be difficult for the child and parents. Aspects that need consideration:

- **Positioning**: it is important to change the position regularly of children in hip spicas to avoid skin damage due to pressure. The child may not be able to sit up so needs to be propped up with pillows or on a perch.
- **Hygiene and dressing**: this can be difficult as the child is not able to be bathed and clothing may not fit so needs to be adapted (e.g. using Velcro fastenings).
- **Feeding**: the previously independent child may need assistance.
- **Sleeping**: may be disturbed as the child's usual sleeping position will be difficult to achieve.
- **Moving and handling**: parents will need to be given instruction on the best way to carry the child.
- **Mobility**: the child in a spica will not fit into a normal pushchair. Older children will need to adapt to the use of crutches if in lower limb casts.
- **Travelling**: the child may not fit into a car seat.

On discharge, the child and parents should be given advice both verbally and in writing on what to observe for and how to care for the cast.

89 Traction care

Figure 89.1 Fixed traction

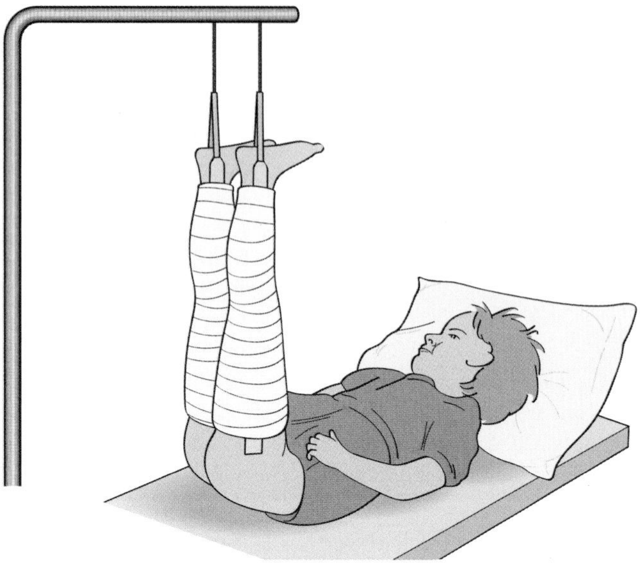

Figure 89.2 Types of balanced traction

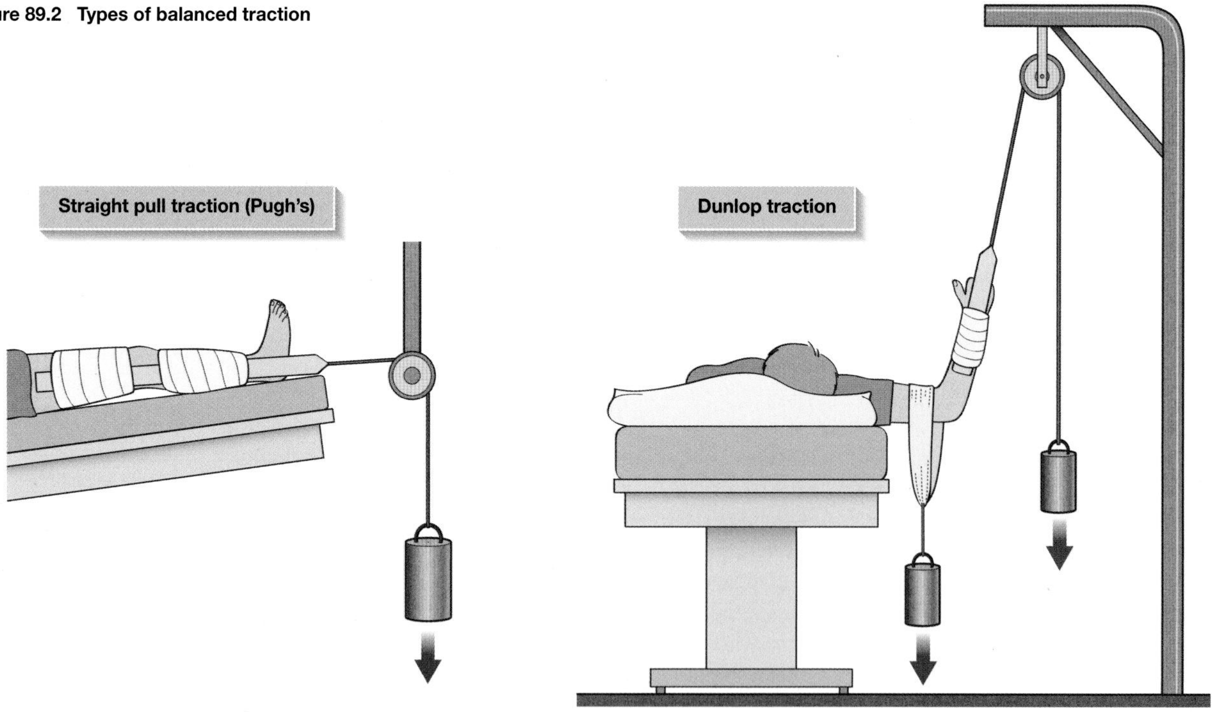
Straight pull traction (Pugh's)
Dunlop traction

Children and Young People's Nursing at a Glance, First Edition. Edited by Alan Glasper, Jane Coad, and Jim Richardson.

What is traction?

Traction is the application of a pulling force that requires counter traction in order to be effective. This follows the principles of gravity. Counter traction can be achieved by the child's body weight or by elevating the end of the bed. This pulling force is applied to the child's limb with a resultant pull on the bone and soft tissues.

Why is traction used?

- To reduce a displaced fracture
- To maintain alignment of a fracture
- To reduce muscle spasm
- To relieve pain
- To prevent or correct deformity caused by contracture of the soft tissues
- To immobilize inflamed or injured joints
- To aid reduction of a dislocated joint (e.g. developmental dysplasia of the hip).

Types of traction

The type of traction selected is determined by the age of the child, the type and position of the fracture, the amount of displacement, the condition of the skin and soft tissues and the desired outcomes. The traction should be used to maintain the fracture position until there has been sufficient healing to enable the limb to be immobilized in a plaster cast until complete healing has occurred.

Fixed

This is achieved by the pulling force being exerted between two fixed points. Examples of this type of traction are the application of a Thomas splint and Gallows.

Gallows traction (also known as Bryant's traction) is used for the conservative treatment of fracture of the shaft of femur in children under the age of 2 years or not weighing more than 16 kg. It is also used for preoperative positioning prior to hip surgery. It is a type of fixed traction. The child's legs are suspended from a Balkan beam attached to the cot by skin extensions. The child's body weight is used to provide counter traction. This is achieved by the child's buttocks being raised off the bed. It is therefore important to check that this is maintained. The traction is applied to both legs. Neurovascular observations need to be undertaken as vascular impairment is a complication of this traction. The child usually adapts quickly to the traction but involvement of the family and the play therapist to provide distraction is essential.

Balanced (sliding)

This is where the pulling forces are balanced to provide traction and counter traction between two mobile points – the use of suspended weights and the child's own body weight. This is achieved by elevating the end of the bed so the child moves in the opposite direction to the applied traction.

Methods of applying traction

- **Skin:** adhesive or non-adhesive skin extensions are applied to the limb and bandaged into place.
- **Skeletal:** involves the insertion of a metal pin through the bone which is then attached to a stirrup. The traction cord is attached to this. This type of traction may also include the use of a Thomas splint and a Pearson knee flexion piece.

Care of the traction

- Check the traction a minimum of once per shift and after repositioning of the child. This includes ensuring the frame and attachments are tight, any pulleys are running freely and the cords are securely knotted and not frayed.
- Check the weights are securely fastened and are free of the bed or floor and that the correct weight (as documented in the medical notes) is applied.
- Ensure correct alignment of the child and the cords to ensure the pulling forces are maintained.
- Ensure that counter traction is maintained.
- Ensure skin extensions are in the correct position and bandages have not become loose or slipped.
- The bandages should be removed at least once daily to enable the skin to be checked.
- If a Thomas splint is used then this needs to be checked for correct fitting. The area around the ring should be checked for pressure and swelling.
- For skeletal traction the pin sites should be checked for signs of infection and that the pin has not slipped. The ends of the pins should be covered to prevent injury to the other limb.

General care considerations

Traction restricts the child's independence and movement. Young children may regress in their development and adolescents need to adjust to loss of control over their environment. The abnormal positioning required can cause difficulty with the child's activities of living; however, they adapt quickly. Involving the child as much as possible in their care can help with their adjustment as well as encouraging parental participation.

- **Analgesia:** ensure the child receives adequate pain relief.
- **Skin care:** as well as checking the skin for irritation from the traction, areas prone to pressure due to immobilization should be assessed. Changing the child's position is important. Once settled the child will move position him/herself.
- **Eating and drinking:** this can be difficult because of the position of the child so he/she may need assistance. Adequate nutrition and fluids are required to aid healing and prevent bladder and bowel problems.
- **Elimination:** the child will not be able to go to the toilet so will need to use a bedpan. Urinary stasis may lead to urinary tract infections and the reduced level of activity can lead to constipation. Previously toilet-trained children may regress to bed wetting.
- **Care of pin sites** (see Chapter 87).
- **Neurovascular observations** (see Chapter 90).

90 Neurovascular observations

Figure 90.1 Position of pulse points

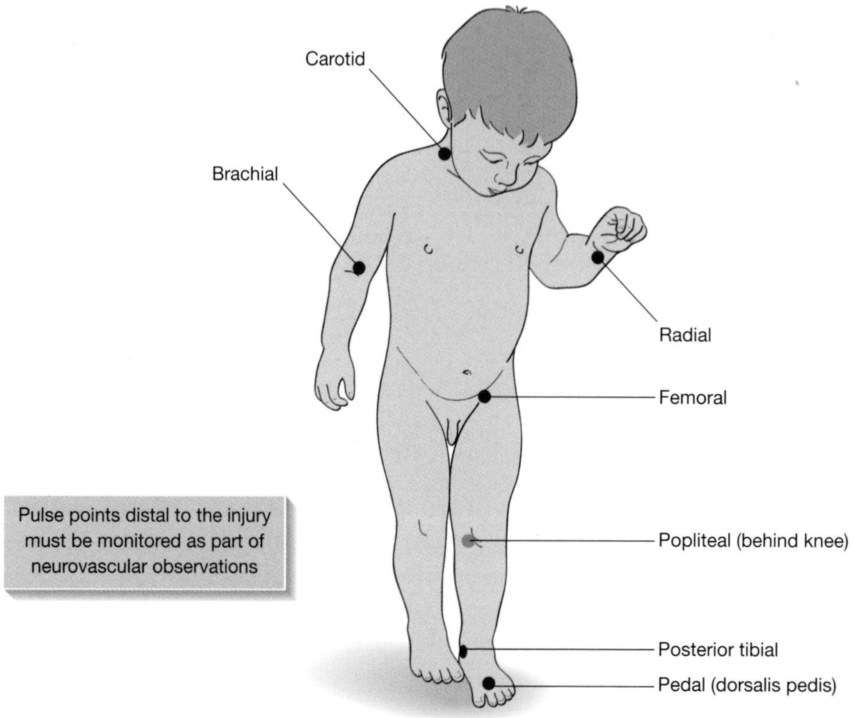
Carotid
Brachial
Radial
Femoral
Pulse points distal to the injury must be monitored as part of neurovascular observations
Popliteal (behind knee)
Posterior tibial
Pedal (dorsalis pedis)

Figure 90.2 Pain assessment

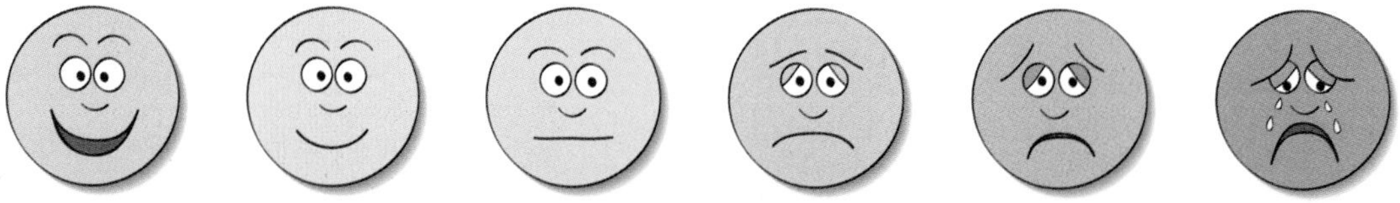

Wong-Baker FACES pain rating scale	**0**	**1**	**2**	**3**	**4**	**5**
	No hurt	Hurts little bit	Hurts little more	Hurts even more	Hurts whole lot	Hurts worst
Alternate coding	**0**	**2**	**4**	**6**	**8**	**10**

Children and Young People's Nursing at a Glance, First Edition. Edited by Alan Glasper, Jane Coad, and Jim Richardson.

For any child or young person who has traction or a cast applied following acute injury or orthopaedic surgery it is essential that neurovascular observations are monitored and recorded to assess the risk of developing complication of recovery (GOSH 2011).

Compartment syndrome, neurovascular deficit and vascular impairment are rare complications of injury and surgery that, if not detected early or left untreated, may result in disability or death of the child or young person (Wright 2009; GOSH 2011). Compartment syndrome usually becomes apparent in the first 72 hours after injury or surgery but may be as soon as 48 hours or as late as 6 days (GOSH 2011). Although there is evidence to suggest that in children it may occur 8 hours after injury (Ferlic et al. 2012).

Compartment syndrome

Muscle, bones and nerve fibres are surrounded by strong non-elastic fibrous tissue – fascia – creating individual compartments that join together to form one. When pressure rises within these compartments the fibrous tissue is unable to accommodate this by stretching which could result in decreased blood flow to the area causing the cells to be starved of oxygen and subsequent ischaemia and death to the tissue. Rise in pressure within the compartments may also be caused by direct injury which would induce an inflammatory response resulting in decreased supply of blood to the tissues and swelling of the limb. This is further impacted with the presence of cast or traction which prevents the skin from swelling, putting further pressure on the structures inside. If compartment syndrome is not noticed quickly it soon leads to necrosis of tissue which can result in amputation of the limb.

Neurovascular observations

By close contact and monitoring of the child or young person, the children's nurse has optimal opportunity to assess for risk by carrying out neurovascular observations (Wright 2009).

Neurovascular observations should include monitoring of numbness or pins and needles, discoloration of toes or fingers. Warmth of extremities should be checked and comparison made between affected and non-affected limb as well as movement of toes, fingers and, if appropriate, the affected limb. An effective tool for neurovascular observations is the five P's (Dykes 1993):

- Pain
- Pallor
- Paraesthesia
- Pulselessness
- Paralysis.

Pain

Pain that is inconsistent with the nature of the injury is an early indicator of damage or risk. Children and young people should have their pain assessed regularly using an age and ability appropriate tool and managed accordingly (RCN 2009).

Pallor

Colour and warmth of the skin of the affected limit is an indicator of good perfusion and circulation. It is essential for the nurse to compare the affected limb with the unaffected limb where applicable. Good colour and warmth are provided by a healthy blood supply to the area but it is important to consider the limb that is overly warm compared with the opposing limb – this could be an indicator of poor venous return caused by obstruction. A cool pale limb could be indicative of poor blood supply.

Peripheral perfusion may also be assessed by measuring capillary refill time by pressing on a digit for 5 seconds and releasing. The digit should recolour within 2 seconds to indicate good perfusion.

Paraesthesia

Sensation of the limb and digits is best performed when the child has their eyes closed or is not watching. Light touch by the finger of the nurse on the affected limb or digits and sensation as described by the child or young person should be compared with the non-affected limb. Any numbness or pins and needles could be indicative of nerve damage as well as reduced perfusion.

Pulselessness

Pulses distal to the injury should be assessed to ascertain circulation compromise. Pulselessness is a late sign of potentially irreversible damage to the limb but it is also important for the nurse to be aware of a strong bounding pulse which could indicate peripheral obstruction to blood flow.

Paralysis

Where limbs, feet or hands are not restricted by casts or traction, flexion and extension of these should be assessed. Even if the child or young person is sleeping, movement should be assessed passively and documented as such. If cast or traction is restricting full movement of foot or hand then digits should be monitored in the same way to assess nerve function.

Further considerations of neurovascular observations

Oozing: it is essential to monitor any blood or fluid loss from the wound, marking the cast where appropriate, during wound care.

Swelling: new or inappropriate swelling could be an indicator of compartment syndrome.

Consent: as with all nursing procedures, it is imperative to explain to the child or young person and parent the purpose of the observations and how these will be carried out. Time must be taken to assist the child with their descriptions of sensation so vital cues are not missed.

Documentation

There is no universal tool that is used to document neurovascular observations but it is the duty of the nurse to ensure documentation is clear, accurate and informed (NMC 2008).

91 Neurological problems

Figure 91.1 The ICF framework

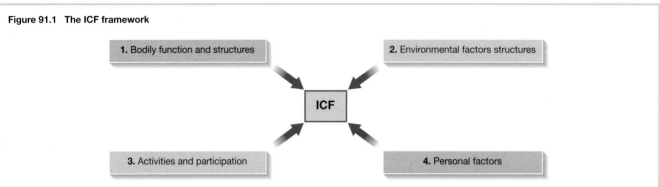

1. Bodily function and structures

2. Environmental factors structures

ICF

3. Activities and participation

4. Personal factors

The International Classification of Functioning, Disability and Health (ICF) provides a standardized and validated framework on which to base assessment of children with multiple needs, particularly those with neurological or developmental deficits. The ICF is used to measure all aspects of health throughout the child's life and focuses on health and functioning rather than on disability.

The ICF can be used for several areas involving clinical, research and policy development issues. This can be at the individual level (e.g. what interventions could maximize functioning), at the institutional level (e.g. what health care services are needed) and at the social level (e.g. is the child eligible for social benefits).

The ICF describes four main elements; these elements are described in detail and incorporated with information about the child's environment to provide a thorough and standardized method of holistic assessment and documentation and include the following conditions.

Cerebral palsy

Cerebral palsy occurs in 2 per 1000 live infants with a higher incidence in males (Forsyth and Newton 2007) and is one of the most common causes of childhood disability and a major cause of severe disability in children. Cerebral palsy is an umbrella term describing a group of disorders that occur during the development of the fetal or infant brain and result in disorders of movement and posture. Dependent on the cause of cerebral palsy, disturbances of sensation, cognition, communication, perception or seizure disorder can also occur.

Some 80–90% of children will survive into adulthood, causes of death being mainly attributed to seizures and respiratory infections (Forsyth and Newton 2007). Management requires interdisciplinary care and therapy and is based on the needs of the individual child, with the focus on enabling functional activity and participation for individuals as well as with other clinical conditions. Outcomes are influenced by personal and environmental factors, including families' socioeconomic status, all of which can serve as barriers or facilitators to functioning.

Headache

Headache is not uncommon in children. The symptoms are dependent on the child's age and the type of headache. The majority of headaches in children are not sinister and are secondary to a viral illness or sinusitis. Differential diagnosis can include tension or cluster headaches and migraine. Less commonly, the cause may be raised intracranial pressure, hypertension, trauma, cerebral haemorrhage or serious infection such as meningitis.

The diagnosis of aetiology of headache is clinical. However, further investigations including radiology should be considered if the symptoms continue and worsen over days to weeks, with or without associated vomiting, or are associated with other physiological changes suggestive of raised intracranial pressure or serious infection, or neurocognitive deterioration, including behaviour.

Treatment is based on potential causes and includes identifying and avoiding triggers, the use of appropriate pharmacology and behavioural and cognitive approaches.

Stroke

Stroke can be defined as a focal neurological deficit with a vascular basis, which lasts over 24 hours and typically presents with hemiparesis and often a visual defect. Transient ischaemic attack (TIA) is similar but lasts under 24 hours.

Headaches, seizures, drowsiness and neck pain are common symptoms associated with paediatric stroke. Stroke affects hundreds of children each year in the United Kingdom and is a common cause of childhood death (Fullerton et al. 2002). Some 50% of children will have a separate medical condition such as sickle cell or cardiac disease and two-thirds of survivors of childhood stroke will have a residual morbidity (Ganesan et al. 2003). Causes of paediatric stroke are arterial ischaemic stroke (AIS), as a result of blood embolus or dissection of an intracerebral artery, vasculopathic (e.g. moya moya syndrome), thrombotic, post varicella, idiopathic; haemorrhagic stroke; venous infarction.

Investigations include CT or MRI scan within 48 hours, or more urgently if the child is deteriorating, echocardiography within 48 hours, cerebrovascular imaging to exclude dissection and investigations for underlying procoagulation tendency. For children with sickle cell disease, exchange transfusion should be undertaken to HbS% <30%.

Treatment for radiologically confirmed AIS is aspirin 5 mg/kg/day, if no haemorrhage or sickle cell disease is present. Treatment for central venous thrombosis is anticoagulation with low weight heparin although the role of thrombolysis is not clear. Prevention of secondary deterioration (e.g. due to seizures) must be initiated, and early rehabilitation commenced. Paediatric stroke guidelines can be found at www.rcplondon.ac.uk/pubs/books/childstroke.

Seizures

A seizure is an abnormal electrical discharge and may produce changes in motor, sensory and cognitive functions. Seizures are of various classifications and require different management protocols (http://www.gosh.nhs.uk/clinical_information/clinical_guidelines/cpg_guideline_00036). Causes include infection, pyrexia, metabolic, trauma, hypoxia, ischaemia, toxicity and electrolyte disorder.

Treatment is based around ABCDE to include termination of seizure, maintenance of vital functions and elimination of any precipitating cause where possible.

Neuromuscular or neuropathic conditions

These can be due to toxins, inflammatory disorders, infection and genetic causes and can include hypotonia, abnormal gait, weakness, fatigue, delayed motor milestones, abnormal reflexes and muscle weakenss. Investigation and diagnosis can be based on investigations including nerve biopsy, radiology, muscle enzyme analysis, genetic testing and tests specific to the potential diagnosis.

Muscular dystrophies

Progressive muscle wasting with joint deformity and decreased mobility occurs but the spectrum varies widely, with Duchenne's muscular dystrophy being one of the most severe types. Treatment is aimed at controlling the onset of symptoms to optimize the quality of life and corticosteroids can be beneficial. The genetic mutation in Duchenne's is carried by the mother and passed mainly to male children. Diagnosis is made by DNA testing and muscle biopsy. Cardiomyopathy and respiratory failure are common and life expectancy is around 25 years of life.

Myasthenia gravis

This autoimmune disease often follows a sudden illness with pyrexia and results in a disorder of neuromuscular transmission (involving acetylcholine) with resulting muscle weakness, fatigue and ptososis. Diagnosis is made by clinical examination, electromyography, Tensilon test (short trial of anticholinesterase) and ice pack test (for evaluation of ptosis). Treatment includes the administration of anticholinesterases for mild cases, pyridostigmine for moderate cases, and plasmapheresis and intravenous immunoglobulins (IVIG) for severe cases. Plasmapheresis (therapeutic plasma exchange) describes the process of separating the patient's blood cells and plasma, and returning the cells to the patient with diluted fresh plasma or a substitute, the aim being to eliminate antibodies from the patient's plasma. IVIG are proteins produced by the immune system, taken from multiple donors and given to the patient intravenously, with the aim of suppressing the inflammatory process. Occasionally, a thymectomy may be required in cases where associated malignancy of the thymus is suspected.

With treatment, children with myasthenia gravis have a normal life expectancy.

Guillan–Barré syndrome

This rare condition is an acute inflammatory demyelination polyneuropathy that occurs following a viral infection. The ascending paralysis spreads rapidly over hours to days and results in respiratory failure. Treatment is supportive plus the administration of plasmapheresis and IVIG. Most children recover after a few weeks although a few may be left with severe disability, involving severe proximal motor and sensory axonal damage.

Metabolic and neurodegenerative disorders

Microcephaly, macrocephaly, developmental delay, hypertonia, hypotonia, abnormal eye signs and cerebellar signs are amongst the many symptoms that should alert the paediatrician to the possibility of metabolic or neurodegenerative disorders in children. Radiology, electromyleography and opthalmology are among the diagnostic tests undertaken. Treatment is mainly supportive, with a poor life expectancy in these patients.

92 Brain injury and coma

Fig 92.1   CT scan demonstrating Extradural Haematoma (EDH)

This can constitute a neurosurgical emergency and result in death unless the haematoma is evacuated promptly. Less severe EDH's can be managed conservatively.

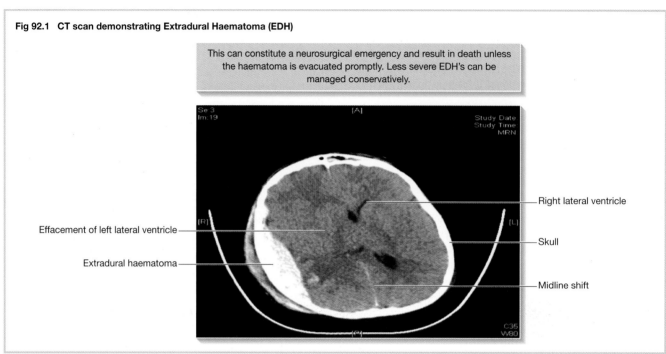

- Effacement of left lateral ventricle
- Extradural haematoma
- Right lateral ventricle
- Skull
- Midline shift

The uncertainty that exists about potential prognosis following traumatic brain injury (TBI) is encapsulated in the Hippocratic aphorism: 'No head injury is so serious that it should be despaired of nor so trivial that it can be ignored.'

Most paediatric head injury is mild; however, head injury remains the most common cause of disability and mortality during childhood, with a mortality rate of 19 per 100 000 in children under 18 years old (Ragheb 2008). Head injury accounts for 5% of all paediatric hospital admissions, with an estimated 3000 children acquiring significant new neurological or cognitive disability annually in the United Kingdom (Sharples 1998).

The age groups most at risk from traumatic brain injury are newborn infants through to age 4, and teens from 15 to 19 years old. The most common cause is road traffic accidents (motor vehicle, bicycle, pedestrian) followed by falls. The best treatment is prevention. Advances in critical care management and reduction of secondary injuries offers the greatest potential to limit the consequences of TBI.

Classification can be mild (based on a Glasgow coma score (GCS) of 13–15), moderate (GCS 9–12) or severe (GCS 3–8).

Physiology

The infant skull is relatively large in comparison to the body and the cervical spine is highly mobile, therefore all children with a history of head trauma must have the neck stabilized at the scene of the accident and maintained until a cervical injury has been ruled out.

Incomplete myelination and less water content in the infant brain means that the young brain is more susceptible to acceleration and deceleration injuries, diffuse axonal injury (DAI) and extraparenchymal haemorrhage. Autoregulation is poor in infants and management must be provided accordingly.

Primary brain injury

This occurs at the time of injury and includes DAI, brainstem injury, cortical contusions and lacerations.

Secondary brain injury

This can occur as a consequence or independent from the primary injury, minutes to days following the injury as a result of adverse physiology, including cerebral oedema, ischaemia, raised intracranial pressure, hypoxia, hypertension, seizures, pyrexia, hyper- and hypoglycaemia and seizures.

Immediate management: this must be prompt and systematic, following paediatric life support principles. Cervical spine injury may occur with paediatric head injury and the cervical spine must be immobilized as a priority:

A Check and maintain airway

B Ensure good oxygenation levels; intubation and ventilation if required

C Circulation must be maintained and blood pressure and pulse kept within normal ranges

D Disability – neurological examination, assessment and treatment; use of paediatric GCS chartand/or AVPU; management of seizure, electrolytes and glucose.

Evaluation and management of other injuries: the key priorities are to stabilize the child and reduce secondary injury. NICE (2007) published evidence-based guidelines for the management of children with head injury, including pre-hospital management, inpatient management and discharge.

Coma

Coma is the most severe impairment of arousal and is defined as an inability to speak, open the eyes to pain or obey commands. It occurs with head injury, secondary to diffuse changes in the cerebral hemispheres and/or dysfunction of the brainstem, electrolyte imbalance and/or seizure activity. Treatment is by management of the underlying cause (e.g. raised intracranial pressure, cerebral oedema) and supportive care (e.g. elective mechanical ventilation).

Pharmacologically induced coma may be required for management of children with severe TBI.

Rehabilitation

Rehabilitation may be appropriate in the home setting with community input, but occasionally prolonged inpatient stay is required. Placement at a specialized paediatric rehabilitation centra may be available or appropriate for some children.

Prognosis

The effects of brain injury in the young child may not become obvious until affected skills are called upon, for example during early school years or during the move to senior school. During these early years the immature brain begins to process more complex information including sensory information.

Long-term deficits may be physical and neurocognitive, the latter including changes in behaviour, mood, speech, memory, learning, attention and executive functions.

Key points

• Accidental head injury is uncommon in infants under 2 years old, therefore the possibility of non-accidental head injury must be considered in this age group and appropriate measures taken.
• The cervical spine should be immobilized as a priority in children with a severe head injury.
• The child with serious head injuries must be transferred to a paediatric intensive care unit where neuroprotection and neurosurgery can be provided if required.
• Rehabilitation can be a long process with an uncertain outcome and should be commenced as soon as possible.

93 Seizures

Figure 93.1   First aid care for a child having a convulsion

- Keep safe, place on side, place something soft under head
- Maintain dignity
- Time seizure, 5-minute duration, contact medical assistance and follow APLS guidelines
- Once seizure has finished, reassure and reorientate child
- Determine possible cause and treat accordingly

Figure 93.2   Types of seizure

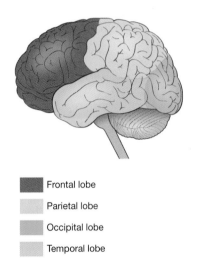

Generalized seizures

Rapid onset and spread of abnormal neuronal activity to the brain resulting in a tonic clonic seizure, child becomes unconscious, a vocal noise may be heard, he/she may fall as limbs become stiff (tonic) and convulse in clonic jerking movements.

Focal seizures

Presentation dependent on lobe of location of abnormal neuronal activity:

Frontal lobe: hypermotor movements

Temporal lobe: altered consciousness, oral and hand automatisms, strange smells, tastes and epigastric rising

Occipital lobe: the seeing of flashing lights, vomiting

Parietal lobe: tingling to hand and face

- Frontal lobe
- Parietal lobe
- Occipital lobe
- Temporal lobe

Children and Young People's Nursing at a Glance, First Edition. Edited by Alan Glasper, Jane Coad, and Jim Richardson.
© 2015 John Wiley & Sons, Ltd. Published 2015 by John Wiley & Sons, Ltd. Companion website: www.ataglanceseries.com/nursing/children

Causes of seizures

Convulsions present as altered consciousness, change in body motor movements, including tonic (stiffening) and clonic (jerking) movements). Potential causes of convulsions need to be considered when nursing the child presenting with seizures:

- Febrile convulsions, usually observed in the child under 5 years with sudden onset of pyrexia, often associated with viral illness
- Metabolic imbalance, including hypoglycaemia (low blood sugar)
- Head trauma: a seizure may indicate increase a rise in intracranial pressure
- Infection, encephalitis or meningitis
- Syncope; a faint caused by a decrease in blood pressure
- Breath holding, hypoxia or reflex anoxic seizures present with tonic movements in response to a sudden painful stimulus
- Alcohol or drug toxicity
- Congenital brain abnormality or tumour may present as focal seizures
- Epilepsy.

Epilepsy

Epilepsy affects 1 in 240 children in the United Kingdom (Epilepsy Action 2013). Epilepsy being the reoccurrence of seizure of primary cerebral origin. The clinical presentation of a seizure may show as a generalized or focal seizure with different observed or experienced symptoms dependent on where in the brain the abnormal activity occurs. A very small percentage of children who experience febrile convulsions will go on to gain a diagnosis of epilepsy. Management of condition will be dependent on cause, type of seizure seen and epilepsy syndrome.

Nursing care

When caring for the child presenting with seizures, it is essential to ensure safe surroundings, protecting them from injury and use a ABCDE approach, timing of seizure, ensuring patent airway; this can be assisted by placing the child on his/her side. If the convulsion has duration of 5 minutes, their own rescue plan or local advanced life support (APLS) guidelines should be followed. It is important to terminate the seizure as soon as possible to reduce the risk of status epilepticus, a continuous seizure of 30 minutes' duration or a cluster of seizures in which the child does not regain consciousness. It should also be acknowledged that many seizures will terminate before admission to the acute setting. In determining the reason for the seizure occurring, a good history from the primary caregiver or a witness is essential; trigger, presentation and recovery from seizure should be obtained. Birth and family history, educational attainment, psychosocial and developmental concerns are also relevant.

Further investigations

Further investigations that may be required to ascertain a diagnosis or to reduce risk of further convulsions are blood and urine tests to rule out infection or metabolic imbalance. A initial blood sugar (BM) test should be completed to rule out hyperglycaemia. ECG to look for cardiac abnormalities and EEG may be useful in aiding or excluding diagnosis of epilepsy, but it is important to be aware that an EEG may be normal in a person with epilepsy and abnormal in a person without epilepsy. Findings should be added to the presentation of seizure history. An EEG would not be indicated in a child with febrile convulsions. An MRI or CT scan would look for brain abnormalities in a child presenting with focal seizures. NICE guidance informs good practice for diagnosis, treatment and appropriate referral to tertiary centres (NICE 2012).

Treatment

Antiepileptic medication (AED) should only be commenced on consultation with a expert practitioner; this would rarely be indicated following the first convulsion. The prescribing of correct AED will acknowledge potential reason for seizure and epilepsy syndrome, with the aim of controlling seizures, on a good dose with minimal adverse effects to medication. Other treatment for refractory, difficult to treat seizures:

- Epilepsy surgery
- Vagal nerve stimulation (VNS)
- Ketogenic diet.

Follow-up care

On discharge, education for the patient and family is very important. An emergency care plan should be discussed if potential risk of prolonged seizure is present, a seizure of duration of 5 minutes and over. A family should be educated in the use of benzodiazepine buccal midazolam, rectal diazepam and first aid information should be offered for people involved in the care of the child, including education. Daily management of risk should be acknowledged including close supervision around water, bike helmets when cycling and a good sleep pattern. It should also acknowledge support offered for comorbidities of learning difficulties and psychosocial anxiety.

94 Meningitis

Figure 94.1 Recognizing symptoms in babies and young children

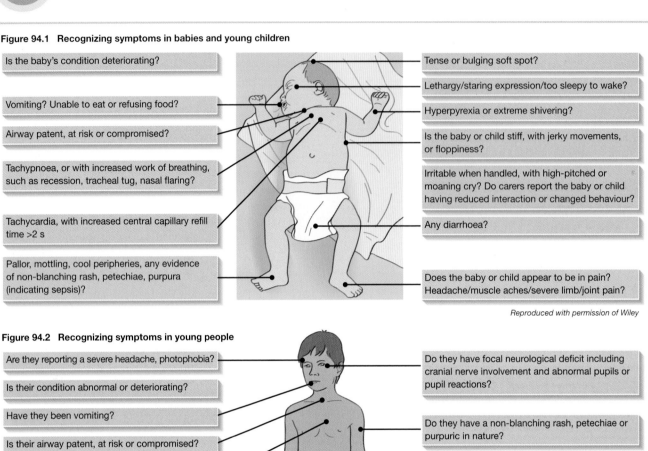

Is the baby's condition deteriorating?

Vomiting? Unable to eat or refusing food?

Airway patent, at risk or compromised?

Tachypnoea, or with increased work of breathing, such as recession, tracheal tug, nasal flaring?

Tachycardia, with increased central capillary refill time >2 s

Pallor, mottling, cool peripheries, any evidence of non-blanching rash, petechiae, purpura (indicating sepsis)?

Tense or bulging soft spot?

Lethargy/staring expression/too sleepy to wake?

Hyperpyrexia or extreme shivering?

Is the baby or child stiff, with jerky movements, or floppiness?

Irritable when handled, with high-pitched or moaning cry? Do carers report the baby or child having reduced interaction or changed behaviour?

Any diarrhoea?

Does the baby or child appear to be in pain? Headache/muscle aches/severe limb/joint pain?

Reproduced with permission of Wiley

Figure 94.2 Recognizing symptoms in young people

Are they reporting a severe headache, photophobia?

Is their condition abnormal or deteriorating?

Have they been vomiting?

Is their airway patent, at risk or compromised?

Are they tachypnoeic, do they have increased work of breathing?

Are they tachycardic, do they have a increased central capillary refill time >2 s?

Do they appear confused, delirious, are they exhibiting signs of deteriorating consciousness or altered mental state?

Are they in a toxic moribund state? Teenagers may be combative, confused or aggressive – you may suspect drug abuse, drunkenness

Do they have focal neurological deficit including cranial nerve involvement and abnormal pupils or pupil reactions?

Do they have a non-blanching rash, petechiae or purpuric in nature?

Are they exhibiting paresis – muscular weakness caused by nerve damage or disease?

Have they had a seizure?

Are they exhibiting Kerning's sign – extension of the knee on a flexed hip at 90° causes restriction and pain?

Are they exhibiting Brudzinski's sign – such as reflex flexion of a lower extremity on passive flexion of the opposite extremity?

Figure 94.3 Signs of acute raised intracranial pressure

The Cushing reflex

Symptoms include:

- Increasing blood pressure and decreasing heart rate due to medullary brain ischemia
- Pupil dilatation
- Coning: the herniation of brain contents: symptoms include worsening bradycardia, hypertension respiratory depression, bilateral papillary dilatation, decerebrate posturing. These will eventually cause death

Figure 94.4 Tumbler test for septicaemia

If a glass tumbler is pressed firmly against a septicaemic rash, the marks will not fade

You will be able to see the rash through the glass. If this happens get medical advice immediately

It is harder to see on dark skin, so check paler areas

Remember someone who is very ill needs medical help even if they have no rash or a rash that fades

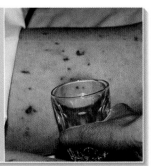

Courtesy of the Meningitis Trust

Children and Young People's Nursing at a Glance, First Edition. Edited by Alan Glasper, Jane Coad, and Jim Richardson.
© 2015 John Wiley & Sons, Ltd. Published 2015 by John Wiley & Sons, Ltd. Companion website: www.ataglanceseries.com/nursing/children

Meningitis remains the leading infectious cause of death in early childhood; it is most common in infants from 1 month to 5 years, or young adults, and affects approximately 2–6 per 100 000.

Meningitis causes an inflammation of the meninges and cerebrospinal fluid, due to a viral or bacterial infection. While viral meningitis is most common, it is usually self-limiting, therefore the focus will be on the management of bacterial meningitis which has an overall mortality rate of 5–10% of cases. Once the central nervous system is infected an inflammatory response is stimulated, this may result in vasculitis, thrombosis, infarction and oedema which may cause raised intracranial pressure (RICP), brain damage and death.

Common causes
- Meningococcus – serotypes A, B, C, Y and W135
- *Pneumococcus*
- *Haemophilus influenzae*
- Rarer causes include tuberculous meningitis, leptospirosis, sarcoidosis, adverse effects of medications such as trimethoprim.

Early recognition, diagnosis and effective management are vital to improve morbidity and mortality outcomes.

Prevention
Introduction of immunizations has led to a rapid reduction in meningitis cases. Under the UK NHS vaccination programme, all children are eligible to receive vaccines against:
- *Haemophilus influenzae* type b (Hib)
- Meningococcus serotype C (Men C)
- Pneumococcus.

Introduction of the Men C vaccine in 1999 decreased the number of people under 20 years diagnosed with serotype C meningitis by 99%. Serotype group B meningococcus is now the most common cause of bacterial meningitis as a vaccine is not yet available.

Assessment
It is essential that children's nurses are able to rapidly assess and recognize any baby, child or young person who presents with the symptoms of meningitis or meningococcal septicaemia (Figures 94.1 and 94.3). Following a subjective and objective A–E structure allows effective assessment of the child. A good assessment is one that is holistic, inclusive and that does not miss anything. This is important as the child may present at any stage of the illness from simply being feverish and irritable to being in decompensated distributive shock.

Planning care
Planning care must focus on the effective management of the problems identified during the assessment process and assisting with investigations to confirm diagnosis.

Primary care
If meningitis is suspected the child should be immediately transferred to an acute hospital environment. If urgent transfer is not possible the GP may initiate antibiotic treatment in accordance with NICE (2013) recommendations.

Secondary care
Effective communication with both the child and family is vital to allow them to make informed decisions regarding care and treatment.

Diagnosis
- History, subjective and objective A–E assessment, consider whether any signs of RICP, or septicaemia such as spreading purpuric rash or 'shock'.
- Bloods for full blood count, CRP, coagulation screen, urea and electrolytes, blood cultures, blood glucose, blood gas and a polymerase chain reaction (PCR) test looking for *Neisseria meningitides*.
- Consider lumber puncture; **contraindications** include the child who is respiratorally, cardiovascularly or neurologically compromised or unstable, this includes any signs of RICP, seizures, shock or extensive or spreading purpura.

Management of bacterial meningitis
NICE (2013) recommend immediate administration of:
- Under 3 months – IV Cefotaxime plus either amoxicillin or ampicillin
- Over 3 months – IV Ceftriaxone plus corticosteroids as per NICE (2013) guidance.

Management of fever and pain
Inflammation of the meninges causes pain, headache, irritability and photophobia. All children with meningitis will also be pyrexial. Treatment with antipyretics and anti-inflammatories is recommended.

Monitoring should be in accordance with the patient's condition; this may be every 30 minutes to 1 hourly initially. It is essential to report any abnormalities immediately. Monitoring must include:
- Patency of airway, respiratory rate and work of breathing
- Manual pulse/apex if under 2 years, use of a cardiac monitor
- Capillary refill time – this should be taken centrally
- Blood pressure
- Oxygen saturation if not peripherally compromised
- Conscious level (AVPU), interaction with carers
- Paediatric Glasgow coma score (PGCS)
- Blood glucose
- Temperature
- Completion of Paediatric Early Warning Scores (PEWS)
- Check for new or developing purpuric rash, spreading purpura as this will indicate the development of septicaemia.

Neurological monitoring
Constant monitoring using the PGCS is recommended.
- Any fluctuation or reduced level of consciousness, a PGCS of less than 15 or a drop of 3 points or more **must** be reported immediately, as a CT scan may be urgently required.
- Changes that indicate RICP **must** be observed for these include reduced or altered interaction with carers, altered tone, altered posture, a high-pitched cry, neck stiffness, back rigidity or photophobia.
- Long term follow up will be required following discharge to identify any late onset issues such as hearing loss, neurological or orthopaedic or psychosocial effects.

Potential complications
The bacteria causing meningitis can also result in septicaemia, a life-threatening systemic disease. As with meningitis, the infection triggers an inflammatory response which includes an acute vascular and cellular response, stimulating an immune response. This results in increased vasodilatation and cell permeability as the neutrophils attempt to reach the site of infection. this may result in distributive or septic shock. Close monitoring is vital to allow early recognition and treatment of septic shock (see Chapter 95).

95 Septicaemia

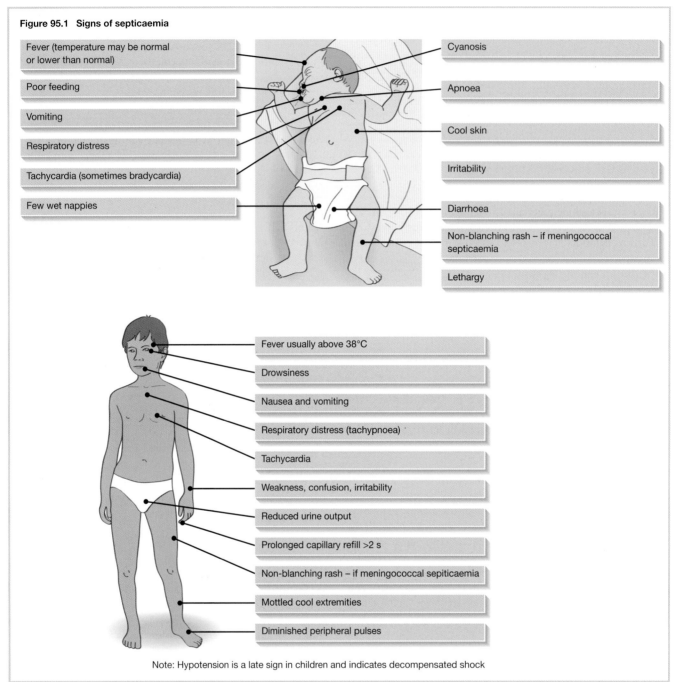

Figure 95.1 Signs of septicaemia

Fever (temperature may be normal or lower than normal)

Poor feeding

Vomiting

Respiratory distress

Tachycardia (sometimes bradycardia)

Few wet nappies

Cyanosis

Apnoea

Cool skin

Irritability

Diarrhoea

Non-blanching rash – if meningococcal septicaemia

Lethargy

Fever usually above 38°C

Drowsiness

Nausea and vomiting

Respiratory distress (tachypnoea)

Tachycardia

Weakness, confusion, irritability

Reduced urine output

Prolonged capillary refill >2 s

Non-blanching rash – if meningococcal sepiticaemia

Mottled cool extremities

Diminished peripheral pulses

Note: Hypotension is a late sign in children and indicates decompensated shock

Children and Young People's Nursing at a Glance, First Edition. Edited by Alan Glasper, Jane Coad, and Jim Richardson.
© 2015 John Wiley & Sons, Ltd. Published 2015 by John Wiley & Sons, Ltd. Companion website: www.ataglanceseries.com/nursing/children

Definition

Septicaemia is defined as the presence of numerous bacteria in the blood that are actively dividing. This results in a systemic response to the infection leading to organ dysfunction. It can be complicated by circulatory collapse, myocardial depression, increased metabolic rate and perfusion abnormalities.

Other terms

Systemic inflammatory response syndrome (SIRS): two of the following four criteria present:
1 Core temperature >38°C or <36°C
2 Severe tachycardia or bradycardia
3 Tachypnoea
4 Raised or reduced leukocyte count.
Sepsis: SIRS in the presence of a proven or suspected infection.
Severe sepsis: sepsis plus one of the following: cardiovascular organ dysfunction or acute respiratory distress syndrome or two or more other organ dysfunction.
Septic shock: sepsis and cardiovascular organ dysfunction.

Management principles

• Recognition of decreased perfusion and altered neurological status
• Assessment needs to follow a logical approach
• Goal of treatment should be resolution of the primary problem, improvement of tissue perfusion and oxygenation
• Need to assess, reassess to determine response to therapy, identify need for changes and detect any deterioration.

Maximize oxygen delivery

• Assessment of airway and breathing
• Is the airway patent?
• Is there respiratory distress?
• Monitor respiratory rate and work of breathing
• Administer high flow oxygen to help with oxygen delivery
• Monitor oxygen saturations (consider where to place the probe in light of poor perfusion)
• Monitor acid–base balance: acidosis can affect oxygen delivery as well as oxygen utilization.

Reduce oxygen demand

• Treat fever
• Treat pain
• Eliminate needless stress.

Optimize cardiac output

• Assess circulation – heart rate, capillary refill, colour
• Correct any acid–base imbalance or electrolyte disturbance as this will affect the ability of the heart to pump
• Give fluid – 20 mL/kg (usually 0/9% saline) as a rapid bolus, then reassess. Use 20 mL/kg increments. May need up to and over 60 mL/kg in the first hour
• Neonates: 10 mL/kg as a rapid bolus then reassess. Use increments of 10 mL/kg
• May need intraosseous access
• Goal is to restore normal perfusion
• May have ongoing fluid requirements
• May need to seek advice from a tertiary paediatric centre.

General considerations

• Appropriate antibiotics
• Care of the family
• Skin care in light of poor perfusion
• Maintain blood sugar within normal limits
• Mouth care
• Prevention of secondary infection
• Nutrition.

⬛ **For specific management of meningococcal septicaemia refer to NICE Guidelines.**

96 Respiratory problems

Figure 96.1   Assessment of the child with a respiratory problem

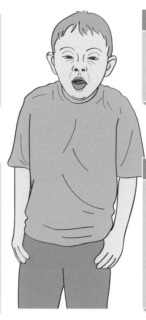

Assess: Sounds and extra noises

- Grunting, heard on expiration
- Stridor, heard on inspiration
- Wheeze, heard on expiration
- Auscultation, crackles, poor air entry

Assess: Other indicators of respiratory problems

- Pulse oximetry
- Blood gas analysis
- Peak flow
- Chest X-ray, microbiology and virology

Assess: Airway and respiratory rate, depth and effort

Look for signs of increased effort which could include:

- Increased respiratory rate and depth
- Mouth pursing
- Grunting
- Nasal flaring
- Head bobbing
- Use of accessory muscles including intercostal, supraclavicular and subcostal recession
- Tracheal tug

Assess: Physical appearance and cardiovascular system

- Skin colour, lips, nails, limbs and warmth
- Does the child look relaxed or anxious
- Capillary refill
- Weak cry
- Heart rate and pulses
- Symmetry of chest movement
- Level of conciousness

History of the presenting complaint	Past history relating to the respiratory problem	Family and social history
• Age of child • Was the onset sudden or was there a preceding illness? • Is there a cough, wheeze or stridor? • Are there difficulties with feeding? • Are there other symptoms than respiratory? • Is there associated vomiting? • Is there a fever? • Is the child using any medication? Has any medication been administered?	• What is the neonatal history? • Has the child had any similar episodes? • Does the child have a diagnosis of asthma or another recent respiratory illness? • Are the child's immunizations up to date?	• Any history of atopy in the family such as asthma, hay fever, eczema? • Are there any siblings or other family members with similar illnesses? • What are the family's living conditions? • Is the child exposed to tobacco smoke? • Do the family have any pets?

Respiratory assessment

Undertaking a comprehensive respiratory assessment is key in deciding the diagnosis and therefore determining the management of a child who presents with a respiratory problem. The key elements of a comprehensive respiratory assessment are:

- History of the presenting complaint
- Past history relating to the respiratory problem
- Family and social history
- Physical assessment of the child.

Once a comprehensive respiratory assessment has been undertaken a diagnosis can be established and treatment and supportive measures instigated.

Bronchiolitis

Bronchiolitis is a seasonal disease which most commonly affects infants aged 3–6 months. The infant presents with breathing difficulties, poor feeding, irritability, wheeze and, in the very young, apnoea. The symptoms of bronchiolitis are coryzal, a harsh cough, wheezing and tachypnoea. Only a small number of infants will require hospitalization. The most common cause of bronchiolitis is respiratory syncytial virus (RSV) which accounts for over 50% of cases. The effects of the virus are to cause inflammation in the small airways which leads to air trapping and a prolonged expiratory phase. Treatment for bronchiolitis is supportive and includes oxygen therapy and feeding support, either enteral or intravenous. Non-invasive ventilation may be required if the infant has persistent apnoea.

Upper airway obstruction

Upper airway obstruction can occur in children of all different ages and there are a variety of causes. It is characterized by stridor which occurs on inspiration. Symptom progression and severity is assessed in relation to the stridor. Stridor on exertion > stridor at rest > recession on exertion > recession at rest > exhaustion, respiratory failure.

Laryngotracheobronchitis

This is the most common cause of upper airway obstruction in children aged 6 months to 6 years. It most commonly occurs in the 1–3 year age group and is usually viral in origin. The main causative virus is parainfluenza. It is characterized by subglottic inflammation and narrowing. The symptoms are usually worse at night. It is usually benign in course but some children will need treatment. This can either be oral steroids, usually dexamethasone, or nebulized budesonide. Both of these treatments have been shown to be effective. It is very important to reduce both the child's and the parents' anxiety.

Epiglottitis

This is a relatively rare respiratory bacterial infection but it is life-threatening. It tends to occur in older children aged 3–6 years and the stridor is accompanied by drooling and a high temperature. The treatment is endotracheal intubation to bypass the obstruction, and intravenous antibiotics. It is important to note that if you suspect epiglottitis you must not extend the neck or place the child in the supine position unless someone is present who can intubate the child as doing either of these things will often precipitate complete airway obstruction.

Foreign body inhalation

The main diagnostic difference between foreign body inhalation and the other causes of upper airway obstruction is the absence of fever or other systemic symptoms. The child will present with stridor and difficulty in breathing but there will be no preceding history and the child will normally have been fit and well beforehand. Treatment of foreign body inhalation involves the identification and removal of the object, usually by bronchoscope.

Respiratory infections

Most respiratory infections of childhood are viral in origin and on the whole self-limiting. However, it is important to consider bacterial infections in children who have persistent symptoms. Bacterial pneumonia should be considered in children who have a persistent or repetitive fever of 38.5°C or above and symptoms of respiratory distress. Treatment is with antibiotics, usually oral.

Common respiratory interventions

Much of the treatment and nursing care that children with respiratory problems receive is focused on assessment and support. The most common respiratory interventions are oxygen therapy, suctioning and positioning.

Oxygen therapy

When choosing the method for administering oxygen the following factors need to be taken into consideration:

- Age of child
- Clinical condition of child
- Percentage or flow rate of oxygen prescribed
- Compliance of child.

Head boxes, nasal cannula and face masks can be used to deliver oxygen to children effectively. Head boxes are most useful in infants and can be used to deliver high concentrations of oxygen. They must always be used with humidification. Nasal cannula can be used to deliver lower flows of oxygen no more than 2 L and are good for children who may need longer term oxygen therapy or short-term postoperative oxygen. Face masks are the most effective method of delivering high concentrations of oxygen to older children who are acutely unwell.

Suctioning

Suctioning is often required for children with respiratory problems. Suctioning can be traumatic for children and it can also cause clinical distress with decreased oxygen saturations and increased work of breathing. Indications for suctioning:

- The child's breathing becomes difficult because of vomiting or excessive secretions, in the oropharynx or nasopharynx.
- The child's skin may look pale, blue or grey, particularly around the mouth or nose.
- The child is coughing excessively and unable to clear secretions.

Positioning

Optimal positioning of children and infants can improve oxygenation and decrease respiratory workload. Positions that can improve work of breathing include:

- Prone positioning
- Sitting upright
- Lying over someone's shoulder.

97 Asthma

Figure 97.1 What is asthma?

Symptoms

- Wheeze
- Cough day and night (night time cough is significant in diagnosis)
- Difficulty in breathing
- Tightness in the chest

Diagnosis

Asthma affects children of all ages and with differing degrees of severity. Diagnosis in the under-3 age group is particularly difficult to give a definitive diagnosis because of the immature smooth muscle in the lungs and therefore its capacity to respond to bronchodilator medication. Diagnosis at any age can be problematic as there is no one definitive gold standard test that can be carried out to confirm this. Diagnosis should be based on:

- Full history, including atopy and other allergies
- Physical examination, bloods for IgE and rast levels
- Results of spriometry
- Consideration of differential diagnosis
- Response to treatment with a bronchodilator

Physiology

In response to asthma allergens or triggers, the lining of the bronchioles become swollen, inflamed and oedema is present within the bronchial tissue. As the inflammation becomes persistent, a number of changes happen in the airway including epithelial cells sloughing off the airway wall which mixes with mucous resulting in thick plugs being formed. This increase in mucous and narrowing of the airway results in bronchoconstriction, characterized by wheeze, cough, shortness of breath and difficulty in breathing. Airways can become permanently narrowed as a result of numerous repeated asthma attacks.

What happens to the airways during an asthma attack?

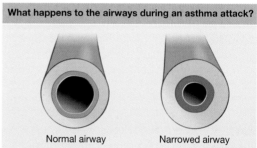

Normal airway   Narrowed airway

Asthma is triggered by a number of environmental factors:

- Grass pollen
- Viral infections, coughs and cold
- Smoking, passive smoking
- Household dust mite
- Hair and dander from pets and animals
- Stress and anxiety
- Exercise
- Chemicals, perfumes, paint
- Changes in humidity and temperature
- Exhaust fumes, pollution
- Sawdust

Goals of treatment

- Abolish symptoms during night and day
- Reduce the number of attacks and reduce school absences
- Adequate control with minimal medication, reviewed regularly, stepped up and down regularly
- Prevent hospital admissions, manage condition at home through evidence-based practice, self-management plans, peak flow measurement, education and support. This can be achieved by utilizing the resources within school nursing and specialist nursing roles both within the hospital and primary care settings.

Treatment

The British Thoracic Society and Scottish Intercollegiate Guidelines (2009), updated in 2012, advise on appropriate treatment for children and young people according to age. Treatment usually consists of use of a bronchodilator using a spacer device as and when needed. If this is required on a regular basis, a preventer inhaler (inhaled steroid) will be prescribed to be taken in the morning and at night using a spacer device. Treatment is stepped up and down as symptoms improve or deteriorate. Regular review of symptoms is essential via primary care and a full table of prescribing is available via the above guideline.

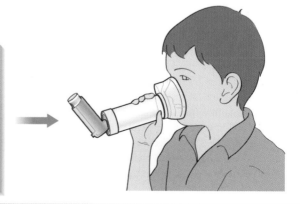

Children and Young People's Nursing at a Glance, First Edition. Edited by Alan Glasper, Jane Coad, and Jim Richardson.
© 2015 John Wiley & Sons, Ltd. Published 2015 by John Wiley & Sons, Ltd. Companion website: www.ataglanceseries.com/nursing/children

Asthma

Asthma is the most common chronic disease in childhood, with a child being hospitalized every 7 minutes in the United Kingdom. The disease has a genetic predisposition combined with environmental factors. There is also a link to related conditions which include hay fever, eczema and allergy and it is common for children to be on several different medications to control each of the related conditions. There are estimated to be over 1.1 million children with the condition, with an average of two children in every school class. Asthma attacks all age groups but often starts in childhood. It is more common in boys than girls until puberty is reached. The disease is characterized by recurrent episodes of breathlessness and wheezing which vary in frequency and severity from person to person. The condition is due to inflammation of the lining of the bronchioles in the lungs and affects the sensitivity of the nerve endings in the airways so they become easily irritated. During an asthma attack the lining of the small passages swell causing the airways to narrow and reduce the flow of air into the lungs.

Psychosocial impact of asthma

As with any chronic long-term condition, asthma can have a dramatic impact on the quality of life and career choices of many young people. Children with asthma have sometimes been reported to be bullied in school and can have frequent episodes of absence due to poorly controlled asthma. For some children this can lead to academic failure resulting in low self-esteem. In addition to this, exercise is a known trigger for asthma and poor control of symptoms and incorrect use of inhalers prior to sport and physical exercise can also lead to poor performance impacting further on a sense of failure. Stress and emotions can also trigger asthma so in some areas of asthma care cognitive behavioural therapy (CBT) is now being used. This has encouraged children and young people that the concept of CBT combined with good asthma management support from parents, school nurses, primary care health professionals and teachers can lead to a positive approach that can improve performance, quality and psychological well-being.

Role of Asthma UK

Asthma UK is a charitable organization that provides advice, education, information and support for families and professionals on all aspects of asthma care from diagnosis throughout life. Information is evidence-based on current research and findings and the organization is seen by all professionals as an excellent and reliable source of information for children, young people and their families. Their website is updated regularly and information can be requested free of charge in most cases for a variety of information. In particular, resources for school staff with regard to education about the condition itself have been particularly useful in promoting good asthma management in schools. Due to several high profile deaths of school-aged children with asthma over recent years there has been an increase in the demand for information available within schools to promote good asthma care. Asthma UK regularly carries out research with young people who have the condition and acts in an advocacy role in promoting the needs of children with asthma.

Treatment and management

There are many different types of treatment for asthma but most treatment consists of the use of different types of inhalers. In most instances the child will be prescribed a bronchodilator (also known as a reliever inhaler) which relaxes the smooth muscle in the small airways making it easier for the child to breathe. This is taken on an as needed basis and its use should be monitored by a health care professional. If the reliever is required on a regular basis a second inhaler is usually prescribed and this acts as a protector. This inhaler provides protection to the bronchioles and, if taken regularly morning and night, this will help to reduce the inflammation in the lungs and control symptoms such as night time coughing and recurrent attacks. This type of inhaler is an **inhaled steroid** and the use of this drug should be regularly reviewed by a health care professional. There are many other types of inhalers including combined or long-acting inhalers and also oral medication can be used in combination with inhalers. Inhalers are also referred to as metered dose inhalers (MDI). The British Thoracic Society (2008) and Scottish Intercollegiate Guidelines (2009) updated in 2012, provide evidence-based guidance for prescribers on all aspects of drug therapy, investigation, diagnosis and symptom management.

Review

Regular review of symptoms and completion of symptom diaries to include use of inhaler can be a useful tool for members of the primary care health team in managing asthma. Self-management plans are advocated for all with clear instructions and guidance around when to act on an increase in symptoms and how to manage this avoiding hospital admission and minimizing risk to the patient. Treatment should be stepped up and down according to symptoms. with minimal medication being taken.

Peak flow measurements are also seen as a useful tool in assessing lung function within the hospital, home or school setting and can be used as an additional tool of assessment for some children who are able to manage to use the peak flow monitor appropriately. This should always be considered along with the severity of symptoms in an attack or prior to an attack. One of the most significant methods to improve the delivery of drug through an MDI is to use a plastic spacer device to deliver the drug. This can enhance the effectiveness of the drug by delivering the full dose and with good technique can ensure that the drug reaches the lungs rather than being swallowed. A face mask can also be used with the spacer so it can be used for infants and young children.

Inhaler technique should always be checked and reinforced at every opportunity along with continued education about the condition itself, avoidance of exposure to triggers and a reminder about the different uses of each type of inhaler or medication prescribed.

Emergency management

This should be discussed and reinforced at every opportunity by the health care professional. In an emergency, one puff of the child's blue reliever should be given via the spacer, with one puff per minute given for 10 minutes or continued until help arrives. The inhaler should be shaken between each puff.

98 CPAP and BiPAP

Figure 98.1 Causes of respiratory failure

Category of impairment	Examples
Impaired ventilation	
Upper airway obstruction	• Laryngospasm • Foreign body aspiration • Epiglottitis • Tumour of the upper airways
Weakness or paralysis of the respiratory muscles	• Drug overdose • Injury to the spinal cord • Poliomyelitis • Guillain–Barré syndrome • Muscular dystrophy • Disease of the brainstem
Chest wall injury	• Rib fracture • Burn eschar
Impaired matching of ventilation and perfusion	• Chronic obstructive lung disease • Restrictive lung disease • Severe pneumonia • Atelectasis
Impaired diffusion	
Pulmonary oedema	• Left heart failure • Inhalation of toxic materials
Respiratory distress syndrome	• Respiratory distress syndrome in the neonate

Figure 98.2 Causes of respiratory distress

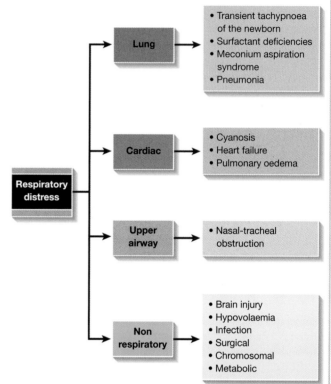

Respiratory distress

Lung
• Transient tachypnoea of the newborn
• Surfactant deficiencies
• Meconium aspiration syndrome
• Pneumonia

Cardiac
• Cyanosis
• Heart failure
• Pulmonary oedema

Upper airway
• Nasal-tracheal obstruction

Non respiratory
• Brain injury
• Hypovolaemia
• Infection
• Surgical
• Chromosomal
• Metabolic

Figure 98.3 CPAP/BiPAP mask

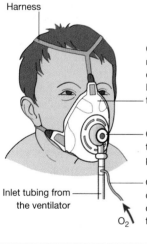

Harness

CPAP/BiPAP masks cover the nose and mouth. A nasal mask or prongs may also be used. Ensure that the mask is correctly fitted to create a good seal

Outlet valves may determine the expiratory positive airways pressure

Inlet tubing from the ventilator

Oxygen is entrained into the circuit. Therefore the F_iO_2 cannot be set only the O_2 flow rate (L/min)

O_2

Figure 98.4 Non-invasive ventilator

• Explain the procedure to the child
• Ensure the pressures are set accurately and that the back-up rate is set
• Ensure the correct size mask is used

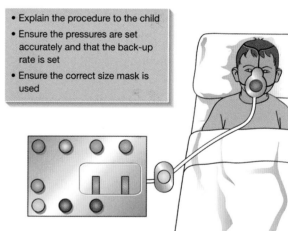

Children and Young People's Nursing at a Glance, First Edition. Edited by Alan Glasper, Jane Coad, and Jim Richardson.
© 2015 John Wiley & Sons, Ltd. Published 2015 by John Wiley & Sons, Ltd. Companion website: www.ataglanceseries.com/nursing/children

Respiratory failure

Continuous positive airway pressure (CPAP) and bi-level positive airway pressure (BiPAP) are commonly utilized methods of non-invasive ventilation used to treat both acute (in hospital) and chronic (in the home) respiratory failure in children. Respiratory failure can occur acutely in children who were previously well, or chronically, as a result of lung or chest wall disease.

Respiratory failure is not a specific disease and occurs when the lungs are unable to oxygenate the blood adequately or are unable to prevent carbon dioxide retention, even at rest. There are three types of conditions that contribute to the hypoxia in respiratory failure: **hypoventilation, impaired diffusion across the alveolar-capillary membrane and mismatching of ventilation and perfusion.**

The causes of respiratory failure can be summarized according to each category (Figure 98.1).

Continuous positive airway pressure and bi-level positive airway pressure

The aims of both CPAP and BiPAP are to prevent worsening respiratory failure and respiratory distress, and to alleviate the child's discomfort. Causes of respiratory distress are not always due to a primary respiratory problem or disease (Figure 98.2).

CPAP and BiPAP can be delivered via a face mask, nasal mask or prongs. When considering which mode to use, it is vital to understand the ways in which they work.

CPAP promotes respiratory function by preventing airway collapse and loss of lung volume. The functional residual capacity is increased, thereby increasing the surface area available for gas exchange and so reducing the work of breathing. It is most commonly used for infants with bronchiolitis, apnoea or children with obstructive sleep apnoea, for weaning from mechanical ventilation or upper airway obstruction. **CPAP is contraindicated in the child who has a reduced level of consciousness and who is not spontaneously breathing.**

BiPAP combines the benefits of CPAP with keeping the lungs open throughout the entire respiratory cycle. Both the inspiratory and expiratory pressures can be manipulated on BiPAP machines, along with rate and a back-up breath rate. Using BiPAP can improve minute ventilation and oxygenation, thereby reducing the work of breathing.

CPAP and BiPAP may not be well tolerated by children, causing agitation, cardiovascular instability, confusion and further exacerbating the hypoxia. The need for sedation and pain relief should be considered. Further complications include gastric distension or perforation, therefore a nasogastric tube should be inserted and kept drainage free; increased airway resistance; and pulmonary air leaks (pneumothorax).

It is crucial to monitor the ECG and SaO_2 continuously and to document the vital signs hourly. Hourly documentation of the pressure settings and respiratory rate and effort should also be undertaken while the child is receiving CPAP or BiPAP. Blood gas assessment should be undertaken regularly, and senior medical help should be close by at all times.

Further considerations

Ensure accurate sizing of the mask or prongs. The equipment and settings should be checked hourly and documented. Appropriately sized emergency airway equipment and suction should be at the bedside.

Position changes to relieve the pressure of the nasal prongs or mask should be part of the routine care of the child and trying to cluster the cares can reduce the oxygen demand and minimize their distress.

The use of CPAP or BiPAP for acute respiratory failure should be carried out in a paediatric high dependency setting and only those members of staff who are trained and assessed as being competent should be involved in caring for the child receiving CPAP or BiPAP.

If a child requires CPAP or BiPAP, their condition could become worse at any stage and may precipitate the need for invasive ventilation. Therefore, close monitoring, documentation and communication with the tertiary referral centre (paediatric intensive care) is essential. Treatment of the underlying pathology is crucial.

99 Cardiovascular assessment and shock

Figure 99.1 Cardiovascular assessment

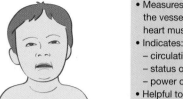

Currently, there is no reliable technology to provide exact values for cardiac output or its components. However, assessments can be performed to provide a picture of the child's cardiac output state.

ECG

- Indication of the electrical current moving through the heart muscle to make it function
- Always associate the trace with feeling for a pulse
- *Beware*: pulseless electrical activity (PEA) is when the ECG can appear normal yet the patient no longer has a cardiac output

Pulse

- Feeling for a pulse will provide more sensitive information about cardiac output than a rate alone
- Assessing the quality of the pulse (whether it is bounding or thread or not) will give an indication of:
  – power and regularity of heart beat
  – patient's volume status
  – peripheral perfusion along with patient's colour and warmth of limb
- Good sites to feel for pulses in children are:
  – brachial
  – femoral
  – radial

Blood pressure

- Measures pressure exerted by blood on the walls of the vessel during contraction and relaxation of the heart muscle
- Indicates:
  – circulating volume
  – status of the vessel walls
  – power of the heart muscle
- Helpful to an overall picture of a child's cardio-vascular status
- *Beware:* a low BP is a late sign, suggesting the child is no longer able to maintain their cardiac output

Capillary refill

- Performed by depressing an area of the sternum or a fingertip for 5 seconds and then observing the time it takes for blood to be restored to the area
- Normal is less than 3 seconds
- Note: when assessing a fingertip, it is important that the finger is either in-line or above the heart to ensure it is the power of the heart that is being assessed and not gravity
- *Beware:* capillary refill may be influenced by the environmental temperature

Urine output

A reduction in perfusion to the kidneys causes a chain reaction in the rennin-angiotensin pathway which governs the production of urine. This results in not only increased sympathetic activity and systemic vascular resistance, but also causes the body to retain water to optimize circulating volume. The obvious result of this is a reduction in the child's urine output. Assessment of urine output will also provide further indications of his/her cardiovascular status

Children and Young People's Nursing at a Glance, First Edition. Edited by Alan Glasper, Jane Coad, and Jim Richardson.
© 2015 John Wiley & Sons, Ltd. Published 2015 by John Wiley & Sons, Ltd. Companion website: www.ataglanceseries.com/nursing/children

Cardiac output

The primary function of the cardiovascular system is to transport oxygen, nutrients and substrates around the body, thus ensuring that the appropriate amounts of these products are present to meet the metabolic demands within the cells.

The prime determinant of efficacy of the transport system is cardiac output. Cardiac output is the amount of blood that is ejected from the heart every minute and is the product of the equation:

$$\text{heart rate} \times \text{stroke volume}$$

Stroke volume is the amount of blood that is ejected from the heart with each beat. Stroke volume is determined by three factors:

1 *Preload:* affected by the volume status of a patient
2 *Afterload:* impacted by the systemic vascular resistance
3 *Contractility:* the power created by the heart muscle to pump the blood around the body.
An analogy to describe this is a hosepipe with an adjustable nozzle.

1 *Preload:* the water flowing through the hosepipe
2 *Afterload:* degree of nozzle adjustment, which will either cause the water to leave the hosepipe in a spray or a narrow jet
3 *Contractility:* amount the tap is turned to allow water through the hosepipe.

These factors of heart rate and stroke volume (encompassing preload, afterload and contractility) adjust to maintain the cardiac output to meet the metabolic demands. Children, in particular, are unable to adjust their contractility in the same way that adults can to maintain their cardiac output. A sudden reduction in preload cannot easily be corrected by the body and alterations to afterload will have a limited affect by itself. Therefore, the only means younger children have of maintaining cardiac output when compromised is to increase their heart rate.

An increase in heart rate can be very effective in improving cardiac output; however, the heart requires time to fill and eject blood. Therefore, an increased heart rate results in less time for filling and ejection to occur. After the heart rate has reached an optimum point, as it increases further, cardiac output will actually begin to reduce. This means children's nurses should carefully consider the cause of tachycardia, as this is the main compensatory mechanism used to maintain cardiac output. Eventually, an increased heart rate will not effectively maintain cardiac output and the child has no other mechanism to compensate for this.

Shock

Shock is the body's inability to maintain its cardiac output (low cardiac output state), resulting in inadequate delivery of oxygen, nutrients and substrates to meet the body's metabolic demands. The consequence is anaerobic respiration causing tissue damage and cell death.

Shock is divided into categories that indicate the cause; however, it is more important to recognize that the patient is shocked first rather than focus on the cause.

Hypovolaemic shock

• Inadequate blood volume in the body.
• Preload is the component of cardiac output that is affected.
• Management is primarily focused on giving fluid to improve the child's volume status.
• Examples of hypovolaemic shock are children with diarrhoea and vomiting or trauma.

Cardiogenic shock

• The heart muscle is not able to generate enough power to pump blood out of the heart effectively.
• Contractility is the component of cardiac output most affected.
• Management focuses on giving drugs to improve the contractility of the heart and where possible reducing the work the heart has to do.
• *Beware:* giving fluid may make the heart work harder so will cause these patients to get worse. As a result it must be given with caution while assessing the impact on the cardiac output.
• Examples are diseases of the heart muscle (cardiomyopathy) or post cardiac surgery.

Distributive shock

• Tone of the vascular system allows for blood volume to be distributed into the wrong areas.
• Afterload is the component of cardiac output most affected
• Management focuses on:
  giving fluids to replace the volume that has moved into the surrounding tissue
  encouraging fluid back into the intravascular space
  improving blood vessels' tone with drugs or cooling so volume will not leak out. Examples are septic shock and anaphylaxis.

100 Inflammatory bowel disease

Figure 100.1   Main inflammatory bowel diseases

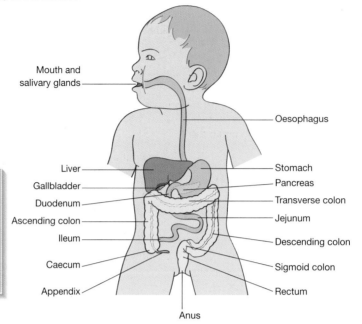

Mouth and salivary glands

Oesophagus

Liver

Stomach

Gallbladder

Pancreas

Duodenum

Transverse colon

Ascending colon

Jejunum

Ileum

Descending colon

Caecum

Sigmoid colon

Appendix

Rectum

Anus

Ulcerative colitis only affects the colon, also known as the large intestine (ascending, transverse, descending, sigmoid colon, rectum and anus). The inflammatory process involves the lining of the bowel causing superficial ulceration

Crohn's disease can affect any part of the gastrointestinal tract, from the mouth to the anus. The inflammation process is described as patchy transmural inflammation (the bowel lining and the deeper layers maybe affected)

Figure 100.2   Signs and symptoms of inflammatory bowel disease

- Abdominal pain
- Diarrhoea
- Urgency to use the toilet
- Passing blood or mucous per rectum
- Blood in stool
- Nausea
- Vomitting
- Loss of appetite
- Weight loss
- Tiredness and lethargy
- Delay in growth and puberty
- Mouth ulcers

Extraintestinal symptoms include skin rashes (erythema nodosum), inflammation of the eye (iritis or uveitis) and joint problems

Figure 100.3   Treatments for inflammatory bowel disease

- Aminosalicylates (mesalazine and sulfasalazine), available in oral and rectal preparations
- Corticosteroids (available as intravenous, oral and rectal preparations)
- Exclusive liquid diet (first line treatment for Crohn's disease)
- Immunosuppressants (azathioprine, 6-mercaptopurine, methotrexate and ciclosporin)
- Biologics (infliximab and adalimumab)
- Surgery (different procedures will be used for ulcerative colitis and Crohn's disease)

Treatment choices will be dependent on the disease activity, extent and distribution. These treatments maybe used on their own or in combination

Children and Young People's Nursing at a Glance, First Edition. Edited by Alan Glasper, Jane Coad, and Jim Richardson.
© 2015 John Wiley & Sons, Ltd. Published 2015 by John Wiley & Sons, Ltd. Companion website: www.ataglanceseries.com/nursing/children

Inflammatory bowel disease (IBD) comprises two lifelong chronic diseases characterized by episodes of remission and relapse: ulcerative colitis and Crohn's disease. It is important to recognize that IBD is not the same as irritable bowel syndrome (IBS) and is not infectious. The cause for IBD remains unknown but it is thought to be the product of a complex interaction of multiple factors: a genetic predisposition and an abnormal reaction of the immune system to certain bacteria in the intestines, possibly triggered by something in the environment. Triggers such as viruses, bacteria, diet and stress have been identified but there is no evidence that any one of these factors is wholly responsible (Crohn's and Colitis UK 2011).

IBD and children

It is understood that the incidence of IBD has been steadily increasing over recent years. Up to 25% of IBD patients are diagnosed below the age of 18 years (Beattie 2010). IBD is commonly diagnosed during adolescence and puberty, a vulnerable time for growth, as well as psychosocial development and education. It is therefore essential that a multidisciplinary team approach is taken when caring for children and families diagnosed with IBD.

Diagnostic tools

Prior to any invasive investigations it is important that a comprehensive clinical history and examination are completed. This will enable the clinician to make a differential diagnosis of IBD before proceeding. Although blood tests are not diagnostic, they can give some indication to whether an inflammatory process is occurring. It is essential that stool cultures exclude any infective source that may be contributing to the child's symptoms. The IBD Working Group of BSPGHAN (2008) suggest that all children suspected of having IBD should have an upper and lower gastrointestinal endoscopy with intubation of the terminal ileum and multiple biopsies from all segments of the intestinal tract should be taken for histological diagnosis. Following this, it is important to establish the extent of the disease process (small bowel and pelvis if clinically indicated) for future care planning; this will be completed with the use of MRI. By using a variety of clinical tools, the clinician is able to build a road map of disease extent and activity; this is essential when planning the child's treatment.

Considerations for children and families diagnosed with IBD

Although IBD can be treated with medical and surgical interventions there is no cure. Being diagnosed with a long-term chronic condition is hard for both the child and family to come to terms with, so it is important that appropriate support is offered via a variety of services (specialist nurse, psychological help and patient support groups). Support systems encourage the child and family to take ownership of the condition; this has a major impact on compliance and concordance to treatment plans.

The aim of treatment for children with a long-term condition is to manage their illness in such a way that they can achieve lifetime goals and make a positive contribution through appropriate education. It is therefore vital that effective communication occurs between health and education services. Teachers need to be aware of the special needs that a child with IBD may have and a school care plan constructed to include points such as easy and discreet access to the toilet. Teachers need to be aware of the issues that could prime bullying, for example prolonged absences from school, delayed growth and puberty, rapidly changing body image depending upon disease activity and treatments (steroid treatment can often cause excessive weight gain, spots and mood swings).

During the childhood years it is commonly the parent's responsibility to ensure compliance and concordance with medication and treatment plans. Adolescence is a tricky time of life for everyone and increasingly so for those with long-term medical conditions. Transitional care programmes are essential for the effective transfer of information, aiming for lifelong support and thus compliance and, ultimately, patient safety. Mamula et al. (2003) predicted that a transitional care programme would improve compliance with medical therapies, effective planning of long-term life goals, independent living skills and improve health-related quality of life, not just in the short term but lifelong.

101 Gastro-oesophageal reflux

Figure 101.1   Gastro-oesophageal reflux

1. Common symtoms of reflux

- Vomiting (projectile, bile or blood)
- Excessive crying
- Refusal to feed
- Abdominal distension
- Severe constipation
- Bloody or dark stools
- Weight loss, or poor weight gain
- Lethargy
- Choking or blue spells

2. Diagnostic investigations

- Endoscopy (upper gastrointestinal)
- Barium swallow and follow through
- Multichannel intraluminal impedance (MII) PH/impedance studies
- Oesophageal manometry

3. Non-medical treatments for reflux

- Elimination of cow's milk and cow's milk protein
- Thickening milk
- Avoid over-feeding
- Wind the baby frequently before, during and after feeding
- Keep the baby upright for at least 30 minutes after feeding
- Where possible try not to lay infant flat – and angle greater than 30° is recommended for sleep time and when changing the babies nappy
- Avoid using car seats immediately after feeding

4. Medical treatments

- Infant Gaviscon
- Histamine-2-receptor antagonists (H2-blockers)
- Proton pump inhibitors (PPI)
- Prokinetic agents (motility drugs)
- Vitamin and mineral supplements

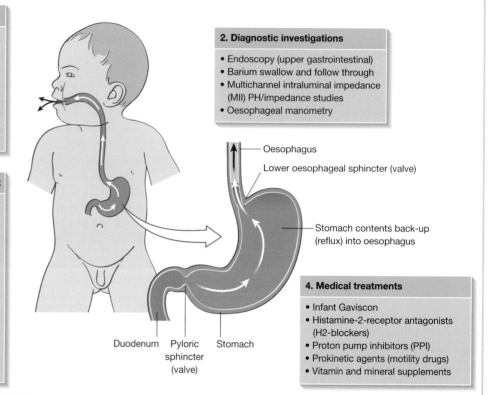

Oesophagus

Lower oesophageal sphincter (valve)

Stomach contents back-up (reflux) into oesophagus

Duodenum   Pyloric sphincter (valve)   Stomach

Children and Young People's Nursing at a Glance, First Edition. Edited by Alan Glasper, Jane Coad, and Jim Richardson.
© 2015 John Wiley & Sons, Ltd. Published 2015 by John Wiley & Sons, Ltd. Companion website: www.ataglanceseries.com/nursing/children

What is reflux?

Gastro-oesophageal reflux (GOR) is the passage of gastric contents into the oesophagus. This occurs normally in all infants, children and adults during and immediately after meals. It is considered physiological when symptoms are absent or not troublesome, and in most cases resolves spontaneously.

Gastro-oesophageal reflux disease (GORD) is present when there are symptoms that are troublesome, severe or chronic, or when there are complications arising from GOR. The most common complication is tissue damage or inflammation to the oesophagus (oesophagitis).

What causes reflux?

GOR occurs as a result of transient lower oesophageal sphincter relaxation. There are several anatomical and physiological features that make infants (younger than 1 year of age) more prone to GOR than older children and adults: having a short narrow oesophagus; delayed gastric emptying; shorter lower oesophageal sphincter that is slightly above the diaphragm; having a liquid diet and high calorie requirement which can put a strain on gastric capacity; and having a larger ratio of gastric volume to oesophageal volume.

It is also important to consider that GOR and GORD may be caused by an allergy to cow's milk protein.

How is reflux diagnosed?

In the first instance, reflux is usually diagnosed by symptoms alone. The main symptoms identified are frequent and troublesome vomiting or regurgitation (this may occur up to 2 hours after feeding), as well as frequent and troublesome crying, irritability or back-arching during or after feeding. This may also be accompanied by refusing feed.

In order to confirm and assess the severity of reflux, and to rule out any abnormalities that could be at the root of the reflux symptoms, specialists may consider conducting diagnostic investigations.

Multichannel intraluminal impedance (MII) PH/impedance test is one of the most commonly used of investigations. The test is conducted by passing a tube with multichannel sensors through the nostril of the child. The tube has a sensor that sits in the stomach and one that sits just above the lower oesophageal sphincter. The advantage of this test is that it is able to detect both acid and alkaline reflux travels, and investigates the correlation between symptom association, meal times and patient position (e.g. nocturnal symptoms which may be exacerbated when lying down flat).

Treatments for GOR and GORD

Non-medical therapies for GOR have been proven to be effective in many cases. Thickened feeds, the elimination of cow's milk and cow's milk protein (from the mother's diet in the case of breastfed infants) as well as other recommended methods should be trialled for 2–3 weeks. If successful, these should be continued for 3 months or until weaning.

Medical treatments include Infant Gaviscon which helps thicken the milk; histamine-2-receptor antagonists (H2-blockers), such as ranitidine, work by blocking or preventing the production of gastric acid; proton pump inhibitors (PPI), such as omeprazole or lansoprazole, work by stopping gastric acid production at its source. Prokinetic agents, such as domperidone, work by speeding up the emptying stomach and helping close the lower oesophageal sphincter.

Do infants grow out of GOR?

Most infants showing signs of GOR will grow out of it between the ages of 12 and 15 months. As young children grow, most cases of reflux will settle when mixed feeding is introduced and when there is an increased effect of gravity on infants as they become more upright and ambulant.

Key points

- GOR is the physiological passage of gastric content into the oesophagus.
- GORD is classified when reflux symptoms become troublesome causing complications such as oesophagitis.
- Most children will grow out of GOR between the ages of 12 and 15 months.

102 Coeliac disease

Figure 102.1 What causes coeliac disease?

Coeliac disease is an autoimmune condition that is caused by an abnormal immune reaction to the protein gluten found in foods such as cereal, bread, pasta and biscuits

Figure 102.2 Common symptoms

- Diarrhoea, excessive wind and constipation
- Persistent or inexplained gastrointestinal symptoms (e.g. nausea and vomiting)
- Stomach pain, cramping or bloating
- Iron, vitamin B12 or folic acid deficiency
- Weight loss
- Lethargy
- Mouth ulcers
- Poor growth

Figure 102.3 The Crossed Grain symbol

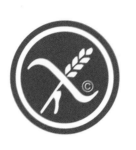

Created by Coeliac UK and promoted by coeliac organizations worldwide – is a food labelling symbol that confirms that a labelled food product is gluten-free

Figure 102.4 Medical treatments

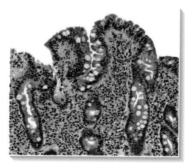

Endoscopy image of person with coeliac disease, showing scalloping of folds and 'cracked-mud' appearance to mucosa

Figure 102.5 Normal villi and damaged villi in coeliac disease

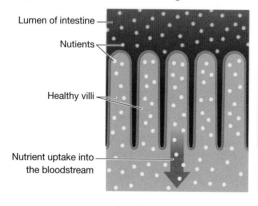

Lumen of intestine — Nutients — Healthy villi — Nutrient uptake into the bloodstream

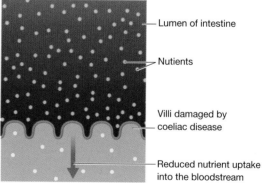

Lumen of intestine — Nutients — Villi damaged by coeliac disease — Reduced nutrient uptake into the bloodstream

Children and Young People's Nursing at a Glance, First Edition. Edited by Alan Glasper, Jane Coad, and Jim Richardson.
© 2015 John Wiley & Sons, Ltd. Published 2015 by John Wiley & Sons, Ltd. Companion website: www.ataglanceseries.com/nursing/children

oeliac disease is an immune-mediated systemic disorder in which the immune system in a person's gut reacts to a protein gliadin that makes up gluten. The antibodies produced against gliadin cause inflammation to the surface of the gut. The damage and inflammation to the gut lining flattens villi that are present in the small bowel.

The villi work by increasing the surface area of the gut and aid to digest food more effectively. However, in the case of coeliac disease, the flattened villi are unable to work this way, resulting in the inability to digest nutrients from foods, leading to symptoms such as diarrhoea and weight loss.

What causes coeliac disease?

It is not fully understood why people develop coeliac disease or why some people's symptoms are more severe than others. However, there are a number of contributing factors that are known to increase the risk of developing coeliac disease, such as family history, environmental factors and other pre-existing health conditions.

Who should be tested for coeliac disease?

Children with coeliac disease present with a variety of non-specific signs and symptoms. Therefore, it is important to identify and diagnose those children who have a less clear clinical picture in order to reduce and prevent negative health consequences caused by the disease:

- **Symptomatic children and adolescents** with otherwise unexplained symptoms and signs that suggest coeliac disease such as chronic or intermittent diarrhoea.
- **Asymptomatic children and adolescents** who have an increased risk of coeliac disease due to pre-existing medical conditions such as type 1 diabetes mellitus, Down's syndrome, autoimmune thyroid disease and those who have a first-degree relative with coeliac disease.

How is coeliac disease diagnosed?

Screening for coeliac disease involves a two-stage diagnostic process. **Blood tests** to identify coeliac disease specific antibodies should be the first diagnostic tool used. The initial tests are IgA class anti-TGN, IgG anti-TGN and IgG anti-DGP. However, in some cases it is possible to have coeliac disease despite negative blood results. It is therefore important to confirm diagnosis with a **histology biopsy**. Biopsies are obtained during gastroscopy and should be taken from the duodenal bulb and the second and third part of the duodenum. NB. Coeliac disease will only be identified from intestinal biopsy if the person being tested is eating gluten regularly.

How is coeliac disease treated?

Once coeliac disease has been diagnosed, the treatment is a strict gluten-free diet. Children and adolescents should be referred to a dietitian for support and advice in adjusting to the new gluten-free diet and ensure that a balanced diet containing nutrients is maintained. By sticking to this strict diet symptoms should improve considerably within weeks.

Untreated or undiagnosed coeliac disease can cause long-term complications:

- Osteoprosis
- Malnutriton
- Lactose intolerance
- Cancer.

Key points

- Coeliac disease is a common digestive condition where a person has an adverse reaction to a protein in gluten.
- The antibodies produced against gluten cause damage and inflammation to the surface of the gut.
- Coeliac disease can be diagnosed with blood tests and histology biopsies.
- Treatment for coeliac disease is a strict gluten-free diet.

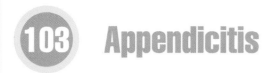

103 Appendicitis

Figure 103.1 Signs and symptoms of appendicitis

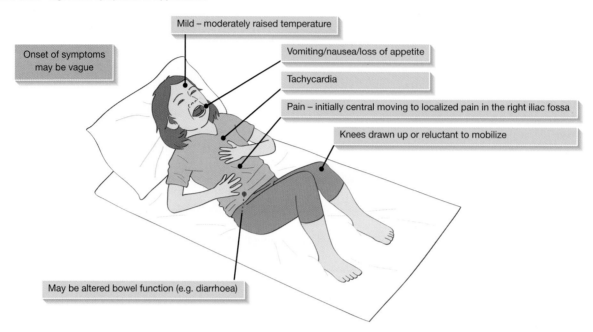

Onset of symptoms may be vague

Mild – moderately raised temperature

Vomiting/nausea/loss of appetite

Tachycardia

Pain – initially central moving to localized pain in the right iliac fossa

Knees drawn up or reluctant to mobilize

May be altered bowel function (e.g. diarrhoea)

Figure 103.2 History and assessment

- Previous hospital admissions or issues with episodes of abdominal pain?
- How long has the child been unwell?
- Any history of vomiting or diarrhoea or recent gastroenteritis in the family?
- Has the child been pyrexic?
- Any strong smell of the urine?
- Where and when did the pain start?
- Has the child already had analgesia and if so what and when?
- When did the child last eat or drink?
- Any signs of dehydration (e.g. dry mucous membranes, skin, sunken eyes, lethargy)?
- If a female adolescent, has menstruation started and date of last menstrual period?

Figure 103.3 Key observations and investigations

- Temperature, pulse, respirations, blood pressure
- Urinalysis (and culture if positive result to exclude urinary tract infection)
- Pain assessment using an appropriate tool
- Blood tests: for urea and electrolytes, full blood count (usually elevated white cells), C-reactive protein (elevated), group and hold (in the event of needing a transfusion)
- Ultrasound scan of abdomen
- Pregnancy test if female and menstruation has commenced
- Weight

Children and Young People's Nursing at a Glance, First Edition. Edited by Alan Glasper, Jane Coad, and Jim Richardson.
© 2015 John Wiley & Sons, Ltd. Published 2015 by John Wiley & Sons, Ltd. Companion website: www.ataglanceseries.com/nursing/children

The appendix is a narrow tube that is attached to the end of the caecum. Appendicitis, or inflammation of the appendix, is a common childhood condition, often caused by an obstruction associated with a kink in the bowel, a faecolith or a foreign body. Subsequent inflammation causes an accumulation of purulent exudate within the lumen of the bowel. As the appendix swells, the blood supply may become compromised and cause the appendix to become gangrenous. Perforation may occur, resulting in peritonitis and the potential for septicaemia. Sudden relief of pain is usually an indication that perforation has occurred.

Principles of care

As with any aspect of children's nursing, care should be family centred. Involving the child and family in decisions and negotiating care in accordance with their wishes will help to build trusting relationships and a sense of control over what is a stressful (and, for some, a new) situation. Good communication, a calm, caring and unhurried approach, will help to alleviate anxiety. Accurate documentation by all involved and good multidisciplinary working is key to quality care. Treatment involves appendicectomy and associated preoperative and postoperative care.

Preoperative care

The aim of preoperative care is to prepare the child and family for appendicectomy safely and effectively. Information should be given to the child in a developmentally appropriate and caring manner. The play specialist has important role in preparing the child for what will happen. Written consent must be obtained by medical staff from the parent (or person with parental responsibility or young person if they have reached the age of consent). Assessment of the child should be ongoing and any change reported to the surgical team. Baseline observations should be recorded for comparison postoperatively and the child's identity checked. Pain relief should be administered according to local policy and clinical guidelines and the effect evaluated and documented. Preoperative fasting is required in accordance with local policy. The Royal College of Nursing guidance (RCN 2005) suggests that water may be given up to 2 hours, breast milk up to 4 hours and solids up to 6 hours preoperatively, although this is currently being reviewed. Intravenous therapy will be commenced (see Chapter 77). The child should be encouraged to pass urine preoperatively and all jewellery, hairpins and prostheses should be removed and stored in a safe place. Make-up and nail varnish should also be removed so that perfusion can be assessed during and after the procedure. These details, along with the child's weight, any allergies or loose teeth/crowns, etc. should be recorded on the preoperative checklist. In many cases, parents are permitted to accompany the child into the anaesthetic room.

Postoperative care

The nurse should accompany the child and parent(s) back to the ward and set out clearly what will happen. The aim of postoperative care is to provide support, minimize pain and to monitor the child's condition, while being vigilant about potential postoperative complications. Oxygen and suction should be available if needed and the child should be advised not to get out of bed unaccompanied. Bed sides should be used if appropriate and a call bell should be left within easy reach if the parent is not present. Postoperative observations, such as temperature, pulse, respirations, blood pressure and pulse oxymetry, should be recorded in line with local policy and any anomalies reported to medical staff. A rapid thready pulse, accompanied by a falling blood pressure and a restless child, may indicate the presence of shock or haemorrhage. Paediatric Early Warning Systems (PEWS) should be in place to detect signs of the deteriorating child. Morphine, either patient or nurse controlled, is normally used for pain relief. Accurate ongoing pain and fluid assessment and management is key during the postoperative period. Intravenous antibiotics may also be required. The commencement of oral fluids should be based upon direction from the surgical team and this is normally detailed in the operation notes. Once tolerated, a light diet may then be offered. Intravenous therapy is discontinued as directed by medical staff. The wound should be observed for signs of infection (redness, swelling, exudate, local tenderness) or dehiscence. Discharge advice should include information about the recovery period and a wound check by the community team.

Key points
* Good communication with the child and family and other professionals is key to the provision of safe and effective care.
* Preoperative checks and the use of PEWS are essential to minimize risk in the perioperative and postoperative periods.
* Pain and fluid balance assessment and management should be an ongoing process.

Acknowledgement: The author would like to thank Sr Roisin McCartan (Southern Health and Social Services Trust) for her comments on an earlier draft of this chapter.

104 Constipation

Figure 104.1 Differential diagnosis of chronic constipation

- Hirschsprung's disease
- Anorectal anomalies (e.g. anal stenosis)
- Spina bifida
- Neuromuscular disease
- Hypothyroidism
- Hypercalcaemia

Figure 104.2 Diagnostic criteria for constipation

Two or more of the following characteristics during the last 8 weeks:
- Frequency of bowel movements <3 per week
- >1 episode of faecal incontinence per week
- Large stools in the rectum or palpable on abdominal examination
- Passing of stools so large they may obstruct the toilet
- Display of retentive posturing and withholding behaviours
- Painful defecation

Figure 104.3 Chronic constipation

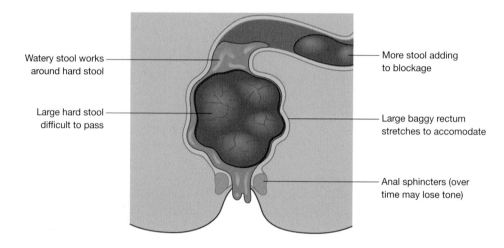

Watery stool works around hard stool

Large hard stool difficult to pass

More stool adding to blockage

Large baggy rectum stretches to accomodate

Anal sphincters (over time may lose tone)

Figure 104.4 (a) A three-pronged approach is needed to manage functional constipation

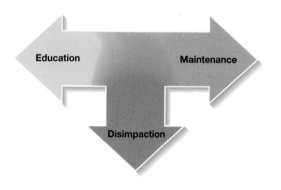

Education

Maintenance

Disimpaction

(b) Managing constipation

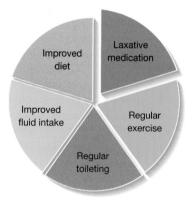

Improved diet

Laxative medication

Improved fluid intake

Regular exercise

Regular toileting

Constipation in children is a common complaint which presents many therapeutic challenges, depending on the age and presentation of the child. It can be associated with faecal soiling, and can happen at any age. The term 'faecal impaction' is also used to describe the condition.

In most cases it is functional (has a non-organic aetiology) and can be diagnosed with a careful history and thorough examination.

Criteria for a definition of functional constipation are mostly based on a variety of symptoms relating to reduced frequency, faecal incontinence and a change in consistency of the stools. A Paris Consensus on Childhood Constipation Terminology (PACCT) working group published a simplified terminology to standardize and define the diagnostic criteria (Figure 104.2).

There are many causes of functional constipation which can be interlinked and thereby make finding an obvious precipitating factor difficult. An understanding of normal bowel physiology that underpins the normal defecation process helps identify possible causes and helps direct appropriate treatment.

Children and Young People's Nursing at a Glance, First Edition. Edited by Alan Glasper, Jane Coad, and Jim Richardson.
© 2015 John Wiley & Sons, Ltd. Published 2015 by John Wiley & Sons, Ltd. Companion website: www.ataglanceseries.com/nursing/children

The constipated child

At the centre of childhood constipation is stool staying in the colon for longer than it should. This can happen for a variety of reasons and the cause and effect can be intertwined:

- Poor diet and/or low fluid intake
- Fear of pain – passing a hard stool in the past can lead to a delay in toileting or toilet avoidance
- Incomplete rectal evacuation
- Distraction – video games 'finish this level'
- Embarrassment.

Up to 63% of children with constipation and soiling have had a history of painful defecation that began at less than 3 years of age (Partin et al. 1992; Borowitz et al. 2003; Benninga et al. 2004). When stool is retained in the large bowel it adapts and stretches to accommodate the extra load. Being able to hold more means the pressure needed instigate the urge to defecate is increased. So chronic constipation can be a cause of constipation (Figure 104.3). This accommodation means that large hard stools may be passed –'toilet blockers' which may lead to pain or rectal bleeding. Overflow diarrhoea or soiling is caused when there is watery faeces flowing around the hardened faeces that are being kept in the rectum and colon by a contracted external sphincter (Loening-Baucke 1996). Sometimes it is this overflow diarrhoea that proves a hurdle in getting a child or family to accept a diagnosis of constipation; 'He can't be constipated. He has loose stools every day!'

Management of the child with functional constipation and faecal impaction

The management of functional constipation in children is not just about laxative medication. A three-pronged approach of education, disimpaction and maintenance is needed (Figure 104.4). The authors' experience is that if one facet is missing, the therapy rarely succeeds.

Drugs used in constipation

Laxatives are are generally classified according to their mode of action. The BNF divides them into five groups:

1 *Bulk-forming laxatives* generally increase faecal mass and thereby stimulate peristalsis
2 *Stimulant laxatives* increase intestinal motility
3 *Faecal softeners* lubricate or soften the stool to try to avoid painful defaecation
4 *Osmotic laxatives* increase the volume of water in the large bowel. They act as a softener and have a wash-out effect
5 *Bowel cleansing solutions* are used to prepare the bowel for radiological investigations, surgery or colonoscopy.

It is highlighted in the BNF for Children that 'for children with chronic constipation it may be necessary to exceed the licensed doses of some laxatives'.

Disimpaction

Clearing a blockage or backlog of hard faeces is a vital component of the management strategy. It must be done prior to establishing a maintenance therapy and the medication used may form part of that maintenance plan in a lower dose.

Local policy and consultant choice and experience will determine the type of medication used for faecal impaction. NICE Guidelines on constipation were published in 2010.

The oral route is the preferred route of administration as it is better tolerated and less traumatic for the child and parents. Disimpaction can also be achieved using the rectal route, with enemas and suppositories or manual evacuation in theatre. Although these routes may achieve disimpaction sooner, they are poorly tolerated and may exacerbate stool withholding behaviour and prove too invasive and distressing for the child.

Compliance with the treatment option is essential. Involving the child and family in deciding the best course of action is vital to promote an understanding of aims and enlist cooperation.

Evaluation of a child with chronic constipation requires a full medical history. Other causes of constipation are uncommon but need to be excluded. Taking a detailed history is the most important step in managing a child with constipation. It allows facts to be clarified, a diagnosis to be made and a therapeutic relationship to be built up. It enables an informed choice on type and amount of laxative needed if indicated. Doses can often be titrated to reflect results and possible adverse effects. It is important that there is an understanding that symptoms may get worse before they get better as the stool built up will need to be cleared.

Patient education

Giving parents an understanding of bowel physiology and the mechanism of constipation is a vital component in the management strategy. It helps to demystify the condition and aims to promote cooperation and involvement in resolving the problem. It should be explained that this involvement and cooperation is essential and that the process may take some time to resolve. If faecal soiling is a symptom, education will help alleviate blame (i.e. the parents may think their child is 'lazy' or 'dirty' when the child may have no control over the soiling). The educational message may need to be repeated several times during the treatment. Reassurance may be needed to help the parents maintain a positive and supportive attitude. It is also about giving ownership of the problem to the children (4 years and older) and encouraging them to take responsibility. The use of picture books, powerpoint presentations and appropriate language help in getting the message across.

Maintenance therapy

Once disimpaction is achieved the treatment then focuses on the prevention of a recurrence. Laxative medication may be needed for a prolonged period to facilitate bowel emptying and a return of sensitivity to the muscles and nerves of the rectum.

Medication is only one component of the maintenance therapy and here again education is key. Strategies to improve diet, fluid intake, exercise and regular toileting are vital ingredients to promote better bowel emptying. It is these life skills that will facilitate a weening down of the medication after a sustained period of normal stooling with no soiling.

Regular follow up is needed to insure that the treatment is working and assess progress or relapse. Revisiting the education points, evaluating the strategies and offering reassurance and advice are essential for a successful management plan and promote cooperation and compliance.

105 Renal problems

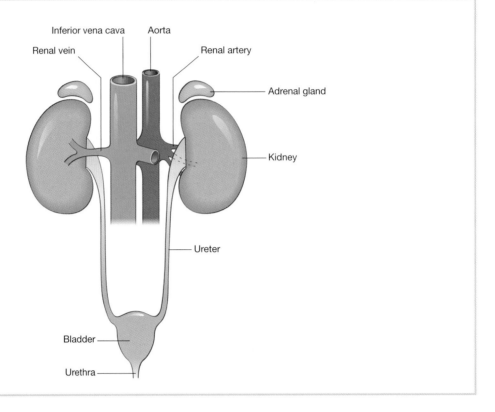

Figure 105.1 Renal problems

- Inferior vena cava
- Aorta
- Renal vein
- Renal artery
- Adrenal gland
- Kidney
- Ureter
- Bladder
- Urethra

Kidney function in children

The younger the child the more likely kidney function is to be immature and relatively inefficient. The kidney:

- Filters blood to remove waste products
- Maintains fluid and electrolyte levels by selective removal (or reabsorption) and elimination
- Helps to maintain blood pressure (renin)
- Helps to stimulate red blood cell production (erythropoietin)
- Regulates calcium metabolism.

Renal function is vital to life

Kidney structure

- The kidneys are a pair of organs situated either side of the spine at the back of the abdominal cavity at the level of T12 to L3 vertebrae
- Partially protected by 11th and 12th ribs and the perinephric fat
- Have a rich blood supply directly from the aorta via the renal arteries. Are very vulnerable to hypoperfusion for any reason
- Superficial renal cortex and innermost renal medulla form 14–16 renal nodes
- These contain the filtering and resorbtion functions at the level of the nephron
- Urine formed during this process is drained into the renal pelvis and via the ureter into the bladder for excretion.

Structural renal disorders

- Prenatal malformation or non-formation can lead to abnormalities such as horseshoe kidney
- Strictures in the renal arteries may lead to hypertension
- Strictures in the renal drainage system can lead to damming back of urine and subsequent pressure damage
- Ineffective vesicoureteric valves can lead to reflux of urine from the bladder back up the ureters, leaving the child vulnerable to disturbed function and infection.

Acquired renal disorders in childhood
Post-streptococcal glomerulonephritis

This is an immune response to a streptococcal infection (e.g. throat or skin infection) leading to renal damage with reduced function. It generally resolves spontaneously but sometimes monitoring and supportive therapy is necessary.

Nephrotic syndrome

- Produced by a number of disease processes
- Leads to damage of the filtering apparatus leading to increased permeability allowing protein to be filtered and lost
- Proteinurea and low blood protein
- Causes fluid shifts in the body leading to the characteristic oedema
- Generally amenable to treatment with corticosteroids.

Children and Young People's Nursing at a Glance, First Edition. Edited by Alan Glasper, Jane Coad, and Jim Richardson.
© 2015 John Wiley & Sons, Ltd. Published 2015 by John Wiley & Sons, Ltd. Companion website: www.ataglanceseries.com/nursing/children

Nursing to include the following:
- Make sure that child and family understand what is happening, what to expect and how they can be involved
- Monitor constituents of the urine – urinalysis
- Monitor weight
- Monitor fluid intake and output
- Integrity of skin and oedematous tissue.

Haemolytic uraemic syndrome
- Rare but important cause of severe kidney damage in childhood
- Often seen in the wake of infection with *Escherichia coli*
- Severely unwell child
- Can lead to acute renal injury and subsequent end-stage renal damage.

Renal tract infection
- Children are particularly vulnerable; the younger the more vulnerable
- Symptoms include fever, pain, vomiting
- May be recurrent, requiring cause to be investigated; diagnostic imaging may be required
- All children with a fever of unknown origin higher than 38°C should have a urine sample tested
- Clean catch or urine collection pad should be used
- Treatment is by appropriate antibiotic therapy.

Acute renal injury (failure)
- Wide range of causative factors (e.g. reduced blood supply (hypovolaemia, hypotension), toxins, physical injury, obstruction)
- As the kidney's vital functions are disturbed or lost the child becomes globally unwell;
    lassitude
    loss of appetite and vomiting
    headache
    disruptions in vital functions – vital signs
- Treatment is based on the underlying cause. May be reversible but may lead to chronic disturbed function.

End-stage renal damage (chronic renal failure)
- Devastating end-point of any of the processes that lead to kidney damage beyond repair
- Severe reduction of glomerular filtration rate for more that 3 months
- Treatment based on which systems are primarily affected
- Long-term supportive nursing is geared to maximal child and family independence in management and minimizing disruption to child and family life and experience.

Renal replacement therapy
Dialysis
Haemodialysis:
- Blood is filtered mechanically to remove waste products and excess water

- Requires venous access
- Requires around three sessions per week, each lasting around 4 hours.
  Peritoneal dialysis:
- Fluid is instilled into peritoneal cavity to use the peritoneum as a filtering membrane
- Adjustment of the composition of the dialysate produces removal of waste products and excess water through osmosis
- Needs to be performed around four times a day with a dwell time of around 30 minutes. Alternatively, may be carried out overnight.

Both forms are vulnerable to complications such as infection. This therapy can be severely disruptive to the child's and family's lifestyle. Both forms still require some restrictions to fluid intake and nutrition.

Kidney transplantation
Kidney function can be restored with a successful renal transplant. Rejection remains a risk as the body's defensive immune reaction to 'foreign' tissue. This requires long-term suppressant medication.

Tumours
- Some, such as Wilm's (nephroblastoma), characteristically occur in childhood
- Affects around 70 children per year in the United Kingdom
- Most often detected as a painless swollen abdomen
- Usually unilateral
- Depending on the stage at detection, the chance of recovery is good; around 90% at 5 years
- Treatment involves surgery and possibly radiotherapy and/or chemotherapy.

Renal injury
- Children are particularly vulnerable due to:
    high level of physical activity
    immature judgement
    risk taking and impulsivity
- May lead to blunt trauma with damage, rupture and haemorrhage (NB Kidneys are highly vascular)
- Early identification and surgical intervention are vital
- May lead to loss of kidney.

Tests used in renal disorders
- Prenatal testing (e.g. structural scan with diagnostic ultrasound)
- Diagnostic imaging, X-ray ± contrast media
- Urinalysis – NB blood, protein
- Blood chemistry – electrolytes, blood protein levels, etc.

106 Haematological problems

Figure 106.1   Easy bruising

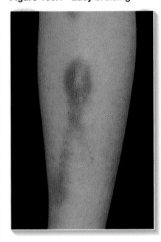

Figure 106.2   Petechial rash

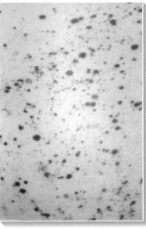

*From Hoffbrand AV, Moss PAH.
(2011) Essential Haematology, 6th edn.
Reproduced with permission of Wiley.*

Figure 106.3   Thrombocytopenia with absent radii (TAR)

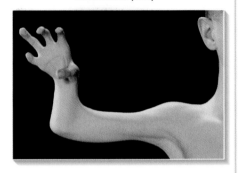

Figure 106.4   Fanconi's anaemia

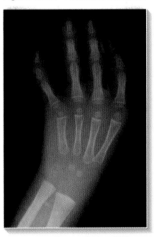

*From Hoffbrand AV, Moss PAH.
(2011) Essential Haematology, 6th edn.
Reproduced with permission of Wiley.*

Figure 106.5   Purpura fulminans

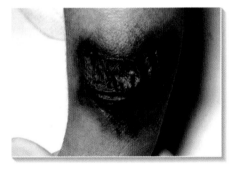

Figure 106.6   Hermansky–Pudlack syndrome

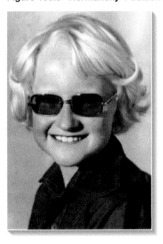

Figure 106.7   Haemophilia

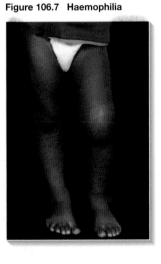

Figure 106.8   Dactylitis

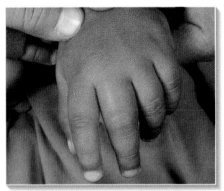

*From Hoffbrand AV, Moss PAH.
(2011) Essential Haematology, 6th edn.
Reproduced with permission of Wiley.*

Figure 106.9   Facial appearance in β-thalassaemia major

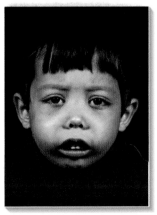

*From Hoffbrand AV, Moss PAH.
(2011) Essential Haematology, 6th edn.
Reproduced with permission of Wiley.*

Children and Young People's Nursing at a Glance, First Edition. Edited by Alan Glasper, Jane Coad, and Jim Richardson.
© 2015 John Wiley & Sons, Ltd. Published 2015 by John Wiley & Sons, Ltd. Companion website: www.ataglanceseries.com/nursing/children

The most common manifestation of haematological disorder in children is a history of easy bruising and/or bleeding. Bruising is easy to see in Caucasian children but much harder to see in children of Asian or Afro-Caribbean descent – in these children lumps may be palpable just under the skin.

Bleeding in neonates and young children is abnormal and should always be investigated. A full blood count and clotting screen will identify abnormalities of platelet count and coagulation. Further specialist investigations should then be undertaken following discussion with a paediatric haematologist.

Some rare haematological disorders present with structural abnormalities, such as missing bones/digits and facial abnormalities that are characteristic of the underlying disorder. These may be present without bruising or bleeding. Abnormalities of haemoglobin (sickle cell anaemia and thalassaemia) are now tested for in routine neonatal screening programmes and are thus often diagnosed before symptoms occur.

Treatment of children with diagnosed haematological disorders usually relies on replacement of missing blood components with blood or blood products such as factor VIII (now manufactured using recombinant technology for children in the United Kingdom) for haemophilia or red cell transfusions for those with sickle cell anaemia or thalassemia. Some of the haematological conditions described can be cured by bone marrow transplantation; others are long-term conditions where management offers good quality of life.

Easy bruising

This is caused by bleeding into the skin. Bruising is a normal reaction to injury (Figure 106.1). Although painful, bruises are not normally dangerous unless they affect vital organs or are a sign of an underlying bleeding disorder. Potential causes: 'normal' childhood trauma, idiopathic thrombocytopenic purpura (ITP), leukaemia, bleeding disorders and bone marrow failure.

Petechial rash

Small purple or red 'dots' caused by capillary haemorrhage under the skin (Figure 106.2). Unlike meningitis in bleeding disorders, the rash does not fade with pressure. Potential causes: ITP, leukaemia, rare platelet disorders and meningitis.

Thrombocytopenia with absent radii (TAR)

This is a rare congenital disorder characterized by thrombocytopenia in infancy, which improves with age, and shortening or absence of the radial bones (Figure 106.3). Babies are born with shortened or absent forearms. This syndrome can also be associated with lower limb abnormalities.

Fanconi's anaemia

This is an autosomal recessively inherited anaemia associated with growth retardation, kidney and skeletal abnormalities which can include TAR or absent thumbs and bone marrow failure (Figure

106.4). Children experience pancytopenia – reduced levels of red and white blood cells as well as platelets – usually presenting with easy bruising, recurrent infections and anaemia.

Purpura fulminans

Purpura fulminans is a skin necrosis caused by occlusion of blood vessels in the skin (Figure 106.5). Potential causes: severe protein C deficiency (inherited or acquired), sepsis and disseminated intravascular coagulation (DIC).

Hermansky–Pudlack syndrome

This is occulo-cutaneous albinism with platelet disorder. An autosomal recessive disorder (both parents carry the gene and are unaffected). Children are fair eyed and skinned and have easy bruising from an early age, often bleed significantly with surgery (Figure 106.6).

Haemophilia

Haemophilia affects 1 in 5000–10000 male infants worldwide. Haemophilia results in joint bleeding that, without prompt or prophylactic therapy, causes early arthritic damage, reduces mobility resulting in disability (Figure 106.7).

Haemophilia A (FVIII deficiency) affects 80% of those with haemophilia. Haemophilia B (factor IX) deficiency is much rarer. One-third of newly diagnosed children have no previous family history.

Dactylitis

Painful swollen fingers seen in children with sickle cell anaemia, this is a genetic disorder of the haemoglobin gene which is found in as many as 1 in 4 West Africans. Sickle cell anaemia (or disease) presents in those who inherit an abnormal gene from each parent. Sickle cell anaemia causes painful crises when blood sickles resulting in occlusion of blood vessels usually related to infection, dehydration and extremely cold weather. Dactylitis is caused by painful infarction in the small bones which in turn leads to fingers of differing lengths (Figure 106.8).

Facial appearance in β-thalassaemia major

This is a genetic disorder of the haemoglobin gene which is found most commonly in people who originate from Mediterranean regions (β-thalassemia) or the far East (α-thalassemia). Carriers of these abnormal genes are not usually affected by anaemia. Inheritance of only abnormal genes in α-thalassaemia is incompatible with life. In β-thalassaemia, severe anaemia occurs within the first few months of life, when red cell destruction also causes hepatosplenomegaly. Bone marrow overgrowth causes bones to expand and causes the typical features of bossing of the skull and face (Figure 106.9).

107 Musculoskeletal problems

Figure 107.1   Congenital talipes equinovarus (CTEV). Also known as club feet

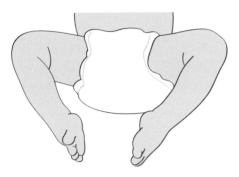

Figure 107.2   Ponseti casting. Note separate leg plaster used for each leg

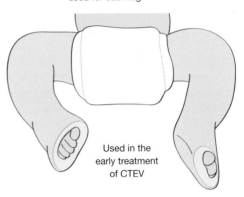

Used in the early treatment of CTEV

Figure 107.3   Denis Browne boots

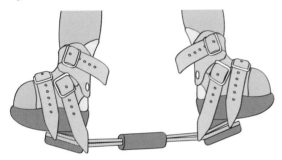

Used following completion of Ponseti manipulation and serial casting

Figure 107.4   Pavlik harness

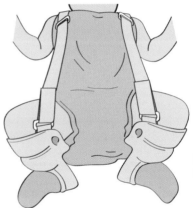

Used for the treatment of developmental dysplasia of the hip

Developmental dysplasia of the hip

Developmental dysplasia of the hip (DDH) is a spectrum of disorders related to abnormal development of the hip at any time during foetal life, infancy or childhood (Clarke and Dowling 2003). It ranges from mild acetabular abnormality and joint laxity to irreducible dislocation of the femoral head. The cause is thought to be multifactorial including heredity with generalized joint laxity and a positive family history; hormonal with increased maternal hormones prior to delivery leading to joint laxity; intrauterine breech position; oligohydramnios (reduced amniotic fluid) during pregnancy and postnatal positioning – babies who are carried with legs swaddled together are more likely to develop DDH. The condition is more common in firstborn babies and females.

Diagnosis is by postnatal screening which includes Barlow's test of instability and Ortolani's sign of reduction. The babies should be examined when warm and comfortable, preferably after a feed. Other signs are extra skin creases, shortening of the limb (Galeazzi's sign), limitation of abduction or differences between sides and limp or waddling gait in older child.

If suspected, the diagnosis can be confirmed by hip ultrasound or an arthrogram. The aim of treatment is to keep the head of the femur in the acetabulum to enable development of the joint. This can be done by the use of an orthosis (Pavilk harness), a hip spica plaster cast, closed or open reduction or by femoral or pelvic osteotomy. The Pavlik harness is a hip flexion–abduction splint that enables the baby to kick while keeping the hips in the correct position. It needs to stay on 24 hours a day initially but as treatment progresses it can be removed for bathing. Regular checks at a clinic are required for 3–4 months.

Congenital talipes equinovarus

This is a congenital deformity in which the foot points downwards and inwards; it is often bilateral. It is also known as club foot. The condition affects boys more than girls.

The cause is unknown but intrauterine moulding, nerve and muscle imbalance and delayed development have been suggested. It can be associated with other conditions. The condition can be detected on antenatal scans.

Treatment should begin as soon as possible with the aim of correcting the deformity and maintaining the correction. The method used for this is the Ponseti technique of manipulation and serial plaster casting (Linehan and O'Sullivan 2011). This is done weekly, with correction usually achieved after 5–8 manipulations. The infant may need surgical intervention in the form of Achilles tenotomy. The final cast is worn for 3 weeks followed by the application of boots attached to a bar such as Denis Browne boots. These have to be worn most of the day for 3 months and during the night for several years. Relapse is more common when this has not been followed. It is essential for the health care team to provide information and support to the parents during this emotional time.

Scoliosis

Scoliosis is a deformity of the spine with marked lateral curvature (Bessette and Rousseau 2012). It can be classified according to the age of onset: infantile, 0–3 years; juvenile, 3–10 years; adolescent, over 10 years. There is often a family history and girls are affected more than boys.

The risk of progression of the curvature is increased during the rapid growth rate of puberty. The physical signs are one shoulder higher, a protruding scapula, one side of rib cage higher, one hip higher and an uneven waist.

An X-ray is undertaken to confirm the degree of spinal deformity. **Treatment:**
* Observation and regular checks
* Bracing and/or plaster casts – these prevent progression but do not correct existing deformity
* Surgery – for curves >40°, fusion of the spine to prevent progression and instrumentation to correct deformity is performed.

Slipped upper femoral epiphysis

This is displacement of the proximal femoral epiphysis on the femoral neck. It is most common in adolescents, with boys affected more than girls. Affected teenagers are usually obese but they can be tall and thin with delayed maturity. It is thought there may be a possible endocrine dysfunction. The child presents with pain and limp. There is a possibility that the other hip will also be affected.

Treatment is by insertion of pins or screws to hold the slipped part of the femur in place.

Perthes' disease

This is avascular necrosis of the femoral head where there is disruption of the blood supply leading to death of the bone causing it to cease growing. There is swelling of the soft tissues of the hip joint. The cause is unknown. It is most commonly seen in those aged 5–9 years but can occur at any age. Boys are affected more often than girls.

The child presents with a limp and hip or knee pain without a history of injury. This pain follows the pathway of the obturator nerve. It is a self-limiting condition. Following the first stage of interruption of the blood supply revascularization occurs, where growth of new vessels occurs and there is bone resorption. New bone formation takes place that is weak, leading to collapse and flattening of the femoral head.

Reossification is the final stage in the process where the head of femur gradually reforms and the necrotic bone is removed.

The aim of treatment is to contain the femoral epiphysis within the acetabulum. This is done by rest and restriction of activity. The child requires analgesia for the pain and is required to be non-weight-bearing. Initially, this may be by traction or splintage. Physiotherapy is required to achieve and maintain the range of movement. If the femoral head is not able to be contained in the acetabulum then surgery in the form of a pelvic or femoral osteotomy may be necessary. All of these conditions may require the use of a plaster cast (see Chapter 88) and traction (see Chapter 89).

108 Reproductive and sexual problems

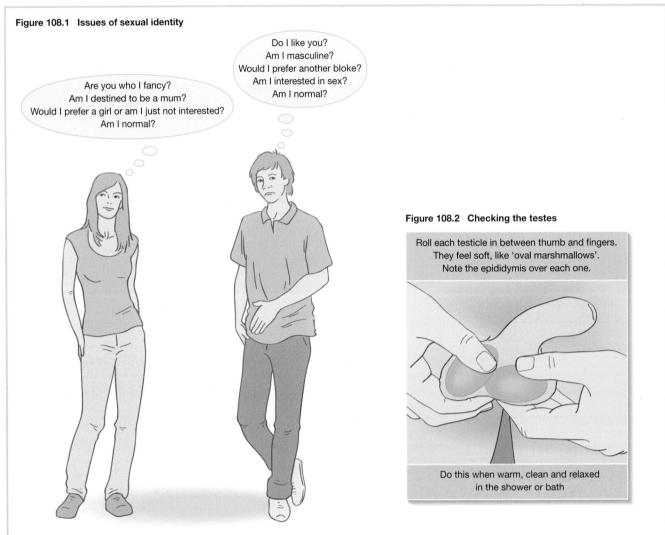

Figure 108.1 Issues of sexual identity

Are you who I fancy?
Am I destined to be a mum?
Would I prefer a girl or am I just not interested?
Am I normal?

Do I like you?
Am I masculine?
Would I prefer another bloke?
Am I interested in sex?
Am I normal?

Figure 108.2 Checking the testes

Roll each testicle in between thumb and fingers.
They feel soft, like 'oval marshmallows'.
Note the epididymis over each one.

Do this when warm, clean and relaxed
in the shower or bath

Structural abnormalities

At birth or in early childhood various anatomical abnormalities are evident within the reproductive, genital or urological organs that result from failures in embryological development: absence of vagina or other parts of the female reproductive tract. Occluded vagina but remainder present and normal in shape; ambivalent or ambiguous genitalia – actual sex determined through chromosomal analysis and endocrine status. In the male micropenis, hypospadias (urethral opening on underside of penis), epispadias (urethral opening on upper part of penis), and cryptorchidism (undescended testis). These are assessed for surgical intervention at an appropriate age in order to protect future function where possible and prevent other problems (e.g. testicular cancer if testes remain undescended) and to protect the child's body image.

Developmental issues

Reproductive and sexual functioning is a combination of mind and body function. Adolescence is when these processes and functions

mature and become a focus of attention. Part of becoming a sexually mature adult may involve difficult decisions about sexual identity. This is not necessarily easier with the modern, open and free views of sexuality as the issue needs to be considered earlier in development. In addition, hormone levels are relatively unstable and interlinked with basic drives centrally controlled within the brain: sleeping, eating, drinking and exercising. The moody, relatively uncooperative and uncommunicative teenager is difficult to establish a rapport with, thus. 'You have an issue – this is a confidential service and we are here to help' facilitates a working relationship.

Signs of puberty may not necessarily be welcomed or understood by the child , despite videos and classroom teaching sessions. Puberty can occur precociously as early as 8 years of age or be delayed beyond 16 years.

Male signs of puberty and potential problems

Signs of puberty are facial, underarm and pubic hair, with increases in glandular activity – sweat = odour; sebaceous gland activity –

potential acne; pubic hair; voice change and break; growth spurts, which = potential acne; the voice changes or breaks; and growth spurts continue until maturity.

Penile and scrotal developmental problems

- **Phimosis:** the foreskin remains too tight for retraction to allow for cleansing underneath glans – failure to do this can result in penile cancer. Surgical division with conservation of foreskin is now preferred to circumcision. Phimosis may also result from infection where identification and appropriate treatment is required in addition to surgery.
- **Balanitis:** swelling of the glans ($\pm$ foreskin). The glans is red and sore as a result of irritation (from for example: accumulated smegma, infection – thrush or sexually transmitted – dribbled urine, highly scented shower gels).
- **Paraphimosis:** occurs if a tight foreskin is retracted round the penis causing the glans to swell and resulting in significant pain. Emergency surgical management and treatment of any infection is required. This can occur at any age, without sexual activity and requires urgent referral. A young male who presents with genital pain **must** be examined.
- **Varicocoele:** swollen veins within pampiniform plexus. Although not a problem in itself, the resultant increases in temperature can cause low sperm counts and male infertility.
- Hydrocoele: painless fluid-filled sacs that enlarge the scrotal contents but feel soft and mobile, these may cause anxiety.
- **Testicular cancer:** the most common cancer in young men, but it is easily treated if detected and diagnosed early. Self-examination of testicles is to be promoted in order to achieve this. If boys know how their testes and epididymis feel, they are more likely to feel the harder rougher shape of a potentially cancerous change (Figure 108.2).
- **Inguinal hernia:** occurs where a section of intestine has prolapsed into the scrotum through the inguinal canal. This requires surgical repair.

Trauma

- **Frenulum breve** ('short'): this may rupture with masturbation or sexual intercourse and can lead to a haematoma under the glans epidermal tissue which will resolve. If pain or trauma continues with sexual activity, further surgical division may be necessary but not circumcision.
- **Testicular torsion** causes acute pain as a result of ischaemia from twisting of the testicle about the spermatic cord.
- **Testicular trauma** causes significant pain.

Female signs of puberty and potential problems

Increase in height and weight, female body shape – breast development, widening hips, hair growth pubic, underarms with increased sweat gland activity – odour, and sebaceous gland activity – potential acne; particularly linked with menstrual cycle post menarche. A girl's menstrual pattern is one of the major indicators for her general as well as reproductive health.

Normal bleeding pattern for established (~1 year) menstruation

- *Frequency:* every 21–35 days
- *Length:* 3–7 days (from spotting to ending with no colour in loss)
- *Amount:* 20–80 mL (up to 4 tampons/day), few, small clots

- **Primary amenorrhoea:** delayed puberty. Investigations commence if there are no signs of puberty by 14 years – examining lifestyle, diet, exercise, family history, and chromosomal analysis if no menarche by 16 years with full endocrine profile.
- **Infrequent or scanty periods (oligomenorrhoea):** most frequently caused by polycystic ovarian syndrome (PCOS), examine for hirsutism and virilism; rarely, congenital adrenal hyperplasia; even less often, androgen secreting ovarian or adrenal tumours. PCOS treatment includes weight loss, metformin to counteract insulin resistance, combined oral contraceptive pill (COCP) when the body mass index is under control to protect endometrium.
- **Excess bleeding (menorrhagia):** dysfunctional bleeding (DUB) is the most frequent diagnosis of exclusion in young women: local (e.g. fibroids, polyps, endometritis or endometrial carcinoma), a clotting disorder or endocrine. Treatment for DUB includes COCP and or non-steroidal anti-inflammatory drugs. Both the latter are also treatments used for the concomitant dysmenorrhoea that precedes and accompanies menstruation if endometriosis is the cause.
- **Pelvic pain:** a good history helps determine potential causes including:
    early pregnancy problems such as miscarriage or ectopic, if sexually active
    pelvic inflammatory disease (STI – chlamydia and or gonorrhoea)
    contraceptive post intrauterine device or termination
    trauma surgical, potential adhesions, infection, consider potential abuse
    menstrual, the first day date for the last menstrual period is vital information and relationship of pain to cycle could indicate endometriosis which often goes undiagnosed and untreated but is a significant cause of distress.
    If COCP or Depo-Provera injection therapy are unsuccessful, specialist treatment centres are now available.

Other pelvic pain causes: ovarian cysts (rupture haemorrhage and torsion), fibroids and gynaecological malignancy are possible but rare in the adolescent age group. Non reproductive tract causes need to be considered such as urinary tract infection, renal calculi, irritable bowel and diverticulitis.

- **Vaginal discharge**s: most are physiological but associated itch, malodour, colour change or consistency may indicate abnormality. Causes could be foreign body (e.g tampon), infection (non STI e.g. Candida or bacterial vaginosis) likelihood of these is increased with excess washing (>1/day) and shaving pubic hair, or an STI.

109 Skin conditions

Figure 109.1 Children's concerns about the reaction of others to their skin conditions

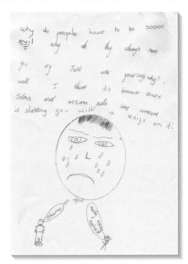

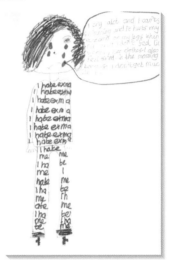

Figure 109.2 Macule

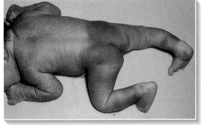

Figure 109.3 Papule

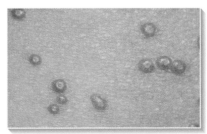

Figure 109.4 Plaque

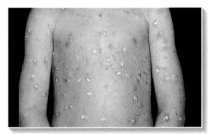

From Miall L, Rudolf M, Smith D. (2012) Paediatrics at a Glance: Evaluation of the Child, Development and Developmental Assessment, 3rd edition. Reproduced with permission of Wiley

Figure 109.5 Wheal

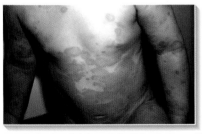

Figure 109.6 Vesicle

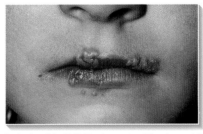

Figure 109.7 Pustule

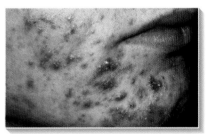

From Miall L, Rudolf M, Smith D. (2012) Paediatrics at a Glance: Evaluation of the Child, Development and Developmental Assessment, 3rd edition. Reproduced with permission of Wiley

Figure 109.8 Crust

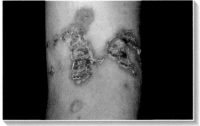

Figure 109.9 Lichenification

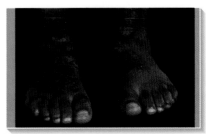

From Miall L, Rudolf M, Smith D. (2012) Paediatrics at a Glance: Evaluation of the Child, Development and Developmental Assessment, 3rd edition. Reproduced with permission of Wiley

Children and Young People's Nursing at a Glance, First Edition. Edited by Alan Glasper, Jane Coad, and Jim Richardson.
© 2015 John Wiley & Sons, Ltd. Published 2015 by John Wiley & Sons, Ltd. Companion website: www.ataglanceseries.com/nursing/children

Skin conditions in children (<14 years of age) comprise about 21% of all those consulting with skin disease; this age group represents 19% of the population (Office for National Statistics 2001). Data from NHS Direct for 2008 showed that 4% of all calls related to skin rashes, with the most common age group being children aged 1–4 years (31.8%), with a further 15.3% of calls relating to children <1 year and 15.1% in the 5–14 years age group (Schofield et al. 2009).

Assessing the child with a rash

The skin should be examined in a warm well-lit room, preferably with natural lighting or artificial lighting that will not change the natural colour of the skin.

Clinical history

- Onset: acute or chronic
- Systemic symptoms (fever)
- Duration of rash
- Change in rash over time: flare and remission
- Symptoms of rash (itching, pain, soreness)
- Family history of skin disease
- Recent contact with individuals with a rash (scabies, chickenpox)
- Drug history
- Allergies
- Other medical history (atopy: asthma, hay fever)
- Does it occur at different times of the year?
- School and hobbies – do they have an impact?
- Medications – applied to the skin, taken by mouth or purchased by the parents
- Previous and present treatments and their effectiveness
- Are there any treatments, actions or behavioural changes that have influenced the condition?

Coping with the skin condition

A great deal can be observed in the child's face and persona, which may give insight to how they feel and are coping with the skin condition. They may be withdrawn, not sleeping or be very conscious about their appearance and the reactions of others; staring, name calling or bullying (Figure 109.1). There are several psychological and disease-specific scores that can measure the impact of skin disease (http://www.dermatology.org.uk/quality/quality-life.html).

Clinical examination

When examining the child, use a gown or sheet to maintain dignity as each area of the skin is exposed for examination. Touching is an important aspect of the examination. It provides information about skin texture and temperature and also breaks down the physical barrier and stigma associated with skin disease. The skin should be examined thoroughly from the scalp to toes including hair, nails and flexures, looking at the following.

Distribution

Is it acral (hands, feet), extremities of ears and nose, in light-exposed areas or mainly confined to the trunk?

Character

Is there redness (erythema), scaling, crusting, exudate? Are there excoriations, blisters, erosions, pustules, papules? Are the lesions all the same (monomorphic, e.g. drug rash) or variable (polymorphic, e.g. chickenpox)? Lesions can further be defined as primary lesions which are present at the initial onset of the disease:

Macule: a flat mark; circumscribed area of colour change: brown, red, white or tan (Figure 109.2)

Papule: elevated 'spot'; palpable, firm, circumscribed lesion, generally <5 mm in diameter (Figure 109.3)

Nodule: elevated, firm, circumscribed, palpable; can involve all layers of the skin, >5 mm in diameter

Plaque: elevated, flat-topped, firm, rough, superficial papule >2 cm in diameter. Papules can coalesce to form plaques (Figure 109.4)

Wheal: elevated, irregular-shaped area of cutaneous oedema; solid, transient, changing, variable diameter; red, pale pink or white in colour (Figure 109.5)

Vesicle: elevated, circumscribed, superficial fluid-filled blister <5 mm in diameter (Figure 109.6)

Bulla: vesicle >5 mm in diameter

Pustule: elevated, superficial, similar to vesicle but filled with pus (Figure 109.7).

Secondary lesions are the result of changes over time caused by disease progression, manipulation (scratching, rubbing, picking) or treatment:

Scale: heaped-up keratinized cells; flaky exfoliation; irregular; thick or thin; dry or oily; variable size; silver, white or tan in colour (Figure 109.4)

Crust: dried serum, blood or purulent exudate; slightly elevated; size variable (Figure 109.8)

Excoriation: loss of epidermis; linear area usually due to scratching

Lichenification: rough, thickened epidermis; accentuated skin markings caused by rubbing or scratching (Figure 109.9).

Shape

Are the lesions small, large, annular (ring-shaped) or linear?

Skin types

With different skin colours and hair types, lesions that appear red or brown in white skin, appear black or purple in pigmented skin and mild degrees of redness (erythema) may be masked completely. Inflammation commonly leads to pigmentary changes – both lighter (post-inflammatory hypopigmentation) and darker (post-inflammatory hyperpigmentation) – which may persist for a long time after the initial skin condition has settled.

Investigations

- Samples of scales, crusts, hair and nails – yeast, fungus, virus, bacteria
- Skin biopsy (blistering rashes or when diagnosis uncertain)
- Blood investigations, depending on diagnosis and assessment.

110 Atopic eczema

Figure 110.1 Eczema can impact on the patient's quality of life

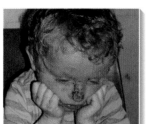

Reproduced with permission of Centre of Evidence based Dermatology Nottingham

Figures 110.2 and 110.3 In some ethnic groups, atopic eczema can affect the extensor surfaces rather than the flexures, and discoid or follicular patterns may be more common

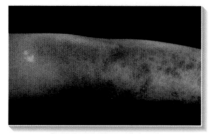

Reproduced with permission of Centre of Evidence based Dermatology Nottingham

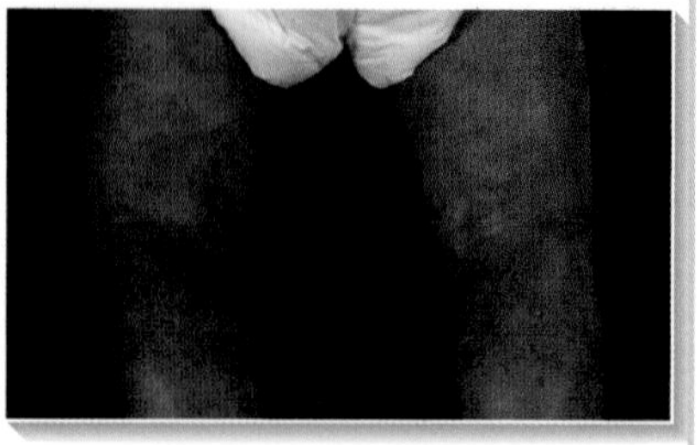

Reproduced with permission of Centre of Evidence based Dermatology Nottingham

Figure 110.4 Facial eczema is common in infants

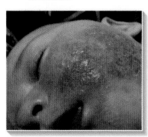

Figure 110.5 Flexural involvement

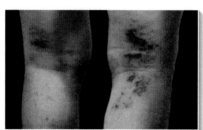

Reproduced with permission of Nottingham CEBD Group

Figure 110.6 Eczema on extensor surface of arms

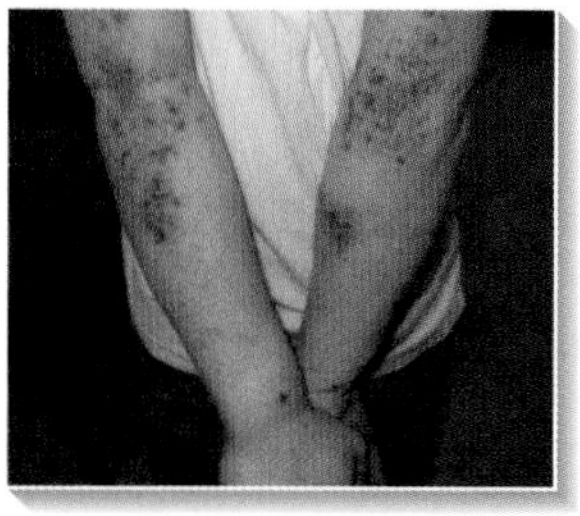

Reproduced with permission of Nottingham CEBD Group

Figure 110.7 Discoid or follicular pattern of eczema

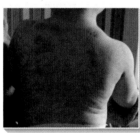

Reproduced with permission of Nottingham CEBD Group

Figure 110.8 Eczema can cause lichenification

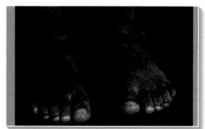

Reproduced with permission of Nottingham CEBD Group

Figure 110.9 Weeping and crusting may be signs of infection

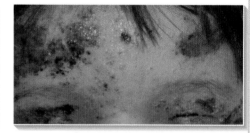

Reproduced with permission of Nottingham CEBD Group

Figure 110.10 Assessing severity of eczema *Adapted from NICE (2007) CG57: www.nice.org.uk/guidance/CG57. Reproduced with permission*

	Skin/physical severity		Impact on quality of life and psychosocial well-being
Clear	Normal skin, no evidence of active atopic eczema	**None**	No impact on quality of life
Mild	Areas of dry skin, infrequent itching (with or without small areas of redness)	**Mild**	Little impact on everyday activities, sleep and psychosocial well-being
Moderate	Areas of dry skin, frequent itching, redness (with or without excoriation and localized skin thickening)	**Moderate**	Moderate impact on everyday activities and psychosocial well-being, frequently disturbed sleep
Severe	Widespread areas of dry skin, incessant itching, redness (with or without excoriation, extensive skin thickening, bleeding, oozing, cracking and alteration of pigmentation)	**Severe**	Severe limitation of everyday activities and psychosocial functioning, nightly loss of sleep

Figure 110.11 Management of eczema

Clear	Emollients					
Mild	Emollients	Mild potency topical corticosteroids				
Moderate	Emollients	Moderate potency topical corticosteroids	Topical calcineurin inhibitors	Bandages		
Severe	Emollients	Potent topical corticosteroids	Topical calcineurin inhibitors	Bandages	Phototherapy	Systemic therapy

Children and Young People's Nursing at a Glance, First Edition. Edited by Alan Glasper, Jane Coad, and Jim Richardson.
© 2015 John Wiley & Sons, Ltd. Published 2015 by John Wiley & Sons, Ltd. Companion website: www.ataglanceseries.com/nursing/children

Atopic eczema (atopic dermatitis) is a chronic inflammatory itchy skin condition which usually develops in early childhood and follows a remitting and relapsing course. It often has a genetic component that leads to the breakdown of the skin barrier. This makes the skin susceptible to trigger factors, including irritants and allergens, which can make the eczema worse. Although atopic eczema is not often thought of as a serious medical condition, it can have a significant impact on quality of life (Figure 110.1).

Diagnosis

Diagnose atopic eczema when a child has an itchy skin condition plus three or more of the following:
• Visible flexural dermatitis involving the skin creases (or visible dermatitis on the cheeks and/or extensor areas in children aged 18 months or under)
• Personal history of flexural dermatitis (or dermatitis on the cheeks and/or extensor areas in children aged 18 months or under)
• Personal history of dry skin in the last 12 months
• Personal history of asthma or allergic rhinitis (or history of atopic disease in a first-degree relative of children aged under 4 years)
• Onset of signs and symptoms under the age of 2 years (do not use this criterion in children under 4 years).

In children of Asian, black Caribbean and black African ethnic groups, atopic eczema can affect the extensor surfaces rather than the flexures, and discoid or follicular patterns may be more common with post-inflammatory hypo- or hyperpigmentation (Figures 110.2 and 110.3).

Assessment

History:
• Time of onset, pattern and severity
• Response to previous and current treatments
• Possible trigger factors (soap, detergents, weather, seasons, skin infections, animal dander, pollens, house dust mite, foods and stress)
• Impact of the condition on children and their parents or carers
• Dietary history
• Growth and development
• Personal and family history of atopic disease
• Take into account the severity of the atopic eczema and the child's quality of life, including everyday activities and sleep, and psychosocial well-being. There is not necessarily a direct relationship between the severity of atopic eczema and its impact on quality of life
• Take into account the impact of atopic eczema on parents or carers as well as the child.

Clinical findings

The appearance of eczema varies and is related to the age of the child, their ethnic background and the presence of infection. The distribution changes with age; the face is a common site in infants (Figure 110.4), followed by flexural involvement (Figure 110.5). It can affect the extensor surfaces rather than the flexures (Figure 110.6), and a discoid or follicular pattern may be seen. It can be localized or widespread (Figure 110.7). There may be dry skin and fine scale, areas of ill-defined erythema (redness), excoriations, lichenification (Figure 110.8), vesicles, weeping and crusting which may be signs of infection (Figure 110.9). Infections may be bacterial or viral (eczema herpeticum).

Assessing severity

To assess severity see Figure 110.10.

Management

Use a stepped approach for managing atopic eczema, tailor treatment step to severity. Use emollients all the time and step treatment up or down as necessary. All aspects should be supported by education and demonstrations (Figure 110.11).

Referral

Refer immediately (same day) for specialist dermatological advice if you suspect eczema herpeticum.

Refer urgently (within 2 weeks) for specialist dermatological advice if:
• The atopic eczema is severe and has not responded to topical therapy after 1 week
• Treatment of bacterially infected atopic eczema has failed.

Refer for specialist dermatological advice if:
• The diagnosis is uncertain
• The atopic eczema is not controlled based on a subjective assessment by the child or parent or carer
• Atopic eczema on the face has not responded to appropriate treatment
• Contact allergic dermatitis is suspected
• The atopic eczema is causing significant social or psychological problems
• The atopic eczema is associated with severe and recurrent infections
• The child, parent or carer might benefit from specialist advice on treatment application.

Refer for psychological advice children whose atopic eczema has responded to management but for whom the impact on quality of life and psychosocial well-being has not improved.

Refer children with moderate or severe atopic eczema and suspected food allergy for specialist investigation and management.

Refer children with atopic eczema who fail to grow at the expected growth trajectory, as reflected by the UK growth charts, for specialist advice relating to growth.

Source: NICE (2007). Adapted from *CG 57 Atopic eczema in children: management of atopic eczema in children from birth up to the age of 12 years*. London: NICE. Available from www.nice.org.uk/guidance/CG57. Reproduced with permission.

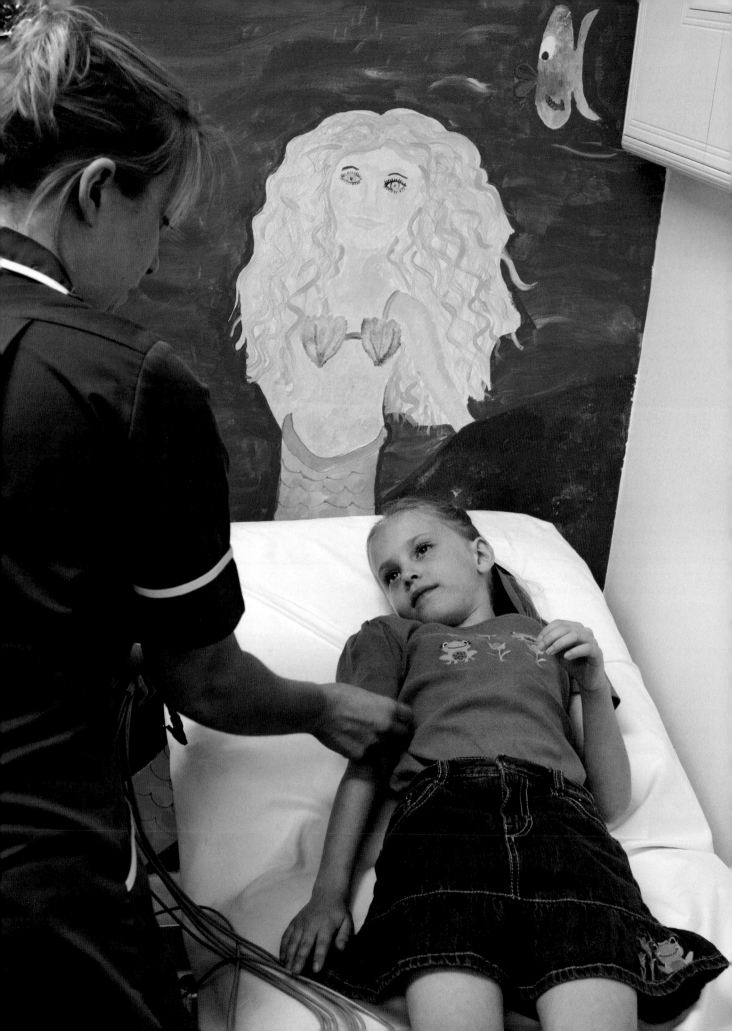

Chronic and life-limiting conditions

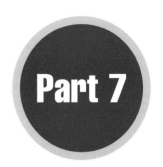

Part 7

Chapters

Don't forget to visit the companion website for this book at www.ataglanceseries.com/nursing/children where you will find over 500 interactive multiple-choice questions to supplement your learning.

111 Living with chronic illness

Figure 111.1 Family challenges

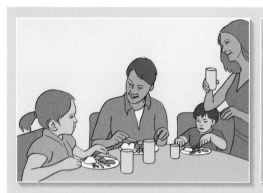

- Learning to integrate the restrictions of disease and treatment with other more routine aspects of their lives
- Developing knowledge and understanding of the child's condition and needs
- Living with uncertainties and knowing how to deal with emergencies
- Continuing to see the child as a child first and foremost
- Practical adaptations: home, location, work, lifestyle, finance
- Avoiding disruption to relationships
- Ensuring that siblings receive the same level of care and attention and feel involved
- Providing the extra time and support needed to help their child cope with the demands of the condition
- Having confidence in receiving support from other carers and professionals
- Finding time for themselves

Figure 111.2 Emotion and problem focused coping strategies

Emotion focused coping strategies Dealing with *feelings* about the situation (adapted from Lazarus and Folkman 1984)	• Not focusing on the condition; perspective seeking • Unburdening and explaining stress • Maintaining an image of the healthy child; normalizing • Thinking positively and clinging to hope • Taking one day at a time and staying calm • Seeing the child happy • Trusting others
Problem focused coping strategies Dealing with child's *needs* (adapted from Lazarus and Folkman 1984)	• Being assertive; taking charge of situations; learning and understanding • Advocating for child • Maintaining family integrity • Talking to other families and developing social support networks • Cooperating with professionals; adhering to treatment • Sharing responsibilities

Figure 111.3 Role of the children's nurse

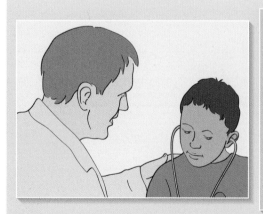

- Sensitive breaking of news to parents; helping parents to see their child as a unique individual who is a child first and the condition or disability as secondary
- Continuing to share evidence-based information at a pace that suits
- Helping the family to understand their emotional responses and coping strategies and coordinate specialist support as appropriate; ensuring sensitive and responsive family centred care at times of challenge or crisis
- Acting as an advocate for the child; ensuring their rights are upheld and they are involved in decisions; working in partnership to prepare the child and family to deal with 'normal' life transitions as smoothly as is possible; enabling the child or young person to self-manage their condition as far as they are able
- Collaborating with other professionals and services to ensure holistic family needs are met (e.g. regarding housing and finance)
- Planning ahead with the young person and family, enabling them to cope with transition from children's to adult services; ensuring well-coordinated and holistic end-of-life care and bereavement support as appropriate

Definitions

Chronic illness in childhood affects a relatively high proportion of the population. Estimates vary but are thought to be around 10–12% (Eiser 1997). The term 'chronic illness' is a generic term that relates to a wide range of long-term conditions including those that have a biological basis and consequent effects on the physical functioning body systems; sensory or physical disabilities; conditions that impact on long-term mental health and well-being; and those that affect cognitive and psychological development, communication and learning. Some children and young people may be affected by more than one condition or disability or have symptoms that affect a number of body systems.

Many conditions present at (or before) birth and others develop during childhood or the teenage years. Common features include the ongoing nature of the underlying disease; wide ranging consequences for the life of the individual child and family; possible limitations in daily living requiring some care in hospital (with continuing care ideally provided at, or closer to home); medication; dietary restrictions or special feeding regimes; special assistance, equipment, mobility aids or adaptations at home. Living with uncertainty may also be a feature, for example for the parents of the toddler who has Down's Syndrome who are unsure how he/she will respond to heart surgery; for the boy who has Haemophilia and is worried he may have a joint bleed during a PE lesson; for the teenage girl who has epilepsy and fears she may have a seizure while out at the cinema with friends.

Impact on the child and family

Learning that a child has a chronic illness will have a very significant effect on parents and must be handled with skill and sensitivity. The professionals involved must recognize that parents may be experiencing shock and grief and will need time and repeated opportunities to ask questions in order to be able to come to terms with the news. Implications may be far-reaching, affecting everyday routines, hopes and ambitions and the relationships between family members (including siblings) and the outside world. These vary, for example from the child who has mild Asthma that is well managed by the GP with few limitations on lifestyle to the young person who has to learn to self-manage Diabetes through daily injections of insulin, blood glucose monitoring and a carefully controlled diet. More extensive restrictions will be experienced by children who are dependent on technologically complex equipment to sustain their lives, for example children who require dialysis due to End-Stage Renal Failure or those who are dependent on assisted ventilation because of a complex breathing problem. Chronic illnesses also include mental health problems such as Anorexia Nervosa and potentially progressive or life-limiting conditions such as Cystic Fibrosis, Muscular Dystrophy and Leukaemia.

For many children and young people with more severe conditions, there will be numerous challenges: the management of symptoms; being active; maintaining optimal health and well-being despite limitations; exercising choice in how care is managed; and participating in as full a life as possible. Professionals will need to consider the support needed by a family learning to integrate the restrictions of disease and treatment with other, more routine aspects of their lives; recognizing the impact of parent's anxiety about the child's condition and well-being and the child's right to as 'normal' a childhood as possible. The reactions and support of brothers and sisters and other family members will also be an important consideration.

Child and young person first and foremost

According to the Children's Act (2004) the child or young person with a chronic illness will be considered to be a child in need of additional support and will require ongoing coordinated services, perhaps involving a number of professionals and agencies working together to ensure that he/she is safe, healthy and achieves his/her full potential. The role of the nurse is central in ensuring that children, young people and families receive the most supportive, responsive and empowering care possible and that this leads to optimal health, well-being and development. It is important to remember that the child who has a chronic illness is a child first and foremost. They share the same rights as healthy children and have similar concerns: about their relationships with other children, siblings and parents; fitting in; their ability to succeed; play and leisure interests; hopes, dreams, ambitions and fears. Life course transitions such as moving from nursery, through school, to further or higher education and employment may present particular challenges. Friendships and intimate relationships, establishing social and financial independence will be challenges for young people with chronic illness too. Transition between services (e.g. paediatric clinic to adult services) may present additional challenges requiring a coordinated and carefully planned approach starting in the early teenage years.

112 Cystic fibrosis management

Figure 112.1 Features of cystic fibrosis

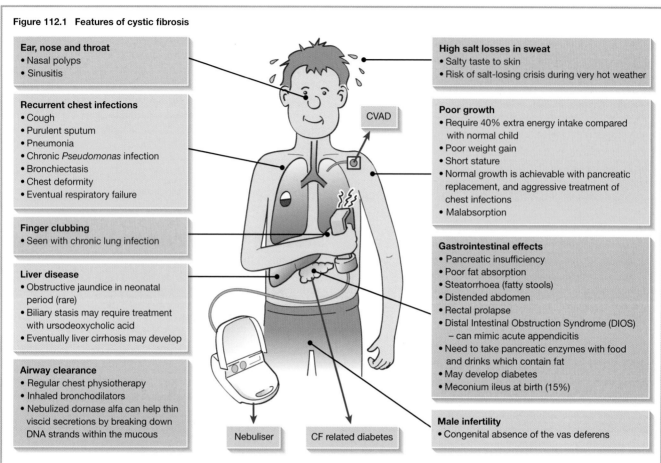

Ear, nose and throat
• Nasal polyps
• Sinusitis

Recurrent chest infections
• Cough
• Purulent sputum
• Pneumonia
• Chronic *Pseudomonas* infection
• Bronchiectasis
• Chest deformity
• Eventual respiratory failure

Finger clubbing
• Seen with chronic lung infection

Liver disease
• Obstructive jaundice in neonatal period (rare)
• Biliary stasis may require treatment with ursodeoxycholic acid
• Eventually liver cirrhosis may develop

Airway clearance
• Regular chest physiotherapy
• Inhaled bronchodilators
• Nebulized dornase alfa can help thin viscid secretions by breaking down DNA strands within the mucous

CVAD

High salt losses in sweat
• Salty taste to skin
• Risk of salt-losing crisis during very hot weather

Poor growth
• Require 40% extra energy intake compared with normal child
• Poor weight gain
• Short stature
• Normal growth is achievable with pancreatic replacement, and aggressive treatment of chest infections
• Malabsorption

Gastrointestinal effects
• Pancreatic insufficiency
• Poor fat absorption
• Steatorrhoea (fatty stools)
• Distended abdomen
• Rectal prolapse
• Distal Intestinal Obstruction Syndrome (DIOS) – can mimic acute appendicitis
• Need to take pancreatic enzymes with food and drinks which contain fat
• May develop diabetes
• Meconium ileus at birth (15%)

Male infertility
• Congenital absence of the vas deferens

Nebuliser   CF related diabetes

Figure 112.2 Professionals involved

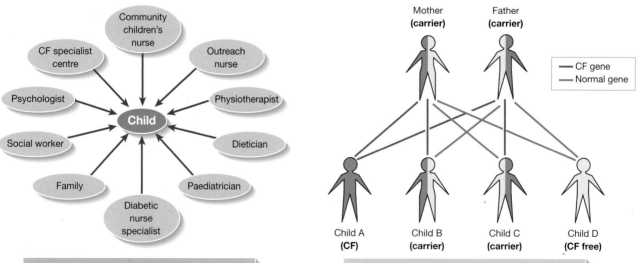

Community children's nurse
CF specialist centre
Outreach nurse
Psychologist
Physiotherapist
Child
Social worker
Dietician
Family
Paediatrician
Diabetic nurse specialist

Mother **(carrier)**   Father **(carrier)**

— CF gene
— Normal gene

Child A **(CF)**   Child B **(carrier)**   Child C **(carrier)**   Child D **(CF free)**

CF therapy:

• Nebulisers
• Physio
• Creon (enzyme)
• Exercise
• Lung function tests
• Cough swab
• Diabetic review

• 'Live a normal life'
• Liver scans
• Blood tests
• Hospital admissions
• Annual review
• 3 monthly local review
• Dietician

Genetic life limiting disorder found on chromosome 7. It affects CF trans membrane regulator. It is a recessive disorder which has thousands of mutations but both parents need to be a carrier for them to have a child which is affected by cystic fibrosis. They have a 1 in 4 chance of their child having cystic fibrosis depending on which mutation the child has will determine the severity of the condition. This condition requires daily intense treatment, can impact on all aspects of life.

Children and Young People's Nursing at a Glance, First Edition. Edited by Alan Glasper, Jane Coad, and Jim Richardson.
© 2015 John Wiley & Sons, Ltd. Published 2015 by John Wiley & Sons, Ltd. Companion website: www.ataglanceseries.com/nursing/children

ystic fibrosis (CF) is one of the most common life-limiting conditions that impacts on the quality of life of the child and their family. The condition can affect multiple organs, not only the lungs. CF affects the transfer of salt between our cells, and where salt goes water follows (osmosis). This alters the environment and effective motility within the organ. Earlier diagnosis improves prognosis.

Detection of CF

Screening of newborn babies for CF was commenced in 2007 and most cases are diagnosed this way. A blood test is carried out at birth with other screening tests.

Other ways in which CF can be diagnosed:
* Meconium ileus, which is bowel obstruction at birth
* Recurrent chest infections
* Failure to thrive and malabsorption.

CF diagnosis can be confirmed if the child presents with the above via a sweat test or a stool sample. Further tests are required to determine the mutation and severity of the condition.

Common problems and management
Chest infections

The lining of the lungs are covered in thick sticky mucous in CF patients, making it more difficult to clear the lungs of the mucous which contains bacteria and fungus. This leads to recurrent chest infections.

Pseudomonas aeruginosa is the most common fungal infection and causes scarring on the lung. It is hard to eradicate and so, once identified using a cough swab, lifelong treatment begins to suppress its growth and prevent scarring. Children with CF have daily prophylactic oral antibiotics to help prevent infection. Oral antibiotics are changed to a treatment regimen when the child becomes symptomatic. If the child remains unwell they will require hospital admission for intravenous antibiotics. It is a constant battle to prevent infection and maintain lung function. Failure to do so results in scarring of the lungs and the eventual need for a lung transplant.

A daily intensive physiotherapy regime also helps to clear the lungs of mucous in conjunction with nebulizer therapy.

Pancreatic insufficiency

Some children with CF have a deficiency in breaking down fatty foods which cause bowel obstructions. In the same way as their lung lining is thick and sticky, the gastric lining is also unable to pass food and break down any waste products. They produce foul-smelling sticky stools and require enzyme capsules (Creon) to aid digestion and absorption of vitamins and minerals. They require a high calorie diet to meet the metabolic demands, as children with CF are constantly fighting infections. If they are unable to maintain a good weight, they may have a gastrostomy device fitted to enable artificial feeding directly into the stomach. They may also need additional salt in their diet to replace salts lost through sweating.

CF-related diabetes

CF-related diabetes can develop as a result of blockages in the pancreas in the same way as the lungs become sticky and do not work efficiently. Some CF children require glucose monitoring and high blood sugars can be controlled by diet or insulin. Most patients with CF who go on to develop CF-related diabetes find it hard having to fit blood glucose monitoring and insulin injections into an already hectic treatment regime. To have both CF and CF-related diabetes can be hard to come to terms with.

Liver

Liver damage can be caused in the same way as the lungs; the bile ducts become sticky and the liver can develop cirrhosis. Patients need annual liver scans to detect any liver damage early.

Infertility

Most men with CF will go on to have problems with infertility and may require interventions to conceive.

Women with CF can have problems with fertility but most can go on to have children. They need to be monitored closely throughout their pregnancy.

Carriers of the CF gene are offered genetic counselling prior to starting a family when the risks are explained.

Impact on family

Diagnosis of CF is a life-changing event that impacts on all aspects of life. The treatment is not a cure but compliance with all forms of treatment can extend life expectancy, currently 38 years.

Everything is a constant battle and young adults find it hard to comply with all the treatment, attending school and taking control of their CF. Families struggle financially and parents become carers.

Segregation is required in CF clinics and on hospital wards to prevent cross-contamination. This helps to prevent infections but results in CF being a very isolating condition where peer support is hard to obtain. Parents can mix but patients are advised not to.

Transitional preparation begins around the age of 10 years and is based on preparing the young person for independent living. Most hospital wards only cater for under-16-year-olds and so CF patients are prepared for taking ownership of the condition, learning their medication routine and knowing when to seek medical interventions. This can be a hard time for everybody as parents have to take a back seat and allow their child to take more control which the child may not be ready for.

The burden and compliance with treatment is not only on the child or young person but the whole family. Every day is impacted by CF, whether the child is unwell or not. Having a child with CF causes constant uncertainty. The biggest uncertainty for the child or young person and their family is living with a reduced life expectancy.

A day in the life of a CF patient

The severity of CF is determined by the particular mutation. Therefore, treatment varies from daily oral antibiotics and physiotherapy, to nebulizers 3 times a day, intense physiotherapy, up to 20 different tablets throughout the day, Creon with every meal and artificial feeds overnight. This is in conjunction with 3-monthly admissions on to the ward for IV antibiotics for 2 weeks at a time, or sometimes 3 weeks. CF patients also attend regular clinics and undertake an annual assessment which involves a whole day of tests and lung function monitoring. Patients with severe CF have 24-hour oxygen therapy and a long wait on the transplant list. The disease is a battle for survival and a normal life.

113 Juvenile idiopathic arthritis

Figure 113.1 Juvenile idiopathic arthritis

Criteria for diagnosis of juvenile idiopathic arthritis (JIA)

- Patient under 16 years
- Arthritis (joint swelling or effusion) or two of the following: limitation of range of movement; tenderness or pain on motion; increased heat in joint
- Duration of 6 weeks or longer
- Exclusion of other causes

Diagnosis is on clinical findings. Antinuclear antibodies, rheumatoid factor, human leukocyte antigen typing or ultrasound aid assessment. X-ray and MRI may be considered

Possible complications

- Joint contractures
- Growth failure
- Leg length discrepancy
- Osteoporosis
- Joint damage requiring replacement
- Blindness from associated uveitis
- Scoliosis (secondary)
- Macrophage activation syndrome and amyloidosis (rare)

Many complications have been shown to be avoided with early recognition and aggressive treatment

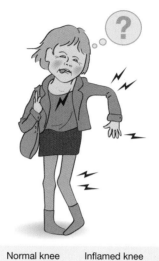

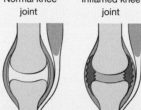

Normal knee joint   Inflamed knee joint

Treatment

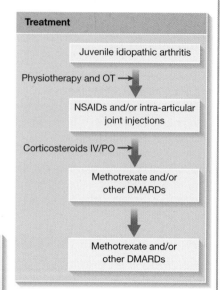

Juvenile idiopathic arthritis

Physiotherapy and OT →

NSAIDs and/or intra-articular joint injections

Corticosteroids IV/PO →

Methotrexate and/or other DMARDs

Methotrexate and/or other DMARDs

Effects of arthritis on joints

- Synovitis
- Pannus formation
- Cartilage and bone erosion

Paediatric rheumatology team

- Consultant
- Specialist nurse
- Physiotherapist
- Occupational therapist (OT)
- Ophthalmologist
- Psychologist
- Orthotist
- Play specialist

Differential diagnosis

- Biomechanical joint pain
- Reactive/post-infectious arthritis
- Septic arthritis/osteomyelitis
- Trauma/haematological disorders
- Malignancy including leukaemia, lymphoma
- Pain problems

Triangle of care

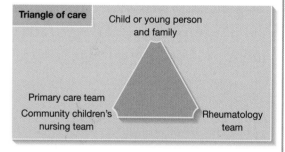

Child or young person and family

Primary care team
Community children's nursing team

Rheumatology team

Disease subtypes	Classification (research purposes)
Oligoarticular JIA (previously known as pauciarticular)	Up to four joints in first 6 months of disease (usually larger joints, e.g. knees, ankles and wrists). After 6 months if more than four joints become affected, classified as extended oligoarticular or if arthritis remains in less than four joints classified as persistent oligoarticular. More common in females (5 : 1)
Polyarticular JIA	Affects five or more joints during the first 6 months of disease. Often includes involvement of large and small joints; may have symmetrical pattern. Classified as rheumatoid factor negative or positive. More common in females (3 : 1)
Systemic onset JIA (previously known as Still's disease)	Arthritis in one or more joints (may not be present initially) with 2-week history of fever (usually quotidian), and one or more of the following: evanescent erythematous rash; lymphadenopathy; hepatosplenomegaly or serositis. Equal incidence in male and female (1 : 1)
Psoriatic arthritis	Arthritis and psoriatic rash or if no evidence of rash, arthritis and at least two of the following symptoms: dactylitis; nail pitting; psoriasis in a first-degree relative. Arthritis is usually asymmetrical
Enthesitis-related arthritis	Arthritis with enthesitis (inflammation where tendons or ligaments attach to bone), or enthesitis with at least two of the following: sacroiliac tenderness and/or lumbosacral pain; presence of HLA B27 antigen; onset of arthritis in a male over 6 years of age; acute anterior uveitis; family history of HLA B27-associated disease. Most common site is calcaneal insertion of Achilles tendon, plantar fascia and tarsal area
Undifferentiated arthritis	Arthritis does not fulfil any of the above subtypes. Can occur with arthritis-associated conditions (e.g. inflammatory bowel disease)

Children and Young People's Nursing at a Glance, First Edition. Edited by Alan Glasper, Jane Coad, and Jim Richardson.
© 2015 John Wiley & Sons, Ltd. Published 2015 by John Wiley & Sons, Ltd. Companion website: www.ataglanceseries.com/nursing/children

Juvenile idiopathic arthritis (JIA) is a term used to describe a group of autoimmune diseases characterized by arthritis. The UK prevalence is 1 in 1000. Subtypes devised by the Paediatric Standing Committee of the International League for Rheumatology (ILAR) are described in the Figure 113.1.

Patient history characteristically includes reports of morning stiffness with gradual improvement during the day. Increasing pain with activity in the absence of morning stiffness is usually indicative of a biomechanical problem. Active joints are usually painful on active or passive movement and can be swollen and warm. Other symptoms include fatigue, increased sleep requirements, increased irritability, loss of appetite and weight loss. These are more common in polyarticular or systemic disease.

Although the ultimate aim of treatment is to obtain disease remission, many children will continue to have flares of arthritis, so with persistent disease the aim may be to decrease the frequency of flares.

Joints commonly affected
- Jaw 30%
- Neck 10–40%
- Shoulder 50–60%
- Elbow 50%
- Wrist 80%.

Management

Aims of management are to prevent joint damage and to maintain joint function in order to promote independence and improve quality of life.

Exercise and physiotherapy are important aspects of treatment, aiming to prevent complications by maintaining full joint range of movement, improve muscle strength and prevent reduction in cardiovascular fitness. Educating families and professionals involved in the child's care about exercise is vital to minimize exclusion from activities and isolation from peers. In younger children, it is important to ensure normal developmental milestones are met. Education should also prepare for the possibility of disease flares and consider pain relief, support and advice for management during these periods.

Occupational therapy support and advice may be required for children with multiple joint involvement including joints of wrists and hands. They can provide handwriting assessment and advice for exams. Therapists can liaise with schools and provide information and guidance for teachers about how children can be supported in school to reach their full potential.

Pharmacological management varies depending on severity of disease (see treatment flow chart). Non-steroidal anti-inflammatory drugs (NSAIDs) and intra-articular steroid injections may adequately control oligoarticular disease, but when multiple joints are involved or if the arthritis reoccurs after joint injection, long-term therapy may be required. Methotrexate is the first choice drug, but if ineffective or not tolerated then other disease-modifying antirheumatic drugs (DMARDs) including biologic drugs are required. Steroids (intra-articular, intravenous or orally) can provide short-term relief or bridging until longer term therapy becomes effective. All drugs used require appropriate monitoring. Support and advice is usually provided by the specialist centre; shared care protocols may facilitate local support for prescribing, administering and monitoring, to minimize disruption to school and family life.

Specialist nurses have a pivotal role in coordinating care, holistic assessment and education, psychosocial support, drug advice and monitoring and liaising with primary and secondary care teams.

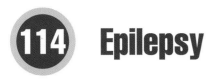

114 Epilepsy

Figure 114.1 Features of epilepsy

Tonic clonic	Absences	Myoclonic jerks	Tonic	Atonic seizures
For a full description of these, see the description below	Children lose awareness of their surroundings which may look like they are asleep, staring into space or their eyes roll back. It usually only lasts a few seconds but they may experience many in a day	Characterized by sudden jerking movements, often of the arms but can be the legs	The tonic stage as outlined, but with no following clonic stage	Characterized by a loss of muscle tone and floppiness

Generalized seizures

Generalized seizures means the whole of the brain is affected and the child loses consciousness

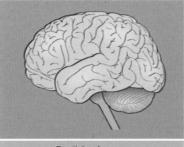

Partial seizures

The term 'partial' is used to describe the type of seizure that begins 'locally' in the brain

Complex

Complex behavioural disturbances

Simple

Small jerking movements, lip smacking

Tonic clonic seizures

This is the most common form of generalized seizure and is also the image many people have when they think of epilepsy. It consists of two stages: tonic and clonic.

At the tonic stage, the child may initially cry out, he/she usually experiences rigidity of the limbs and impaired breathing. The child may also be incontinent. If the child is standing he/she may fall to the ground and if seated will slump in the chair.

At the clonic stage, the child usually experiences generalized jerking throughout the body. This is often followed by a period of unconsciousness and, upon recovery, lethargy and confusion.

The duration of a tonic clonic seizure varies enormously but can range from just a few minutes up to 20 minutes or more.

There is much discrepancy regarding duration in the literature and this figure varies hugely. However, the important aspect to understand is what is typical for the child.

During the clonic stage, the heart is under a huge amount of pressure and often does not function as efficiently as normal so the child's blood supply to the brain may be disrupted.

Children and Young People's Nursing at a Glance, First Edition. Edited by Alan Glasper, Jane Coad, and Jim Richardson.
© 2015 John Wiley & Sons, Ltd. Published 2015 by John Wiley & Sons, Ltd. Companion website: www.ataglanceseries.com/nursing/children

Epilepsy is the most common chronic disabling neurological condition and is where a child has repeated seizures. Seizures occur in the brain and occur when the function of the brain is interrupted or becomes 'disordered'.

It is reported that approximately 1 in 131 people in the general population experience epilepsy but it is more common in the learning disabled population where the prevalence is approximately 1 in 3 and this figure increases as the severity of the learning disability increases (National Epilepsy Society, 2011).

Anyone can have epilepsy and it can develop at any time. However, diagnosis is most common below 20 years old and in older people (above 65 years) (National Epilepsy Society 2011). In children and younger people this is usually due to birth complications, childhood illnesses or infections, genetic conditions and accidents.

Everyone has the potential to have a seizure at different times in their lives and many people do due to illnesses or accidents. One seizure would not result in a diagnosis of epilepsy; a person would experience two or more seizures prior to receiving a diagnosis of epilepsy (National Epilepsy Society 2011). Of those who experience epilepsy, approximately 5% will have photosensitive epilepsy. This is where seizures can be triggered by flashing lights (National Epilepsy Society 2011).

Symptomatic epilepsy can be caused by any damage to the brain. This can be a result of central nervous system (CNS) infections such as meningitis or encephalitis, tumours, neurosurgery or head injury. Many people have idiopathic epilepsy, which means it arises spontaneously and the specific cause is unknown. The UK National General Practice Study of Epilepsy found that 60% of people with newly diagnosed or suspected epileptic seizures had epilepsy with no identifiable cause.

Seizures

During a seizure a person may experience changes in awareness, involuntary movement or confused behaviours. The clinical presentation (what the seizure looks like) depends on a number of factors:

- Part or parts of the brain affected
- Pattern of spread of the disordered activity through the brain
- Cause of the epilepsy
- Age of the individual.

There are approximately 40 different seizure types, so just knowing that a child has epilepsy does not really tell you much about what they experience or what a seizure will look like. To understand that we need to know more about what type of seizure the child has. Although there are 40 different seizure types they are usually divided in two main groups: generalized and partial seizures.

Generalized seizures

Generalized seizures means the whole of the brain is affected and the child loses consciousness. It is really important to remember this – the child is unconscious during the seizure – although in some cases what we see may seem small and insignificant, this is not what the child is experiencing.

Partial seizures

The term 'partial' is used within the literature to describe a type of seizure that begins 'locally' in the brain, in other words in one part of the brain. Partial seizures are often catorgorized as simple or complex. This type of seizure occurs without loss of consciousness; however, consciousness may be impaired and the child will not be in control of what is happening. Although partial seizures can originate anywhere, the most common sites are the frontal and temporal lobes.

Partial seizures can result in the person experiencing abnormalities of taste, smell, auditory and visual hallucinations, changes in pallor, small jerking movements of the limbs, strange mutterings and lip smacking. Additionally, in some cases it can manifest as complex behavioural disturbances. Some children experience a partial seizure that goes on to become a generalized seizure (usually a tonic clonic seizure): this is called secondary generalization.

Treatment

Antiepileptic drugs taken on a daily basis are always the first line treatment option for children with epilepsy but to become seizure-free can be a long process with a range of medication combinations being trialled. This can be a frustrating time for the child and their family and can take many years. Even after many years of medication combinations some people are unable to control their epilepsy and this is referred to as chronic or refractory epilepsy. To enable effective medication regimens, accurate recording of seizure activity is vital.

As well as medication, some people have other treatment options such as epilepsy surgery (brain surgery), vagus nerve stimulation or alternative therapies, such as relaxation techniques.

Status epilepticus

Normally, when a child has a seizure he/she will recover naturally and the seizure will end of its own accord; however, sometimes this is not the case – this is called status epilepticus. Status epilepticus is when the seizure is longer than the normal for that child or the child has several seizures straight after each other. Status epilepticus is an emergency situation as the child is unconscious and the blood supply to the brain can be affected and lead to brain damage.

There are rescue medications available for status epilepticus. The main forms of rescue medication:

- *Clobazam*: usually given orally
- *Diazepam*: most commonly given rectally
- *Lorazepam*: given intravenously, usually in hospital
- *Midazolam*: increasingly being given via the buccal route as this is preferred by carers and the person with epilepsy alike because of the less invasive nature of administration.

Although epilepsy is a chronic condition (meaning that people live with it all their lives and do not 'get better'), some children appear to grow out of it in that their brains develop their own defences. Even if a child does not, there are a wide range of treatment options available and 70% of people with epilepsy have their seizures controlled with medication. Most children with epilepsy live a full and happy life.

115 Childhood cancer

Figure 115.1   Childhood cancer

Cancer is a group of diseases that share common characteristics: uncontrolled cell growth following a genetic mutation

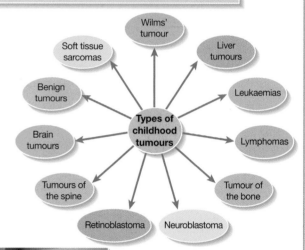

Types of childhood tumours:
- Wilms' tumour
- Soft tissue sarcomas
- Liver tumours
- Benign tumours
- Leukaemias
- Brain tumours
- Lymphomas
- Tumours of the spine
- Tumour of the bone
- Retinoblastoma
- Neuroblastoma

Childhood cancer: the facts

- Cancer in childhood is rare
- Approximately 1700 children in the United Kingdom are diagnosed with cancer each year
- Survival has improved from less than 30% in 1962–1971 to about 75%
- Cancer is the leading cause of death from disease in children and the second cause of death from all causes
- Leukaemia is the most common form of childhood cancer, followed by brain tumours
- Improved survival rates have been attributed to multimodal treatments, a centralized approach to treatment and involvement in clinical trials

Treating childhood cancer

Treatments involve one or more of the following:

- *Surgery:* to excise solid tumour
- *Chemotherapy:* use of cytotoxic agents to eradicate cancer cells, shrink tumour before surgery or for palliative control
- *Radiotherapy:* uses radiation to target tumour cells, or total body irradiation before transplantation
- Children in the UK are treated in specialized regional cancer centres
- Care is often shared with local hospitals
- Protocols are standardized through Children's Cancer and Leukaemia Group (CCLG)
- Duration and combination of treatment modalities is dependent on the child's diagnosis

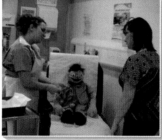

Adverse effects of chemotherapy

Immediate: nausea/vomiting, fatigue, allergic reactions, haemorrhagic cystitis

Short term: alopecia, stomatitis, myelosuppression, immunosuppression, gastrointestinal disturbances

Long term: infertility, growth retardation, secondary cancers, cardiomyopathy

Principles of care

- Centralized approach through CCLG
- Holistic care – biological, psychosocial and spiritual
- Evidence-based care
- Child and family centred approach to care
- Interdisciplinary approach
- Integrated model of care
- Cure with least cost to child
- Long-term follow up

Assessing and addressing the needs of the child and family

Assessment of need is an ongoing process for the nurse caring for the child with cancer and their family, occurring throughout each stage of the illness trajectory. Such need centres on the following areas:

- Physical
- Emotional
- Cognitive
- Social
- Spiritual

Care of the child undergoing chemotherapy

- Information regarding drugs and adverse effects
- Administration of chemotherapy usually via central line
- Minimizing and monitoring adverse effects
- Treatment of adverse effects
- Educating the child and family about minimizing and monitoring adverse effects, safe handling of bodily waste
- Preparation of the child for care during and after investigations (e.g. biopsy, lumbar puncture, MRI/CT scan)
- Supportive care for child (e.g. treating neutropenia, thrombocytopenia and anaemia, with intravenous antibiotics), mouth care, blood or platelet transfusions

Team players – the child with cancer and their family

Quality care for the child or young person with cancer must bemultidisciplinary:

- Oncologist/haematologist
- Psychologist
- Teacher
- Play specialist
- Nurse (CCN, specialist, clinic, ward)
- Radiologist
- Dietitian
- Physiotherapist/occupational therapist
- Dentist
- Doctor
- Laboratory staff
- Pharmacist
- Other families, children
- Voluntary organization
- Social worker
- Hospital chaplain
- Paediatric surgeon

Children and Young People's Nursing at a Glance, First Edition. Edited by Alan Glasper, Jane Coad, and Jim Richardson.
© 2015 John Wiley & Sons, Ltd. Published 2015 by John Wiley & Sons, Ltd. Companion website: www.ataglanceseries.com/nursing/children

Despite improved survival, the diagnosis of a childhood cancer is a life-altering experience for the child and family. As the child and family adapt daily life around the child's condition and necessary treatment, they find themselves in a period of sustained uncertainty in which they hope for cure but are conscious of the ever-present threat of death. Therefore, child and family centred care from the point of diagnosis of a childhood cancer is required from a skilled multidisciplinary team which involves statutory and voluntary services. The children's nurse has a crucial multifaceted role within the team.

Nurse as supporter

On diagnosis, parents can experience a plethora of emotional reactions: guilt, anger, fear and disbelief. The child or young person faces a number of feelings: bewilderment, loss and fear. Emotional support from the nurse is important at this time to help family members develop coping strategies to manage the impact that the condition and its treatment will have. Such impact can centre on psychological, social and financial issues. The nurse is often present while the child and family learn of the diagnosis, and has an integral role in ensuring information is given in a way that is easily understood. Such information provides a platform for decision making and may help to combat some of the stress, anxiety and feelings of helplessness often experienced by parents. Play, as a communication tool, can help the child and siblings express fear and anxieties. It is also a useful mode for imparting information about treatment and care. By assessing on an ongoing basis and recognizing key periods within the illness trajectory, the nurse establishes child and family coping, subsequently providing the required care or referral to specialist support as necessary (e.g. psychologist).

Nurse as physical care provider

Given the expansion of nursing roles in the past two decades, administration of chemotherapy has become a central tenet of the children's cancer nurse's role, following appropriate training. Alongside this the nurse is responsible for the assessment, recording and reporting of the child's physical condition to the medical team, thus enabling an appropriate plan of care. Assessment involves regular recording of temperature, pulse, respirations, blood pressure, fluid balance, weight, urinalysis and elimination. This assessment is of paramount importance to the care of the child and requires the nurse to possess a comprehensive understanding of the individual medical conditions, and the drug-specific adverse effects that may be encountered. The prompt identification of untoward symptoms and subsequent implementation of appropriate care is vital to the success of supportive treatment. Supportive treatment is necessary as the chemotherapy not only affects fast-growing tumour cells, but the body's normally occurring fast-growing cells: healthy blood cells made within the bone marrow; haemoglobin; white blood cells; and platelets. Deficiency of these cells within the body contributes to major adverse effects for the child including haemorrhage, lethargy and fatal sepsis due to lack of infection-fighting cells. During neutropenic (very low neutrophils) sepsis episodes, prompt administration of intravenous antibiotics is required; granulocyte colony-stimulating factor (GCSF, a growth hormone used to help the body produce white blood cells and therefore fight infection), antipyretics, blood product transfusions and nutritional support are essential elements of care to prevent a catastrophic event for the child and family. Fast-growing cells also include mucosal epithelial cells which line the mouth through the body to the anus. Destruction of these cells by chemotherapy commonly leads to electrolyte imbalances and gastrointestinal disturbances alongside increasing the risk of localizing infections. Furthermore, the control of symptoms due to drug administration or disease is also a focus of care for the children's nurse. The administration of antiemetics, analgesia and other supportive drugs help to control these adverse effects, promoting optimum comfort for the child.

Pneumocystis pneumonia (PCP) is a fungus that can be present in healthy people. However, in immunocompromised children it can cause a respiratory infection leading to cough, fever, shortness of breath and, in extreme circumstances, respiratory failure. To prevent PCP, all children with cancer receive prophylaxis during treatment and for 6 months following chemotherapy, usually involving the prescription of oral co-trimoxazole (Septrin) for a locally agreed number of days per week.

Nurse as teacher and educator

The children's nurse must ensure any teaching carried out is family centred, considering any factors that would influence their ability to learn. Teaching involves identifying the signs of infection, the safe handling of bodily fluids, mouth care, immunizations, safety in the sun and the importance of reducing exposure to infection by limiting contact with crowds. Given the family centred approach to care, families may choose to participate in technical aspects of care (e.g. care of their child's central line or nasogastric tube). A nurse-led teaching programme is carried out where parents are supported in the attainment of necessary skills. The nurse educates and assesses parents' ability to learn new skills to care for their child. Teaching and education is a continuous process rather than a one-off activity. A parent's ability to retain the knowledge and skills should be reassessed as appropriate.

Nurse as team player

A diverse team of professionals, with their own specific expertise, provide care to the child with cancer and their family. The composition of the team for each individual child differs according to their diagnosis, condition at a particular time, location and specific family need. Members of the multidisciplinary team include professionals from both statutory and voluntary organizations. Given the amount of time spent with the child and family, nurses often have an in-depth insight into the child and family situation at a given time. Nurses must share knowledge and maintain good levels of communication with the team to ensure best care is provided.

Summary

Children's nurses caring for children with cancer and their families must utilize a range of skills. Compassionate holistic care must be tailored to the unique needs of each child and family unit. A broad range of interpersonal skills is crucial, including the ability to build a therapeutic relationship with the child and family, to use age-appropriate language with the child and siblings and promote communication within families and among the medical team.

116 Cleft lip and palate

Figure 116.1 Cleft lip and palate

Cleft lip and palate can occur as a single abnormality or in association with other congenital abnormalities as part of a syndrome

Incidence
Approximately 1000 babies are born in the United Kingdom each year affected by a cleft lip and/or palate, an incidence of about 1 in 700 live births

Aetiology
- The fusion of the lip and palate happens early in pregnancy (4–11 weeks)
- A cleft lip or palate occurs as failure of this fusion
- A cleft lip can be detected on the 20-week antenatal scan

Causes and contributing factors
- Not known in most cases
- Can happen when a number of genetic and environmental factors occur together
- Smoking
- Alcohol intake during pregnancy
- Medicines taken during pregnancy
- Family history of cleft
- Use of recreational drugs during pregnancy

Associated problems
- Over 400 syndromes associated with cleft
- More likely to occur with an isolated cleft palate (50%)

Most common
- Pierre Robin sequence
- 22q deletion
- Stickler syndrome
- Van der Woude syndrome

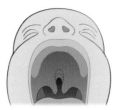

Cleft of the soft palate

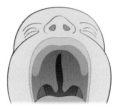

Cleft of the soft and hard palate

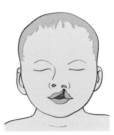

Incomplete cleft

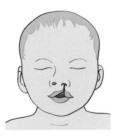

Complete cleft lip

Types of cleft

Types of cleft palate
- Hard palate
- Soft palate
- Hard and soft palate
- Submucous cleft palate

Cleft palate
- Up to 50% of births will be an isolated cleft palate which can involve the hard palate, soft palate or both
- This type of cleft is more common in girls

Submucous cleft palate
Occurs when the skin of the palate is intact but there is a cleft of the underlying muscle

Types of cleft lip
- *Complete:* up into the nose
- *Incomplete:* part of the lip
- *Unilateral:* one side
- *Bilateral:* both sides

Cleft lip
Approximately 20% of referrals will be an isolated cleft lip with or without a cleft of the alveolus (gum)

Cleft lip and palate
- Accounts for approximately 35% of births
- More common in boys
- 25% unilateral
- 10% bilateral

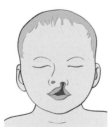

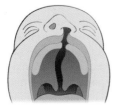

Unilateral cleft lip and palate

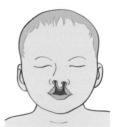

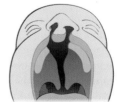

Bilateral cleft lip and palette

Children and Young People's Nursing at a Glance, First Edition. Edited by Alan Glasper, Jane Coad, and Jim Richardson.
© 2015 John Wiley & Sons, Ltd. Published 2015 by John Wiley & Sons, Ltd. Companion website: www.ataglanceseries.com/nursing/children

Cleft lip and palate is a relatively common facial anomaly in babies, which varies in frequency according to racial or ethnic group. The prevalence of cleft lip and palate is highest in native Indians, followed by Chinese and Japanese communities. It is lowest in Afro-Caribbean and Maoris.

Cleft services

Cleft lip and palate is managed by a multidisciplinary team including clinical nurse specialists, paediatricians, surgeons, speech and language therapists, physiologists and orthodontists. Nine regional networks exist in the United Kingdom to facilitate high standards of care based on a hub and spoke principle.

Support and management

Patients with cleft and their families are seen according to nationally agreed standards and care pathways from birth until adulthood. Treatment includes surgical repair of the lip and/or palate, usually in the first year of life. Further treatment includes speech and language therapy, hearing and dental interventions.

Common problems and their management
Feeding management

In an infant without cleft, the uvula and epiglottis lie adjacent to each other which allows fluid to pool safely in the hyperpharynx or oropharynx until the swallowing reflex is triggered. In infants with cleft, the anatomical differences prevent this safety mechanism, resulting in the risk of aspiration if inappropriately fed.

Babies born with a cleft present with a range of feeding difficulties. Poor feeding and growth can lead to increased parental anxiety. The most notable difficulties are insufficient suction, excessive air intake, choking, nasal regurgitation, fatigue, inadequate milk intake and extended feeding duration. The use of soft bottles allows the delivery of milk to the infant who is unable to generate suction to gain adequate nutrition (assisted feeding). Exclusive breastfeeding of these infants may not be possible and many mothers choose to give expressed breast milk.

Although the Department of Health guidelines state that milk alone is a sufficient food for babies up to 6 months of age, babies with cleft may be ready for weaning foods before this age. While weaning foods are not recommended for infants under 17 weeks, most babies enjoy a variety of consistencies prior to the repair of the cleft palate.

Missed diagnosis

There is a 23% incidence of missed diagnosis of a cleft palate in the first 24 hours of birth. This highlights the inadequacy of digital examination of the palate and identifies the importance of visualizing the palate with a spatula and light through to a single uvula. Late diagnosis can result in dehydration, readmission to hospital, faltering growth, increased parental anxiety, early cessation of breastfeeding and litigation.

Otitis media with effusion

Otis media with effusion is almost universal in children with a cleft palate. This high incidence is attributed to eustachian tube dysfunction associated with anatomic and physiological variations of the tensor veli palatini muscle. This results in an accumulation of fluid in the middle ear causing a conductive hearing loss. The treatment includes the insertion of grommets and the use of hearing aids.

Speech

It is recognized that children with a cleft palate are at high risk of both speech disorders and language delay. Approximately 40% of children will require speech and language therapy.

Syndromes

There are over 400 syndromes associated with cleft lip and palate, with approximately 15% of cases affected. The most frequently associated are with an isolated cleft palate, with up to 50% having a congenital abnormality or syndrome.

Pierre Robin sequence

Pierre Robin sequence (PRS) is the most common anomaly associated with cleft palate. It may occur on its own or part of a syndrome, with Stickler syndrome and 22q deletion being the most common. PRS includes the presence of a cleft palate, micrognathia (small jaw) and glossoptosis (a retroverted retroplaced tongue) resulting in respiratory obstruction, which presents on a continuum of severity. The treatment of the obstruction includes positioning, nasopharyngeal airways and continuous positive airway pressure (CPAP).

Reparative surgery for lip and palate

Surgical repair of the lip is undertaken at 3–6 months and repair of the palate at 6–9 months of age. The displaced muscles of the lip and palate are surgically repositioned and joined together. In clefts of or including the hard palate, the palatal selves are brought together. Further surgery on the palate may be undertaken at 3–6 years to improve speech outcomes.

Alveolar bone graft

For clefts involving the alveolus (gum), a bone graft is undertaken at approximately 7–9 years of age.

Postoperative care

The main issues following surgery are breathing, feeding and pain relief. The main emphasis is directed towards protecting the repair, monitoring for excessive bleeding, ensuring adequate hydration and maintaining the airway.

Airway management

Postoperative swelling can result from oedema and the presence of blood or exudate in the respiratory tract. Problems can be caused by an infant used to a large airway coping with a smaller one. Signs of airway difficulties are 'sucking in' of the lower lip on inspiration and sternal, intercostal or subcostal recession. Distress should be acted on promptly as these infants can deteriorate rapidly. Some will benefit from the insertion of nasal airways.

Adequate pain relief is important for both pain management and to facilitate feeding and adequate hydration.

117 Diabetes

Figure 117.1 Type 1 Diabetes

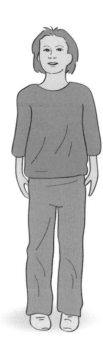

Type 1 diabetes

- Acute presentation due to rapid onset of symptoms over several days or weeks
- Prevalence in children is 1 in 700–1000
- Peak age for diagnosis is 10–14 years; 4% increase in incidence annually, particularly in under-5-year-olds

Diabetic ketoacidosis (DKA)

- Serious life threatening complication
- Presence of ketones
- Hyperglycaemia
- Vomiting and dehydration
- Abdominal pain
- Polydipsia, polyuria
- Kussmaul respiration
- Weight loss

Diagnosis

- Fasting plasma glucose ≥7 mmol
- 2-hour post-prandial level of ≥11.1 mmol
- Polyuria
- Polydipsia
- Weight loss
- Tiredness

Complications

- DKA
- Hyperglycaemia /hypoglycaemia
- Nephropathy
- Neuropathy
- Retinopathy
- Hyperlipidaemia

Hypoglycaemia

- Blood glucose ≤3.9 mmol or below; '4 is the floor'
- Possible causes: missed meals, exercise, alcohol and too much insulin
- Confirmed by blood glucose testing
- Symptom awareness important and prompt treatment is needed
- *Neuroglycopenic*: confusion, irritability, headache, slurred speech, dizziness
- *Adrenergic:* sweating, shakiness, paleness, anxiety, palpitations, hunger
- *Mild:* symptoms recognized and successfully treated with fast-acting and starchy carbohydrate
- *Moderate:* assistance required, consider Glucogel if conscious but airway concerns
- *Severe:* loss of consciousness, risk of seizure, coma and death, give IM glucagon
- Over-treating can result in rebound hyperglycaemia
- Fear can develop, especially regarding nocturnal episodes
- If glycaemic control is good, loss of hypoglycaemia awareness can occur
- Symptoms can occur ≥4 mmol or above if glycaemic control is poor or blood glucose level is falling quickly

Hyperglycaemia

- Fasting blood glucose >7 mmol or 2-hour post-prandial level of ≥11.1 mmol
- Symptoms include polyuria, polydipsia, tiredness, abdominal pain, behaviour change, lack of concentration
- Causes include insufficient insulin, growth spurts, omitted doses, snacking, interaction from other medications, illness, infection, reduced exercise, stress, unhealthy injection sites, if an insulin pump is used there can be problems with insulin delivery
- Increased frequency of blood glucose testing advised
- Test for blood ketones if blood glucose ≥14 mmol; frequency of testing level dependent
- Utilize correction factor
- Use sick day rules advice if concurrent illness, never stop insulin
- Management different if using insulin pump

Type 1 diabetes mellitus is a chronic irreversible condition resulting from a lack of insulin caused by autoimmune destruction of pancreatic beta cells; underlying triggers for this are not yet identified. Early recognition of signs and symptoms is essential as insulin insufficiency results in hyperglycaemia and, if undiagnosed, the life-threatening complication of diabetic ketoacidosis (DKA) occurs. There is short-term impact on and long-term implications to health, due to associated complications.

Type 2 diabetes occurs because of insufficient insulin production or resistance by the body's cells to insulin. Treatment options are determined by the severity and progression of the condition. Management options include diet and physical activity, oral medication and insulin. Incidence within children and adolescents is increasing; rationale for this includes changes in lifestyle and reduction in exercise and obesity.

Other types of diabetes can occur as a result of underlying medical conditions or treatment, and they can also be attributable to genetic factors.

Complications and associated conditions
Hypoglycaemia
Regulation of blood glucose is primarily achieved by the hormones insulin and glucagon. Insulin facilitates absorption of glucose from the blood, allowing its utilization by the body for energy. Glucagon produced by pancreatic alpha cells stimulates glycogen to be released from the liver and muscles, preventing hypoglycaemia. The effectiveness of this glucagon response in type 1 diabetes is suppressed by artificial insulin and it is common for the production of glucagon to become insufficient, consequently episodes of hypoglycaemia will always require treatment according to their severity.

The classification of hypoglycaemia, of which there are three categories, is dependent on the level of impairment to cognitive functioning because the brain is unable to store glucose and is reliant on a continual supply. The symptoms experienced and signs exhibited are unique to the individual and it is important they are able to recognize and treat the episode promptly before it escalates in severity; concentration can be affected for several hours . Frequent hypoglycaemia could indicate insulin adjustments are necessary; wearing medical identity jewellery is advisable. The signs and symptoms of hypoglycaemia can be categorized into neuro-glycopenic (brain or central nervous system response to reduced glucose) and adrenergic (the body's response to the lack of glucose).

Hyperglycaemia
Elevated blood glucose levels can occur and are considered significant if >14 mmol because of the potential for ketone production and development of DKA. There are various causes of raised levels and the insulin sensitivity (how much 1 unit of rapid acting insulin return the blood glucose by) is utilized to return the blood glucose to the target level. If ketones are present, corrections might not be as effective; more insulin will be needed. Rapid-acting insulin can accumulate causing a stacking effect; caution should be applied to frequency of corrections. Insulin pump users should consider infusion set problems or insufficient insulin as potential explanations.

Diabetic ketoacidosis and long term health
Patients with newly diagnosed type 1 diabetes mellitus can present with DKA and there is the potential for those with an existing diagnosis to also develop this condition. As a result of the lack of insulin, the body requires an alternate energy source and produces ketones by utilizing fat and protein. Excessive ketone production causes the pH of the body to become acidic and, accompanied by hyperglycaemia and dehydration, DKA results; cerebral oedema can occur. DKA is a serious preventable medical condition which requires hospitalization and national guidelines dictate management. There is a high mortality and morbidity rate associated with this complication.

Long-term health complications encompass renal failure, blindness and foot problems, with the risk of amputation, heart disease and stroke. Achieving the recommendation for glycaemic control reduces the risk of developing these and screening is undertaken as part of the annual review.

Treatment
Insulin is given using pen devices or infusion pumps and attempts to replicate the body's natural insulin secretion. Regimens are chosen on their suitability and individual appropriateness to optimize glycaemic control. The frequency of insulin administration is dependent on the regimen used.

Psychological and social issues
Appropriate education should be given to staff involved in supporting the individual within the educational setting and care plans should be implemented. The level of support needed will correlate to age and cognitive ability but will also be dependent on the individual's involvement in their practical diabetes care. Attending to health needs during school hours is imperative and must be accommodated.

Many families manage well, however, the diagnosis can be devastating triggering a grief response because of the perceived loss of their healthy child. The incidence of chronic sorrow amongst parents is identified. Although they are not responsible, type 1 diabetes is not preventable, parental guilt is common. The whole family is affected and life changes dramatically for the individual diagnosed. Diabetes intrudes and practical management causes discomfort. Acceptance of the condition can be problematic and resentment can result in concordance issues. Understanding is influenced by cognitive age, and challenges occur at each stage of development, producing added stress. Parents worry about the long-term health implications of sub-optimal control. This can potentially cause conflict, but concern can be interpreted as nagging. Adolescence is a notoriously difficult period, presenting its own unique obstacles, particularly the desire for greater independence and the introduction of risk-taking behaviour. Parents can be reluctant to relinquish control; independence regarding diabetes self-care is not always successful, manipulation is common and diabetes management is often negatively affected during this stage of development.

118 Diabetes management

Figure 118.1 Diabetes management

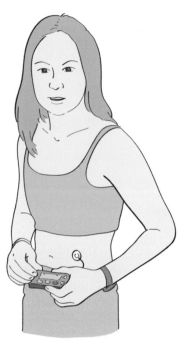

Management

- Secondary health care multidisciplinary team approach
- Achieves best practice tariff requirements
- Identifies a suitable insulin regimen
- Delivers comprehensive education
- Aims to reduce development of the associated complications
- Monitors and reviews glycaemic control
- Prepares young person for transition into adult services. Equips schools/education establishments with the training required to support children and young people with diabetes.

Illness management

- Always give insulin
- Insulin adjustments might be required
- Increase frequency of blood glucose testing
- Test for ketones
- Monitor hydration
- If not eating an alternative source of energy is required
- Early contact with diabetes team for support

Education

- Continual structured programme
- Identified aims and learning objectives
- Considers learning needs and styles
- Provision of supportive literature or written information

Blood glucose testing

- Testing should occur before meals and bed, is advised if participating in physical activity or at any other time if unwell
- Greater frequency of testing if using an insulin pump
- Wash hands with soap and water, dry properly
- Prepare lancet device using a new needle each time
- Prepare blood glucose meter for use
- Obtain blood sample
- Apply to strip
- Result obtained
- Depending on rationale for testing implement action accordingly

Insulin administration basic rules

Injection pens

- Ensure correct insulin and is fit for use
- Use new needle every time and prime before use
- Check correct insulin, correct dose, correct time, correct way
- Dial up required amount and administer into a healthy injection site
- Once plunger depressed fully count for 10 seconds before removing the device
- Dispose of needle in sharps container

Insulin pumps

- Delivered by an indwelling subcutaneous cannula
- Difficulties can be experienced with insulin delivery; troubleshooting required
- Cannulae should be inserted into healthy sites, and are usually changed every 2 days or earlier if problems with insulin delivery are experienced

Insulin regimens

- **BD:** twice daily insulin administration, using a mixed insulin (combination of short and intermediate-acting)
- **TDS:** three insulin injections a day, utilizing a combination of rapid, intermediate and long-acting insulin
- **MDI:** multiple daily injections, minimum of four a day. Combines rapid-acting insulin with food and long-acting insulin usually given once a day
- **CSII:** continuous subcutaneous insulin infusion of rapid-acting insulin. No basal insulin used. Boluses given with food

Different insulin regimes require different eating advice. However, nutritional intake should be healthy and well balanced

Management of diabetes in children and young people is provided by secondary health care using a multidisciplinary approach. The introduction of the best practice diabetes tariff aims to standardize diabetes care nationally to ensure all service provision is equitable. The objective is to equip the individual and their family with the essential practical skills required and the underlying knowledge needed to understand and make informed decisions regarding their diabetes management. Health education includes developing the motivation to succeed, through a programme of structured education addressing self-care, crisis management and lifestyle. Delivery must accommodate cognitive abilities and preferred learning styles. Challenges are encountered, families are asked to question their existing health beliefs and accomplish behavioural changes that are difficult to implement consistently. Specific stages of childhood development present their own management issues. Glycaemic control is determined by the HbA1c. The target is less than 58 mmol/L (7.5%), achieved without frequent or disabling hypoglycaemia. This level reduces the risk of developing the associated complications. Testing for concurrent medical conditions and screening for the associated complications resulting from micro and macrovascular disease occurs as part of the annual review. Blood glucose testing identifies blood glucose levels and these are recorded in a diary and reviewed regularly by the paediatric diabetes specialist nursing team.

Insulin regimens

Insulin therapy endeavours to replicate the natural insulin secretion by the body; however, the endocrine system is incredibly complex and many factors impact on achieving this. A common adverse effect of artificial insulin is hypoglycaemia. The aim is to achieve a preprandial blood glucose level of 4–8 mmol and 2-hour post-prandial levels of no greater than 10 mmol/L. Insulin regimens are chosen for their suitability for each individual child and NICE guidance is provided. Intensive insulin regimens reduce the risk of developing the associated long-term health complications.

Insulin types

Rapid-acting insulin is given immediately before a meal or snack. The dose is calculated by counting the content of the carbohydrate of the food to be consumed and starts working within 15 minutes of being administered, peaks at 30–90 minutes and lasts 3–5 hours.

Short-acting insulin is also given with meals and starts working within 30–60 minutes, peaks at 2–4 hours, lasting for 5–8 hours. **Intermediate-acting insulin** onset occurs after 1–3 hours, peaking at 8 hours and lasts 12–16 hours.

Long-acting insulin starts working after 1 hour and does not have a peak; its duration is 20–24 hours. This is usually given in the evening; however, it can be necessary to halve the dose and also administer it in the morning.

Insulin administration

Insulin is given subcutaneously by insulin pens (prefilled or cartridge) or delivered by an insulin pump. It is absorbed through the underlying fat cells in the skin. Areas for administration include buttocks, thighs, upper arm and stomach; insulin absorption rates are influenced by injection site choice. Injection site rotation is imperative as repeated administration of insulin in specific areas results in lipohypertrophy, a common problem causing erratic insulin absorption. Desensitization to injections in these areas occurs, impacting on willingness to rotate injection sites appropriately. A dose of insulin should never be repeated, additional blood glucose testing is advised if it is unclear if the correct dose or full dose was given.

Nutrition

A healthy well-balanced diet is advocated to optimize growth and maintain a healthy weight. Carbohydrate counting is used with continuous subcutaneous insulin infusion (CSII) and multiple daily injections (MDI) regimens to calculate the insulin to food ratio; a diary is kept and ratios assigned to meal times. Twice (BD) and three times daily (TDS) regimens require regular snacks to prevent hypoglycaemia. Issues can develop regarding attitudes towards food; binging and restricted eating can occur and will impact on blood glucose stability and glycaemic control, intentional hyperglycaemia assists with weight loss. All of these issues will require additional management support by the multidisciplinary team.

Physical activity

Aerobic (low intensity) or anaerobic (high intensity) exercise affects blood glucose. Counter-regulatory hormones released during anaerobic activity can cause a temporary glucose elevation but this can be followed by hypoglycaemia several hours later. Aerobic activity lowers the blood glucose during exercise and afterwards. Prior to the activity additional carbohydrate and increased testing, possibly in conjunction with insulin reductions, can be utilized to prevent hypoglycaemia. If hyperglycaemia is present this could be exacerbated if there is a lack of insulin within the body so it is advisable to check the blood glucose is within target before commencing exercise.

Illness management

A diagnosis of diabetes does not increase the risk of developing illnesses or infections unless blood glucose control is suboptimal. During episodes of illness, control can be affected by insulin resistance because of counter-regulatory hormones increasing, requiring additional insulin doses. However, not all illnesses will result in hyperglycaemia. It is not uncommon for episodes of diarrhoea and vomiting to cause hypoglycaemia due to reduced food intake and increased gut motility resulting in poor absorption, therefore a reduced amount of insulin will be needed.

Irrespective of how the blood glucose is affected during times of illness, insulin should always be given, the frequency of blood glucose and ketone testing should be increased, and hydration maintained. It is advisable to test for blood ketones if the blood glucose level is 14 mmol or above. Blood ketone testing is more accurate; ketone excretion in the urine is delayed potentially impacting on management. If appetite is decreased, carbohydrate will need to be given in the form of drinks. If this is not tolerated and vomiting occurs, medical assessment is advised because of the risk of DKA. Encouraging the individual or their family to contact their health care provider for support at the start of illness could prevent hospital admission and reduce the incidence of DKA.

119 Childhood obesity

Figure 119.1 Childhood obesity

The UK currently has the highest rate of childhood obesity in Europe, with one-third (30.3%) of children aged 2–15 years overweight or obese. Obesity is described as an excess of body fat as indicated through body mass index (BMI) measurement

Relevant publications/initiatives

World Health Organisation (2013)	Childhood overweight and obesity
National Institute for Health and Clinical Excellence (NICE) (2012)	Preventing Type 2 Diabetes: Risk Identification and Interventions for Individuals at High Risk
British Heart Foundation (2011)	Unhealthy food and drink marketing to children
Department of Health (2011)	Healthy Lives, Healthy People: A call to action on obesity in England
Health and Social Care Information Centre (2009)	Children's overweight and obesity prevalence, by survey year, age-group and sex (National Child Measurement Programme)
Department of Health (2006)	Change for Life
National Institute for Health and Clinical Excellence (NICE) (2006)	Obesity: the prevention, identification, assessment and management of overweight and obesity in adults and children
National Audit Office (2006)	Tackling Childhood Obesity – First Steps
World Health Organisation (2004)	A Global Strategy on Diet, Physical Activity and Health

Childhood Obesity – Health Implications

Psycho-social
- Depression
- Low self-esteem
- Eating disorders

Pulmonary
- Asthma
- Low exercise tolerance

Gastrointestinal
- Fatty liver disease
- Gallstones
- Iron deficiency anaemia

Musculoskeletal
- Joint problems
- Flat feet
- Osteoarthritis
- Plantar fasciitis

Sleep apnoea

Cardiovascular
- Heart disease
- Hypertension

Endocrine
- Diabetes Type 2
- Early onset puberty
- Polycystic ovary syndrome

Increased risk of certain cancers

Recommendations Royal College of Paediatrics and Child Health

- All health professionals trained in weight management
- Increase taxation on foods with high fat, sugar or salt content
- Advertising ban on unhealthy foods before 9pm
- Implementation at a local level of plans to increase play and active lifestyle
- Extension of free school meals – these are universally provided in some other European contries

Position statement chilhood obesity (2012)

Causes of childhood obesity

Many children are overweight because they simply eat more calories than they need. Many foods liked by children are high in fat, salt and sugar. From an early age children also pick up poor dietary habits from their parents and family. Excessive portion sizes and insufficient physical activity only serve to compound the issue.

A lack of sleep has also been suggested as a contributory factor. Children going to bed later and getting less sleep has been shown in some cases to increase the levels of the hormones leptin and ghrelin that monitor and act on body fat stores. Other hormone imbalances such as hypothyroidism can have an effect on appetite and body fat, as can some medications.

Current statistics

It is estimated that obesity and its health consequences costs the NHS approximately 4 billion pounds a year; this is set to rise as long-term health implications will manifest for the increasing numbers of overweight and obese children in future years. The current state of affairs in the United Kingdom, and indeed globally, is referred to as the 'obesity epidemic'.

National Child Measurement Programme

The National Child Measurement Programme (NCMP) was launched in England in 2005 and consists of the height and weight measurement of children at primary school in Reception (age 4–5 years) and Year 6 (age 10–11 years). From these measurements the body mass index (BMI) can be calculated using a simple equation:

$$BMI = \frac{weight\ (kg)}{height\ (m)^2}$$

The NCMP is dependent upon parental consent; thus, it could be argued that the results are not representative of the population as a whole as some families do not participate. It is also suggested that there is a higher than average representation of overweight and obese children within those families that refuse consent, and in reality overweight and obesity rates are significantly higher than current figures indicate.

There is also evidence to suggest that parents will consistently under-estimate their child's weight. We are becoming so used to seeing morbidly obese people in the media that we naturally adjust what we think is 'normal' and do not recognize overweight children in many cases.

It is important to recognize that BMI should not be calculated for children in the same way as an adult's BMI. There are specific growth charts for children (WHO centile charts) that indicate a normal BMI range for children of a similar height, age, sex and ethnic background.

Health risks

There are increased intermediate and long-term health risks clearly associated with childhood overweight and obesity. Of mounting concern is the growing body of evidence that many overweight and obese children become overweight or obese adults. Morbidities linked with obesity include heart disease, diabetes, hypertension, fatty liver disease, gallstones, osteoarthritis, early puberty, asthma, sleep apnoea and musculoskeletal problems.

What can be done?

Of key importance to the progress of any weight management programme has to be a wide approach that involves all the family, with gradual changes more likely to be successful. Children's nurses are ideally placed to offer healthy eating advice on an opportunistic basis when working with children and families, but will require further training in order to give up-to-date and effective advice at an appropriate time.

The following suggestions have some merit:

- Avoid snacking – have three regular meals instead
- Eating together at a table instead of in front of the TV
- Reduction of fizzy drinks
- Balanced and varied diet, high in fibre and starchy foods
- Five portions of fruit and vegetables
- Take care with portion sizes
- Healthy snacks if needed
- Avoid fried food.

It is recognized that dietary intake is only a part of the solution as increasing physical activity is crucial to any weight management plan. Children need to be more physically active and spend less time on sedentary behaviours such as computers, video games and television.

Obesity in childhood can also lead to psychological issues and poor self-esteem. Confidentiality and building confidence are important; in particular when working in schools with individual children. Strategies must be discreetly employed and sensitive to the needs and feelings of these vulnerable children. This is also applicable to the implementation of the NCMP.

Change4Life

The Change4Life programme is a government-led initiative aimed at supporting people with healthier choices. It was advised in 2010 that children over 5 years should be engaging in physical activity for at least 60 minutes each day, while children under 5 years should be engaged on a daily basis in active play for 180 minutes. Other Change4Life initiatives include information about healthy snacks, portion control and hidden fats and sugars in everyday foods (launched in January 2013).

Key points

- Reducing the amount of calories eaten is crucial to a successful reduction in weight.
- Successful weight loss programmes must include a range of strategies and an increase in physical activity.
- Changes must be made gradually to increase the chances of success.
- All health professionals have an important role in childhood weight management and should receive appropriate training and support to implement this.

120 Eating disorders

Figure 120.1 Eating issues

Common eating disorders	
Anorexia nervosa (AN)	Inability to eat and maintain body weight. Fixation and anxiety related to body shape, weight and food. Usually affects young girls aged 12–17 years, but approximately 1 boy in 100 of the same age
Bulimia nervosa (BN)	A range of behaviours related to periods of excessive over-eating followed by purging and accompanying feelings of anxiety and self-loathing
Binge eating disorder (BED)	Over-eating to compensate, reduce feelings of poor self-esteem or as a comforting ritual

Risk factors (AN and BN)

- Family history of eating disorders and depression
- Bullying and perceived criticism over eating behaviours, body shape and weight
- Anxiety and desire to be thin due to peer pressure, media or sport needs (e.g. athletics, modelling, dancing, ballet)
- Poor self-esteem, anxiety-provoking triggers such as social situations, obsessive personal and family traits.
- Critical parents, a need to please and always achieve perfection
- Past traumatic experiences including emotional, sexual abuse and neglect
- Fear of failure, adaption, change

Physical symptoms (AN)

The symptoms of AN are those of chronic starvation. In recovery, young people also experience periods of obsessive and checking rituals, self-harm, devious and distracting behaviours (including purging, water loading, hiding food, excessive exercise) in an attempt to reduce feelings of anxiety.

Starvation symptoms include amenorrhoea, diarrhoea, pellagra, lanugo (fine hair), muscle and brain atrophy, poor dental hygiene, oedema, kidney failure, osteoporosis, constipation, acne, cardiac arrest, reduced cognitive ability, electrolyte abnormalities, delayed gastric emptying, endocrine disorders, cold extremities

Summary of recovery treatment for AN and BN

Recovery takes the form of redeveloping a sustainable relationship with food, body image and identity including self-esteem and self-worth

Cognitive behavioural therapy (CBT) aims to help young people rationalize, think and perceive differently. It aims to provide awareness of coping strategies, cognitive drills and new ways of acting

Family therapy aims to explore the nature of dynamics and ways family members can begin to support one another

Individual therapy provides a safe space to build authentic relationships and explore personal issues

Body image work explores personal and wider expectations made about appearance and notions of beauty

Warning signs

- Ritual and routine related to eating in certain places and time
- Wearing oversized and concealing clothing
- Missing meals, claiming to have already eaten
- A denial of sexual development, libido and sexual maturity
- Gives a feeling of mastery, power and control
- Feeling physically defective, socially judged
- Symbolic of becoming invisible, not existing, having low self-esteem

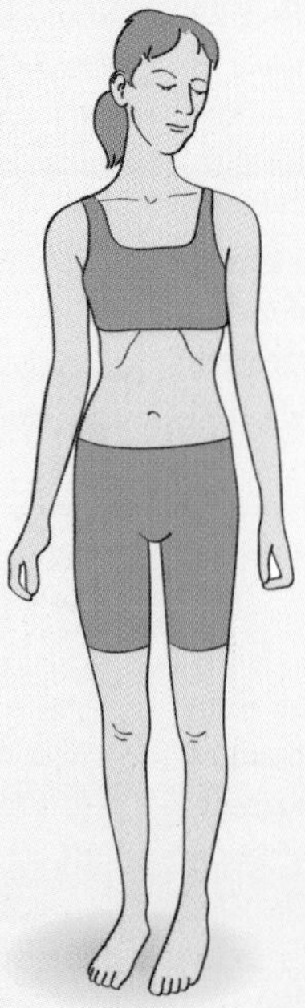

- Ritual and routine related to eating in certain places and time
- Purging, water loading, vomiting, daily/hourly weighing
- Excessive exercising, pre-occupation with body image
- A false and distorted sense of confidence
- ED gives: feelings of control, self-respect and success
- Consumption of only low calorie foods

Children and Young People's Nursing at a Glance, First Edition. Edited by Alan Glasper, Jane Coad, and Jim Richardson.

© 2015 John Wiley & Sons, Ltd. Published 2015 by John Wiley & Sons, Ltd. Companion website: www.ataglanceseries.com/nursing/children

What are eating disorders?

Eating disorders are an abnormal attitude towards food, body image and body weight which transpires in a number of disorder classifications. The primary three are anorexia nervosa (AN), bulimia nervosa (BN) and binge eating disorders (BED).

Anorexia nervosa is when someone attempts to maintain a chronically dangerously low weight by purposefully starving themselves, exercising excessively and purging. It is characterized by an anxious preoccupation with food and body image, with corresponding secretive, ritualistic and manipulative behaviours.

Bulimia is a chronic condition which for some may be constant in their lives. For others it is reactive to stressful events. Bulimia-like binge eating is the attempt to control weight and emotional aspects of life by over-eating and then deliberately being sick or using laxatives (medication to help empty the bowels). Binging is a response to emotional distress, over-compensating, self-esteem issues and difficulty recognizing bodily sensations.

Binge eating disorder is classified as being more spasmodic than bulimia, but no less serious. It is characterized by control and compulsion to overeat.

These eating disorders have a significant impact on the developmental needs of young people, usually during their most significant developmental period (puberty). The direct causes are unknown, but it is known that eating disorders impact not only physically, but also psychologically and on social developmental needs.

Who is affected by eating disorders?

Around 1 in 250 girls and 1 in 2000 boys will experience AN at some point. The condition usually develops around the age of 13–17 years. Based on these figures it can be estimated that 5–10 million people in the United Kingdom at some time will experience some type of eating disorder, ranging from full-blown AN to picky and finicky eating patterns. BN is around five times more common than AN and 90% of patients are female. It is often the case that boys are diagnosed with depression or associated appetite disorders rather than AN or BN.

Causes of eating disorders

The causes of eating disorders are unknown but there is consensus that there are a number of probable causes which include biological, genetic, attachment issues, bullying, media, environmental abnormalities, sexualized trauma, idealized and irrational beliefs about shape, weight and health. These factors appear to be influencing factors in eating disorders in an ever-increasing concern with celebrity, image and issues of thinness.

Treatment
Refeeding program (AN)

It is usual that when a young person's body weight has dropped below a body mass index (BMI) of 13–15 and they are a seriously low weight (e.g. 35–40 kg), they will be admitted for inpatient treatment to local Child and Adolescent Mental Health Services (CAMHS). There is no hard or fast rule regarding these criteria, but a safeguarding decision by professionals regarding the welfare of the young person who is suffering the effects of chronic starvation is the high priority at this point. It might be the case that a young person is admitted against their will on a section of the Mental Health Act (1983), because they are cognitively unable or unwilling to consent to necessary life-saving treatment. Treatment usually takes the form of a two-phase program: refeeding and recovery. The two phases are often blurred because of the long-term and chronic nature of eating disorders (young people can have both AN and BN for a number of years, sometimes past their teenage years). In the first instance, the refeeding program can takes months with the aim of gaining 1 kg/week.

This first refeeding stage involves the establishment of strict mealtime routines, restriction of exercise, a response to increased anxiety and subsequent self-harm, close monitoring at meal times and daily structure. Young people will have increased anxiety because they are either gaining weight as in the case of AN, or being prevented from stress-reducing behaviour of binging, over-eating and purging in the case of BN. This often creates complex multiple dimensions to diagnosis (sometimes referred to as dual diagnosis). In practice, it means young people will experience high levels of **anxiety, depression, self-harm** urges and **obsessive compulsive disorder** (OCD) type symptoms over a period of weeks and months. These vary between individuals, especially in the initial stages of reducing the effects of starvation and gaining weight.

Treatment regimens vary. Some adolescent units focus on weight more than others. This means young people have a 'target weight' (sometimes two weights, a lower and a higher) set and they will work towards attaining and then 'maintaining'. They will be expected to eat all meals at set times, within set time limits and at designated supervised tables. In other units the emphasis is less about weight, measuring out foodstuffs and regular weighing (it is still debated by professionals as to whether young people should even know their weight), and more about health and social implications of change. Yet, target weights are still set and aimed for in preparation for the seamless engagement in the second phase of treatment: recovery. Some young people may also be prescribed medication to help them deal with anxiety, depression and compulsions as they begin to engage with both stages of their treatment.

Recovery program (AN, BN and BED)

The recovery phases of treatment vary according to type and acuteness of the eating disorder. However, it is nearly always the case that a number of interventions are used in combination. When engaging in supportive, psychotherapeutic and self-esteem building interventions, the young person and their families are also being instructed in new ways of relating to food and each other. Some units have facilities that allow for planned meals where the family can eat and plan meals prior to slowly increasing the number of meals expected to be eaten away from the unit. Thus, the mechanics of food preparation and consumption remain at the forefront of treatment, but during the recovery phase there is an expectation of reduced monitoring and surveillance as the young person and family improve and adapt to the disorder. Other interventions that occur during the recovery phase are intended to support and provide skills in maintaining and confronting the triggers that can lead to relapse. They include attendance in body image type therapy, cognitive behavioural therapy (CBT), family therapy and more expressive and creative therapies such as music and art therapy.

Many young people with eating disorders excel in school-based activities and often attempt to distract progress by excessive school work. Recovery is aimed at promoting balance in lifestyle and recognizing relationships with food.

121 Mental health problems

Figure 121.1 Mental health problems

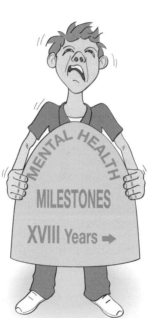

Predisposing influences on mental health

Genetics

Some characteristics such as temperament and intelligence are influenced by genetics. Specific conditions such as autism, Down's syndrome and language disorders

Prenatal and perinatal complications

Maternal impact such as age, smoking, malnutrition, blood type and drug use

Physiological dysfunction

Poorly functioning bodily systems indicative of anxiety, acute psychosis

Parent, family and social factors

Attachment difficulties, neglect, poor parenting, stress, abuse, social disadvantage, chaotic family circumstances, domestic violence, criminality and poor parental mental health, poverty, inadequate role models

Psychological factors

Poor and low self-esteem, deficient cognitive ability, immature defence and coping mechanisms

Developmental milestones

Parenting roles

Safety, care, control, intellectual stimulation, able to take instruction, moral development

Physical

Appropriate physical growth, puberty, sexual maturity

Cognitive

Psychometric intelligence, Piagetian cognitive development, skill acquisition, problem solving, information processing

Emotional

Self-soothing skills, expression and appropriate response to stimuli, curiosity, rudimentary empathy, recognition and anticipation of others, development of temperament toward

Social

Able to engage in creative play, responsive arousal, identity development, autobiographical memory, appropriate adaption to life transitions, language development, ability to self-evaluate and self-regulate, commitment to social values

What is a mental health problem?

There are many factors that contribute to mental health problems for young people and children. Typical statistics suggest that 1 in 10 of children and young people will require professional help at some time in their lives regarding their mental health before the age of 18.

Typically, mental health problems show themselves in two distinct age periods. First, for children aged from 5 to about 12 years and, second, for young people aged 12–18 years. Mental health problems for both groups affect the **emotional, cognitive, educational** and **behavioural** capacity of the patient. The most common mental health problems for children are those associated with inattentiveness and poor social behaviour such as **attention deficit hyperactivity disorder** (ADHD), disruptive behaviour such as **conduct disorders**, and language and emotion type disorders such as **Asperger's syndrome**.

For teenagers, mental health problems include **depression**, **self-harm**, **anxiety disorders**, **social disorders** focused on an inability to cope (including para-suicide), **obsessive compulsive disorders** (OCD), **bipolar disorders**, **psychosis** and **eating disor-**

ders such as **anorexia nervosa**. Unlike adult psychiatry, young people often have complex or dual diagnosis, which means a combination of the above, on their path to achieving their key maturational milestones. According to the World Health Organization (WHO), mental health is 'a state of well-being in which the individual realizes his or her own abilities, can cope with the normal stresses of life, can work productively and fruitfully'. For young people and the family, mental health is not only the absence of mental health problems, but also the accomplishment of developmental milestones that impact and compound difficulties in this life stage.

Types of services

In the United Kingdon, children and young people come under the care of Child and Adolescent Mental Health Services (CAMHS). Every region has access to Tier 3 (community-based specialist teams) and Tier 4 (specialist adolescent inpatient facilities). Both of these tiers have multi-agency specialist professionals (including mental health nurses, social workers, occupational therapists,

Children and Young People's Nursing at a Glance, First Edition. Edited by Alan Glasper, Jane Coad, and Jim Richardson.

consultant psychiatrists, teachers, psychologists, family therapists, art therapists and other therapists) who assess, treat and follow up young people and families in their care.

Most mental health problems take a long time to recover and the need for ongoing support is provided by seamless service delivery and interdisciplinary teamwork. The liaison of Tier 3 CAMHS teams with other health care professionals such as children's nurses usually shows itself in the assessment of risk and evaluation of young people admitted to emergency settings for self-harm, para-suicide attempts and distorted body image issues. It is not uncommon for these young people to be repeat service users as they often come from chaotic and unsettled backgrounds and show their distress through their behaviour.

The role of CAMHS is to respond quickly, provide specialist assessment of mental health status and treatment as necessary, create conditions for seamless service provisions between multi-agency teams, provide specialist knowledge (including that related to the Mental Health Act (1983)) and specify follow up, appropriate monitoring and referral.

Types of mental health problems

Mental health problems in childhood very rarely manifest as a simple single diagnosis as they might in adulthood. Diagnosis is more often dual or complex. What this means is that a child will never present as simply having depression, but rather depression as a symptom of some other conflicting social dilemma confronting the child. Thus, it is common for children with ADHD to show classic signs of inattentiveness, spontaneous outbursts and inability to control their temper as well as having feelings of despair, low mood and anxiety as they get older. Likewise, teenagers with anorexia nervosa will more than likely have periods of anxiety, extreme agitation, low mood and depression as they work through their recovery.

Anxiety disorders (including panic disorders, phobias, PTSD)

These types of mental health problems for children and young people manifest as severe to moderate fear of social situations, objects, people and places. They result in maladaptive coping strategies and triggers including avoidance, physiological responses including panic. Most patients will complain of persistent and constant intrusive thoughts and sometimes the obsessive and compulsive repetition of comforting acts. If the young person is suffering from the effects of past trauma they may be experiencing symptoms of **post-traumatic stress disorder** (PTSD) which include flashbacks, self-harm, fear of losing control and disruption to everyday self-care activities.

Mood disorders

These are sometimes referred to as affective or depressive disorders and relate to a young person feeling either elated (manic) or low (depressed). Most patients recover given time with the use of antidepressant medication. Major depressive episodes have symptoms of withdrawal, suicidal ideation, poor self-care and slowed cognition. Some mood disorders such as **bipolar disorder** may have a physiological and genetic cause that affects the regulation of mood balancing neurotransmitters. **Seasonal affective disorder** (SAD) is thought to be triggered by a response to lack of daylight.

Psychosis

It is rare for children to have psychotic type disorders, including schizophrenia. However, a few young people in their teenage years experience psychotic symptoms associated with distorted delusional thinking, hallucinations (which can be visual, auditory, olfactory or sensory), negative symptoms such as social withdrawal, poor self-care, disrupted thinking patterns and flatness of mood. Psychosis-type disorders can be acute and a one-off as a result of physical or emotional trauma or induced by the use of drugs. For some young people, psychosis can be chronic and need treating with medication or depot injections for a number of years.

Language and learning disorders

There are a number of categories of ADHD, but they all share symptoms of hyperactivity, inattentiveness and impulsiveness. Disruptive behaviour makes it difficult for the child to fit in with their peer group because they are often fidgeting, easily distracted, unable to complete tasks, loud and disruptive. The cause is uncertain, but may be related to anxiety, depression, undetected seizures, emotional trauma or genetics.

Autism and Asperger's syndrome

Autism and Asperger's syndrome are developmental disorders that impact on the ability of the child or teenager to form relationships, emotionally connect, relate to reality, have imagination and socialize. There are different degrees and characteristics, so the disorders are often considered as a spectrum.

Conduct disorders

Children and young people who over a long period of time show an inability to follow rules, display aggressive and violent behaviour out of context may be diagnosed having conduct disorders.

Recognizing problems

The following are behaviours most young people experience at some time in their lives. However, in their chronic state they often accompany a number of mental health problems in childhood and adolescence.

- **Acting out**: expressing distress and over-arousal in inappropriate ways such as tantrums, screaming, running away, self-harm and physical threats, somatic problems, dangerous risk-taking, para-suicide.
- **Withdrawal**: a persistent rejection of company, isolation in bedroom and solitary comfort, elective mutism, phobias, chaotic family systems, special education issues, psychosis, abuse, neglect.
- **Emotional avoidance**: procrastination, seeking risk, desire to question reasonable requests, low self-esteem and pessimistic outlook, seeking destructive relationships, dogged denial, drug and alcohol abuse, engaging in distracting activities, mental and social disengagement, generalized anxiety disorder, PTSD, repetition problems such as ODC, mood disorders, suicide.
- **Attachments and bonding**: affected by neglect, failure to thrive, inconsistent discipline, confused communication patterns, poor protective systems.
- **Physical**: anorexia nervosa, bulimia nervosa, eating disorders, self-harm.

122 Self-harm in childhood

Figure 122.1 Methods of self-harm

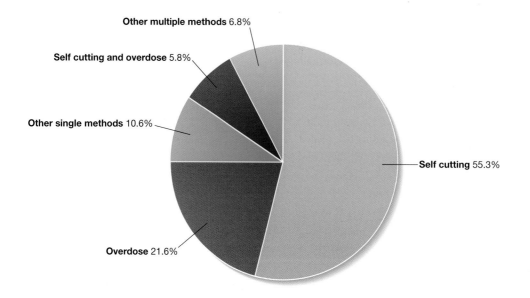

- Other multiple methods 6.8%
- Self cutting and overdose 5.8%
- Other single methods 10.6%
- Self cutting 55.3%
- Overdose 21.6%

Deliberate self-harm is always very serious. It can cause disability and death. It is also serious because it means that a person is seriously emotionally distressed at the time of their injury. Working in an honest and open way with children and their families is always the key to a successful therapeutic relationship.

What is self-harm?

While the term self-harm may at first seem self-explanatory, a universally accepted definition of this phenomenon is not easy to find. Professionals and organizations within which these disciplines work use a range of words to describe this behaviour. Various terminologies have frequently been used in the literature:

- Deliberate self-harm
- Self-injurious behaviour
- Repeated self-injury
- Self-wounding
- Para suicide
- Self-mutilation
- Self-wounding
- Episodic and repetitive self-injury
- Autodestructive behaviour.

Furthermore, definitions can vary from short explanations such as the one offered by the National Institute of Clinical Excellence (NICE) guidelines on self-harm (NICE 2004a: 16) 'Self-poisoning or injury, irrespective of the apparent purpose of the act', to longer definitions, for example the one used by the World Health Organization in 1989 (Platt et al. 1992: 92):

An act with an non-fatal outcome in which an individual deliberately initiates a non-habitual behaviour that, without intervention from others will cause self-harm, or deliberately ingests a substance in excess of the prescribed or generally recognised therapeutic dosage and which is aimed at realising changes which the subject desired via the actual or expected physical consequences.

However, the International Child and Adolescent Self-Harm in Europe (CASE) study group (Madge et al. 2008) utilize a working definition whereby self-harm is seen as an act with a non-fatal outcome in which one or more of the following behaviours are present:

- Ingesting a substance in excess of the prescribed or generally recognized therapeutic dose
- Ingesting a recreational or illicit drug which was an act that the person regarded as self-harm
- Ingesting a non-ingestible substance or object
- Any initiated behaviour that an individual intends to cause harm to self. For example, deliberately cutting oneself, jumping from a height, self-inflicted cigarette burning, wound excoriation and mutilation of the face or other body parts.

A research study conducted by Evans et al. (2005) describes the methods of self-harm school-based adolescents utilized in the previous year (Figure 122.1).

Prevalence of self-harming behaviour

Self-harm is a serious public health problem, and has become increasingly more common among young people. Favazza (1998) describes self-harm behaviour as a morbid form of self-help that is antithetical to suicide. People who deliberately hurt themselves contravene the most basic of human drives – self-preservation. The consequent shaming experience and diminished self-efficacy that may emerge can lead a child's motivation from being self-harming to suicidal. Subsequently, deliberate self-harm is indirectly related to suicide as people who deliberately self-harm are 18 times more likely than the rest of the population to eventually complete suicide. Cooper et al. (2005) reported that there is a 30-fold increase in the risk of suicide for those who self-harm compared with non-self-harmers. In addition, suicide may be an unintended consequence of deliberate self-harm and therefore self-harming behaviours are an ominous sign of the potential to complete suicide (Mangnall and Yurkovich 2008).

Research findings show that self-harm is more common in females (13.9%) than males (4.3%). Young women aged 15–18 years had the highest incidence of deliberate self-harm based on hospital presentations to A&E in 2011, at 589 per 100 000 (NSRF 2011). These rates imply that 1 in every 171 girls presented to hospital in 2011 with a presentation of self-harm. In the United Kingdom, it is one of the top five reasons for acute medical admissions (NHS Centre for Reviews and Dissemination 2000).

What causes self-harming behaviour?

There is no single cause for self-harming activity. However, research suggests that some children may be at more risk of this behaviour than others:

- Young people who are involved in risk-taking behaviours such as alcohol and substance misuse or have addictions
- Those with mental health disorders (e.g. depression, anxiety, eating disorder or schizophrenia)
- Individuals at crisis point or under severe stress (e.g. ongoing family relationship problems)
- Those who have a debilitating or chronic illness
- People who have had experiences of childhood trauma and/or abuse.

Is it just 'attention seeking'?

Some people view self-harming behaviour as 'attention seeking'. This negative attitude is unhelpful to the child as it can leave him/her feeling as though his/her distress and feelings are trivial. Research has shown that children who harm themselves often have great difficulty with asking for help and generally have very poor problem-solving skills. They tend to have memories that overgeneralize their experience and may forget how they solved a similar problem in the past. They can get stuck when trying to solve a current problem. This can lead to feelings of frustration and being out of control. For other young people, self-harm may indicate that they are experiencing symptoms of a mental disorder.

Management and treatment

The primary purpose of intervention is to prevent suicide, prevent any repetition of self-harm and address the worries and issues that are causing this behaviour.

Screening instruments for at risk individuals:
- Beck Hopeless Scale (BHS)
- Child Suicide Assessment (CSA)
- Expendable Child Measure
- Firestone Assessment of Self-destructive Thoughts (FAST)
- Hopeless Scale for Children (HPLS)
- Inventory of Suicidal Orientation 30 (ISO-30)
- Life Attitudes Schedule (LAS)
- Measure of Adolescent Potential for Suicide (MAPS)
- Millon Adolescent Clinical Inventory (MACI)
- Multi-Attitude Suicide Tendency Scale (MAST)
- PATHOS
- Reasons for Living (RLF)
- Suicide Probability Scale (SPS).

Treatment options available for this group:
- Psychological interventions (e.g. cognitive behavioural therapy, dialectical behaviour therapy, problem-solving therapy)
- Behavioural techniques
- Family therapy
- Psychopharmacological interventions
- Group psychotherapy.

Management of self-harm in the paediatric setting

Environmental

Ensure all sharps, ligatures and dangerously ingestible substances are removed from the immediate area. Observe the young person regularly at 15 or 30 minute intervals.

Interpersonal

Provide support to the young person to discuss their concerns, anxieties and low mood.

Behavioural

Consider a behavioural support strategy like a first aid distraction kit. This can consist of a shoe box containing items for soothing or distraction, such as a music device, stress ball and writing materials.

Consider a behavioural contract in conjunction with the multidisciplinary team that will incorporate a commitment to approach staff when they experience the urge to self-harm.

Family

Liaise with the family to assist them to understand self-harm and help them to source community services for ongoing care.

123 What is a learning disability?

A complex way of being

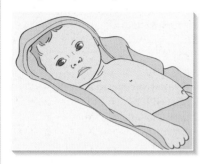

Learning disability is the term that the Department of Health use within their policy and practice documents. In Valuing People (2001), they describe a 'learning disability' as a:

- Significantly reduced ability to understand new or complex information, to learn new skills
- Reduced ability to cope independently which starts before adulthood with lasting effects on development

(Department of Health (2001) Valuing People: A New Strategy for Learning Disability for the 21st Century)

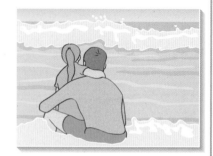

Genetic anomalies

- Down's syndrome
- Edwards syndrome
- Sanfilippo syndrome or mucopolysaccharidosis III (MPS-III)

(http://www.cafamily.org.uk/)

Could be caused **prenatally**

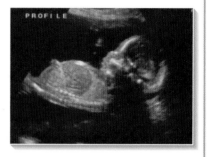

Neonatal anoxia

Could be caused **perinatally**

Precipitated or prolonged labour

- PKU
- Trauma
- Infection
- Or, as in a lot of cases, we just do not know

Could be caused **postnatally**

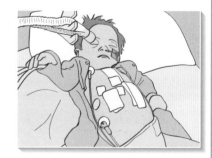

Valued social role

- No-one is born with a disabled identity, it is society that conditions that in an individual, this often happens in the form of a deviant career path
- Deviant career paths – simply put, if life is a career, then as soon as a disability is diagnosed then your 'career' path as a family and an individual is often treated as different or deviant from everyone else
- You should not receive a second-class service just because you have an extra special need
- Human beings

(http://www.nottingham.ac.uk/nmp/sonet/rlos/learndis/babyfirst)

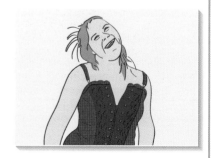

Children and Young People's Nursing at a Glance, First Edition. Edited by Alan Glasper, Jane Coad, and Jim Richardson.
© 2015 John Wiley & Sons, Ltd. Published 2015 by John Wiley & Sons, Ltd. Companion website: www.ataglanceseries.com/nursing/children

What do the words mean?

Often disability, impairment and handicap are used interchangeably but it is important to remember that the WHO makes distinct differences between them and whichever label you see written it is a person first and label second

Impairment: refers to a lack, or loss of some physical or intellectual function. An 'intellectual impairment' suggests the incomplete development (or loss) of mental abilities

Disability: a disability refers to the situation where someone cannot do certain things because of their original impairment. A 'learning disability' refers to someone's restricted, or reduced, ability to learn as quickly, or as readily, as people without impairments

Handicap: a person is handicapped when, because of a disability, she/he has fewer opportunities to take part in everyday life than non-handicapped people. A person with 'learning disability' may have some difficulties in speech or in reading, but the real handicap may be other people's attitudes or prejudice. Handicaps can be reduced through changes in attitude, when people are given more opportunities to take part in the everyday life of the community (http://www.who.int/topics/disabilities/en/)

How do we label a person? Or indeed a family?

Consider what you know about children who have a learning disability and treat this as a reflection or portfolio exercise

• When did you first become aware of people with a learning disability?
• What was the nature of the contact?
• What was the position of your community about these people?
• How much did that influence you?

The right to be yourself!

How do we devalue people who are different? By the imposition of a vicious circle which can reinforce a label and prove to us we were right to have such thoughts.

The vicious circle

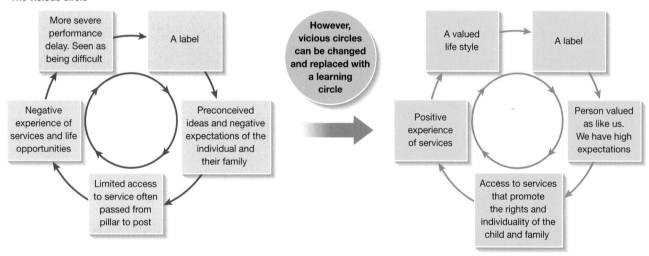

How to reverse the trend?

By measuring people by what they can do, rather than by what they cannot, and using the normalization philosophy in a productive therapeutic way. The concept of being 'ordinary' within your own social sphere is inextricably linked with the **philosophies of normalization** which were developed across Europe and Canada over the last 30 years. Essentially, normalization is a set of guidelines that should ensure that people who are labelled as different get what the rest of us take for granted – a valued social role, and their place in society.

Remember!

• It is a set of values
• A moral code
• Something in which you believe
• It influences how you view people and what you do with them

124 Autistic spectrum disorder

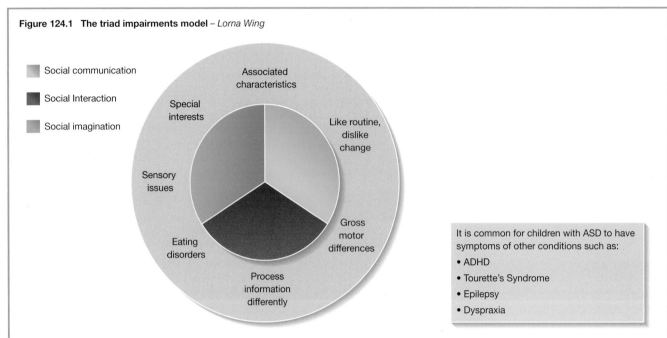

Figure 124.1 The triad impairments model – *Lorna Wing*

It is common for children with ASD to have symptoms of other conditions such as:
- ADHD
- Tourette's Syndrome
- Epilepsy
- Dyspraxia

What is autistic spectrum disorder?

Autistic spectrum disorder (ASD) is a neurobiological disorder of development. It is a lifelong condition; people do not get better from ASD. It is a 'spectrum', which means that while all people with autism share certain difficulties or characteristics, their condition will affect them in different ways and can vary hugely. It includes Asperger's syndrome as well as autism with learning disabilities. It affects how a person communicates with, and relates to, other people. It also affects how they make sense of the world around them. Many people with ASD experience over-sensitivity or under-sensitivity to sounds, touch, tastes, smells and light; this is called sensory hypersensitivity or hyposensitivity.

Autism

The three main areas of difficulty that all people with autism share are sometimes known as the 'triad of impairments':

- Difficulty with social communication
- Difficulty with social interaction
- Difficulty with social imagination.

   Children with ASD do not 'look' disabled. Parents of children with autism often say that other people simply think their child is naughty but this is not the case.

   Autism is a common condition with over half a million people in the United Kingdom, that is around 1 in 100 people. People from all nationalities and cultural, religious and social backgrounds can have autism, although it appears to affect more boys than girls.

Causes

The cause of autism is still not known. However, research suggests that a combination of factors, particularly genetic and environmental, cause changes in brain development. Autism is not caused by the child's upbringing, their social circumstances and is not the fault of the child with the condition or their parents. It is not linked to 'bad parenting' and it is not caused by the MMR vaccination.

Brain differences

Studies have shown that the brains of people with ASD are different in the:

- Frontal lobes
- Limbic system
- Brainstem and fourth ventricle.

   Between 30% and 50% of people with autism have been found to have abnormally high levels of serotonin (a chemical responsible for transmitting signals in nerve cells). Autistic brains have shown to have additional neurons than neurotypical (non-autistic) brains. There are differences in the location of electrical activity in the brain in people with ASD. There are differences in the time course of electrical activity in the brain in people with ASD. Communication between different parts of the brain is reduced in people with ASD. The brain receives a lot of information from the world and people with ASD take more time to process this information.

Triad of impairment

The areas of difficulty in the triad of impairment manifest in different ways in each individual but below is a list of some of the ways it can affect them.

   Impairment of social communication:

- Talk at you
- Incessant communication
- Not true communication (e.g. may not follow the usual rules)
- Concrete understanding
- Do not engage in social chat
- Communication confined to own needs
- Struggle to understand non-verbal communication
- Echolalia
- Repetitive
- Formal speech.

   Impairment of social interaction:

- Abnormal eye contact
- Indifference to others
- Aloofness
- Pay little attention to responses
- Preference for isolation
- Impaired social behaviour
- Empathy issues
- Active but odd
- Passive.

   Impairment of social imagination:

- Rigid inflexible thinking
- Restrictive repetitive play
- Abnormal play; spinning, flapping
- Lack of imagination
- Self-stimulatory behaviours
- Difficulty in generalizing concepts
- Circumscribed interests.

Supporting children with ASD

When supporting children with ASD there are a few key things to remember:

- Think about their sensory sensitivities and try to adapt the environment accordingly
- Remember the triad of impairment and work with it
- Do not try to make the child conform (e.g. do not insist on eye contact), as this is something children with ASD may find difficult
- Remember the autistic brain processes information differently, so allow extra time for this.

125 Communicating with the child who has a learning disability

Figure 125.1 Communication with children who have additional support needs: It's not that difficult

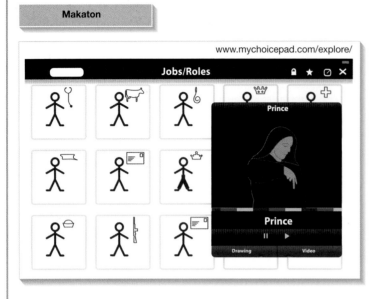

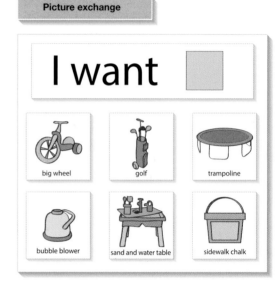

Figure 125.2 Whatever the communication system adopted by the child with a learning disability your responsibility lies in ensuring you listen with your whole self

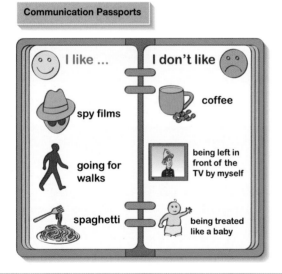

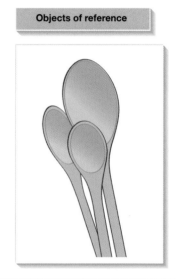

Children and Young People's Nursing at a Glance, First Edition. Edited by Alan Glasper, Jane Coad, and Jim Richardson.
© 2015 John Wiley & Sons, Ltd. Published 2015 by John Wiley & Sons, Ltd. Companion website: www.ataglanceseries.com/nursing/children

Often, the key to establishing a purposeful, mutually satisfying relationship in the care arena involves 'clueing' into the child. This is no different for the child with a profound or multiple disabilities. What does impact on the parameters and rules of that relationship is often our perception of the child and the labels they wear.

The **picture exchange system (PECs)** is an approach that uses pictures to develop communication skills. It is appropriate for children and adults with a wide range of learning and communication difficulties including autism. It involves the individual using the pictures to 'trade' with you for an object, food item or activity. Evolved approaches also include emotions and pain.

A **communication passport** is a book that helps to pass on important information about a child. Communication passports help to enhance the life the child lives and the services they receive and they help to inform you of a child's life and personality, likes and dislikes, reactions and pet words sounds, etc.

Objects of reference: some children prefer real things and learn to use particular objects to symbolize a significant activity. For example, a towel may indicate swimming, or a fork may be used to show that it is time for a meal. This method allows children with communication difficulties to make choices and enables you to tell the child what is going to happen next.

Makaton: being able to communicate is one of the most important skills in life. Almost everything involves communication; everyday tasks such as learning at school, asking for food and drink, sorting out problems, making friends and having fun. These all rely on our ability to communicate with each other. Makaton is a language programme using signs and symbols to help people to communicate. It is designed to support spoken language and the signs and symbols are used with speech, in spoken word order. With Makaton, children and adults can communicate straight away using signs and symbols. Many people then drop the signs or symbols naturally at their own pace, as they develop speech.

For those who have experienced the frustration of being unable to communicate meaningfully or effectively, Makaton can really help. Makaton takes away that frustration and enables individuals to connect with other people and the world around them. This opens up all kinds of possibilities. Makaton uses signs, symbols and speech to help people communicate. Signs are used, with speech, in spoken word order. This helps provide extra clues about what someone is saying. Using signs can help people who have no speech or whose speech is unclear. Using symbols can help people who have limited speech and those who cannot, or prefer not to sign.

Makaton is extremely flexible as it can be personalized to an individual's needs and used at a level suitable for them. It can be used to:

• Share thoughts, choices and emotions
• Label real objects, pictures, photos and places
• Take part in games and songs
• Listen to, read and tell stories
• Create recipes, menus and shopping lists
• Write letters and messages
• Help people find their way around public buildings (http://www.makaton.org/aboutMakaton/).

126 Positive behavioural support

Figure 126.1 Challenging behaviour

Challenging behaviour is defined as: 'Culturally abnormal behaviours of such intensity, frequency or duration that the physical safety of the person or others is placed in jeopardy, or behaviour that is likely to seriously limit the use of or delay access to ordinary community facilities'.

Examples include:

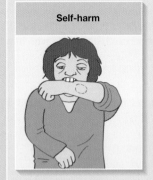

Self-harm

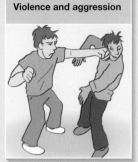

Violence and aggression

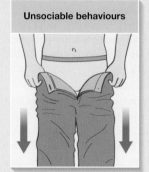

Unsociable behaviours

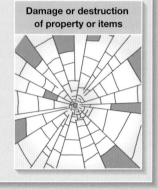

Damage or destruction of property or items

Antecedent

In this box you should write everything that is happening before the child displays the challenging behaviour:

- Who is there
- The date, day and time
- What is happening
- Temperature, noise levels
- What activities are taking place
- Is anything being asked of the child?

Behaviour

In this box you should write a clear description of the behaviour. Try to avoid 'broad' words such as aggression. Different people have different ideas about what aggression is. So be really clear and describe the behaviour.

For example: *'Tom shouted at Rebecca. He called her a fat slob. He then knocked over a chair and walked out of the room slamming the door behind him.'*

This way everyone gets a clear picture of what Tom did which we would not get from 'Tom was aggressive'

Consequence

In this box write everything that happens after the behaviour. Include who says what? Who does what? What does the child do? What changes? What stays the same?

From time to time, children and adolescents may display behaviours that can be described as challenging. The term challenging behaviour is used to represent the challenge the behaviour presents to the service providers and illustrates that it is not intrinsic to the person. Emerson et al. (1987) define it as 'culturally abnormal behaviours of such intensity, frequency or duration that the physical safety of the person or others is placed in jeopardy, or behaviour that is likely to seriously limit the use of or delay access to ordinary community facilities.' It is an umbrella term, which can include socially unacceptable behaviours, destruction of property, self-injurious behaviours and violence and aggression to others.

Challenging behaviours can be life-threatening, such as in cases of extreme self-injury, but in most cases they are not but they have a huge impact on the person's quality of life and the quality of life of those around them. The presence of challenging behaviour is often the reason cited for the breakdown of service provision, resulting in exclusion from services and isolation from families, friends and society.

Children and adolescents do not just decide to suddenly display challenging behaviours. Any behaviour the child is displaying must be occurring for a reason and must be serving a purpose for them. The challenge to staff is to understand that behaviour and work out what purpose it is serving. Any new behaviour may be occurring as a result of many things, such as bullying, emotional disturbances, low self-esteem, mental health problems, physical pain, abuse and neglect, grief, linked to a condition or environmental aspects.

What is positive behavioural support?

Positive behavioural support is about understanding why the behaviour occurs and what maintains it – why does the child continue to do it? Behaviours are 'functional'; that is, they serve a purpose for the child.

In order to understand why challenging behaviours are occurring we need to study other aspects of the child's life. Causes of challenging behaviours are often divided into two main groups: non-biological and biological. Abuse, changes at home and lack of understanding social rules are non-biological causes. Biological causes could be associated with specific syndromes and mental health problems. Many conditions have a predisposition to the manifestation of challenging behaviours. For example, autism is an often cited example of a condition associated with a wide range of behavioural manifestations, including self-injury, aggression, injury to others and socially inappropriate behaviours. Gilles de la Tourette's syndrome is associated with verbal outbursts, obsessive–compulsive behaviour, aggression and self-harm. Challenging

behaviour is also associated with epilepsy in some people as part of their seizures. Phenylketonuria, mental illness and physical pain are additional causes of challenging behaviour.

The first stage with a new behaviour is a full and detailed assessment in order to understand the behaviour. Without an assessment, any interventions attempted may be a waste of time, potentially adding to the problems, leading to frustration for the children's nurse, the child, staff and families. Assessment may involve a combination of more than one assessment tool such as Functional Analysis and the Motivation Assessment Scale as well as more detailed holistic assessments. These assessments are straightforward and easy to use. An example of Functional Analysis is shown in Figure 126.1. When you have completed several of these it is important to analyse them. This means looking for trends and patterns in the behaviour.

- Does it occur at the same time or on the same day?
- Does it occur when the same task is being asked of the child?
- Does the behaviour always occur when a particular other person is around? This may be a sign that the child does not like that person but it can also be a sign that they like the person very much and do not know how to express themselves
- Does the behaviour always manifest in the same way or does the child display different types of behaviour?
- What are the outcomes? Do staff or parents always respond in the same way?

When you analyse the information you may see trends that are reinforcing or maintaining the behaviour which helps us to understand it. Once we have a better understanding of why the behaviour is occurring, we can then introduce strategies to deal with it. Strategies include proactive (preventative) approaches to avoid the behaviours occurring and reactive approaches, how staff or parents will react when the behaviour occurs. Positive behavioural support does not include punishment.

Positive behavioural support needs to contain several key features:

- Values-led: delivers child-centred outcomes
- Based on functional analysis – why, when and how of behavioural analysis
- Focuses on triggers to reduce likelihood of behaviours reoccurring
- Recognizes lack of skills can maintain behaviours, so focuses on skills training, such as becoming better at expressing oneself
- Changes in quality of life used as an intervention and outcome measure
- Has a long-term and multicomponent focus
- Eliminates punishment approaches
- Includes proactive and reactive strategies.

127 Atrioventricular septal defect in children with learning disability

Figure 127.1 Atrioventricular septal defect

Normal circulation

Right | Left

Inferior vena cava → | ← Superior vena cava

Pulmonary veins

To right lung | To left lung

Right atrium | Left atrium

Tricuspid valve | Mitral valve

Pulmonary artery

Right ventricle | Left ventricle

Pulmonary valve | Aortic valve

Aorta

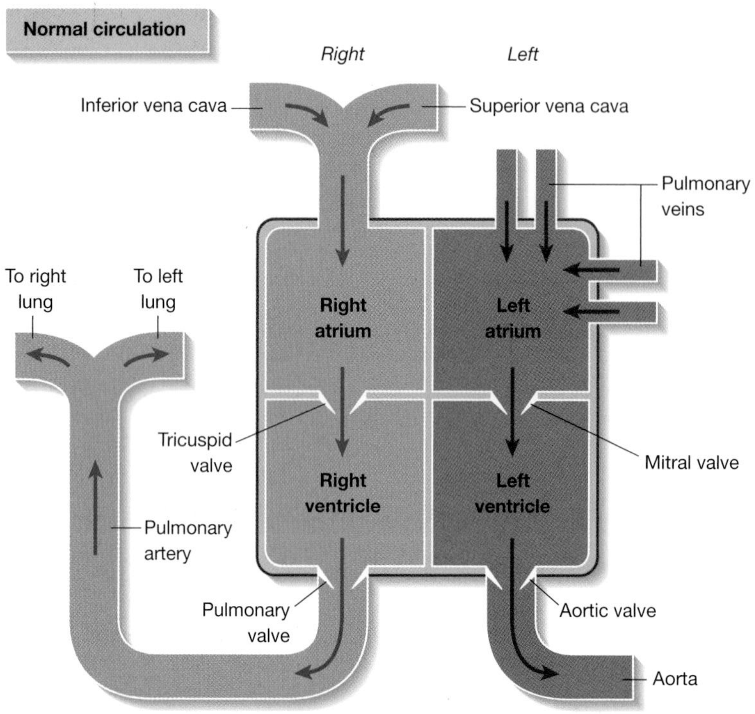

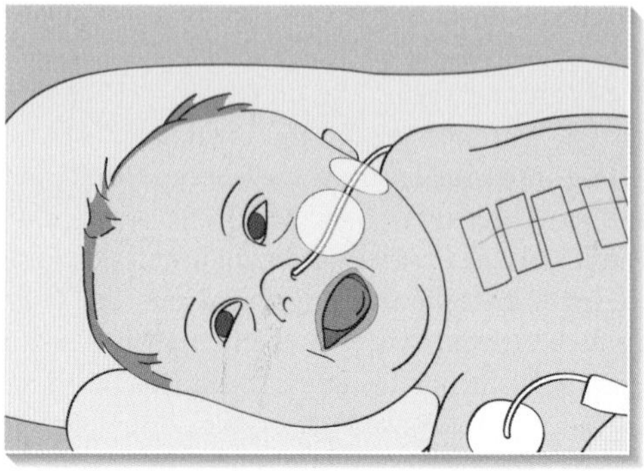

Child born with Down's syndrome and an atrioventricular septal defect

Abnormal circulation

Right | Left

← Abnormal blood flow

Single valve

Atrial septal defect

Ventricular septal defect

Enlarged right ventricle | Enlarged left ventricle

Increased pulmonary blood flow

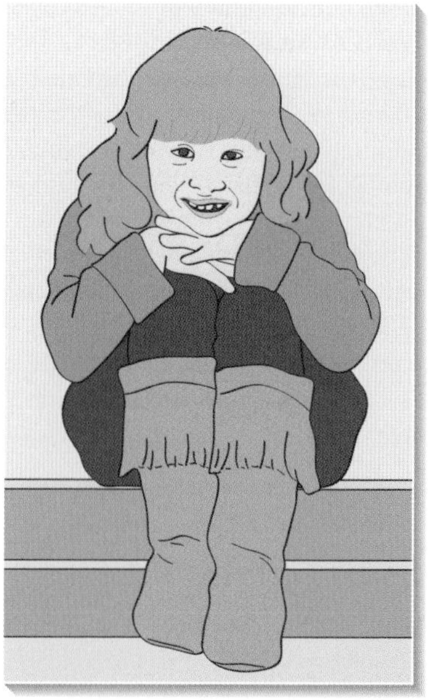

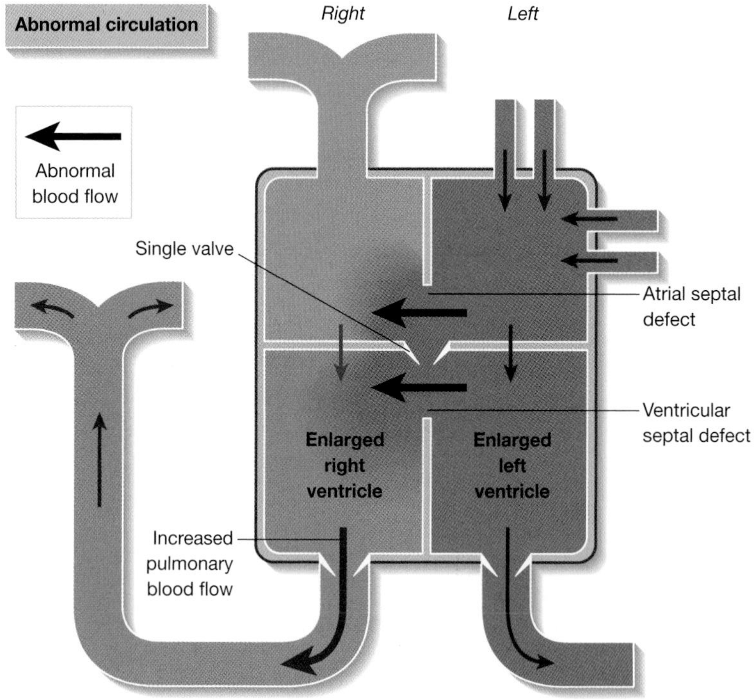

Children and Young People's Nursing at a Glance, First Edition. Edited by Alan Glasper, Jane Coad, and Jim Richardson.

© 2015 John Wiley & Sons, Ltd. Published 2015 by John Wiley & Sons, Ltd. Companion website: www.ataglanceseries.com/nursing/children

An atrioventricular septal defect (AVSD) is the most common congenital heart defect found in children with Down's syndrome, accounting for 50% of the total. In its complete form there is a hole in the wall between the top chambers (atria) and a hole in the wall between the bottom chambers (ventricles), and one common valve between the two atria and the two ventricles. In the partial forms there may not be a hole between the bottom chambers (ventricles) or the mitral and tricuspid valves may not be joined together, but either or both may leak, known as valve incompetence. Because of the high pressure in the left ventricle (needed to pump the blood around the body), blood is forced through the holes in the septum (central heart wall) when the ventricle contracts, thus increasing the pressure in the right ventricle. This increased pressure (pulmonary hypertension) results in excess blood flow to the lungs.

Symptoms

Some of the early symptoms are difficulty in feeding, poor weight gain, fast irregular breathing and a degree of cyanosis (blueness), particularly noticeable around the mouth, fingers and toes. Clinical examination may show an enlarged heart and liver, and a diagnosis of 'heart failure' may be given. This is not as frightening as it sounds – in fact it is the medical term used to indicate that the heart is working inefficiently due to the demands the body is placing on it. Because of the flow of blood from one side to the other, the heart has to work harder than normal. Not all children will exhibit symptoms early in life, and those who do will not necessarily show all of these.

Treatment

Early treatment involves the use of diuretics such as frusemide and spironolactone to control the fluid retention around the body and to reduce the volume of blood in the circulation, thus making the heart's workload easier. These may be used in conjunction with other drugs such as captopril, to make it easier for blood to pass to the body, rather than back through the hole to the lungs. Slow weight gain may lead to the addition of additives such as Calogen, Maxijul or Duocal to a baby's milk to increase calorie intake. Severe feeding problems may necessitate feeding by a nasogastric tube (through the nose and directly into the stomach), so that energy is not used up in obtaining nourishment.

The majority of cases of AVSD are suitable for surgical intervention. This generally takes place within the first 6 months of life. If the condition is left untreated, the increased blood pressure in the lungs causes damage that eventually makes surgery impossible, as the body adjusts to these pressures and could not cope with the surgery.

Follow-up advice

Following surgery there often remains a leaky valve which requires regular monitoring in case more surgery is needed, although in many cases the heart copes very well with the leakage and no further treatment is required. Sometimes, bouts of illness place an additional strain on the leaky valve, but this may be alleviated by treatment with diuretics for a short period. There may be times when chest infections require quite energetic treatment. The repeated use of antibiotics, if used properly, is very helpful and does not reduce the child's resistance to infections.

©Down's Heart Group Revised February 2012.

Acknowledgement: Written in collaboration with the Down's Heart Group.

128 Genetic conditions: Down's syndrome

Figure 128.1 Down's syndrome – dymorphic features

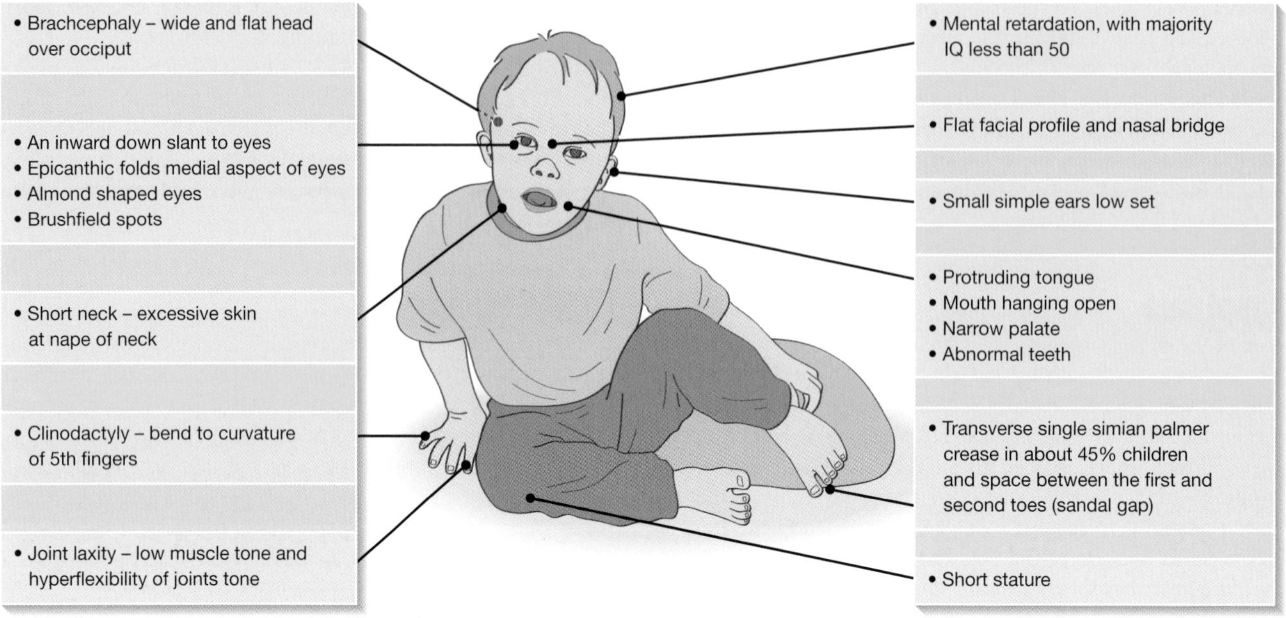

• Brachcephaly – wide and flat head over occiput
• An inward down slant to eyes
• Epicanthic folds medial aspect of eyes
• Almond shaped eyes
• Brushfield spots
• Short neck – excessive skin at nape of neck
• Clinodactyly – bend to curvature of 5th fingers
• Joint laxity – low muscle tone and hyperflexibility of joints tone
• Mental retardation, with majority IQ less than 50
• Flat facial profile and nasal bridge
• Small simple ears low set
• Protruding tongue
• Mouth hanging open
• Narrow palate
• Abnormal teeth
• Transverse single simian palmer crease in about 45% children and space between the first and second toes (sandal gap)
• Short stature

Figure 128.2 Specific medical problems that occur more frequently in people with Down's syndrome

ENT

- Upper airway obstruction
- Chronic catarrh
- Conductive hearing loss
- Sensorineural hearing loss

Cardiac

- Congenital malformations
  - atrioventricular septal defects (AVSD)
  - pulmonary vascular disease (PVD)
- Cor pulmonale
- Acquired valvular dysfunction

Ophthalmic

- Naslolacrimal obstruction
- Cataracts
- Glaucoma
- Nystagmus
- Squint
- Keratoconus
- Refractive errors
- Blepharitis

Endocrine

- Growth retardation
- Diabetes hypothyroidism
- Hyperthyroidism

Endocrine

- Growth retardation
- Diabetes hypothyroidism
- Hyperthyroidism

Immunological

- Immunodeficiency
- Autoimmune diseases, e.g. arthropathy, vitiligo, alopecia

Gastrointestinal

- Congenital malformations
- Feeding difficulties
- Gastro-oesophageal reflux
- Hirschsprung's disease (Marder, 2001)
- Coeliac disegase

Haematological

- Leukaemia
- Neonatal polycythaemia
- Transient neonatal myeloproliferative states
- Neonatal thrombocytopenia

Dermatological

- Alopecia
- Vitiligo
- Dry skin
- Folliculitis

Neuropyschiatric

- Depressive illness
- Autism
- Infantile spasms and other myoclonic epilepsies
- Dementia (adults only)

Orthopaedic

- Metatarsus varus
- Pes planus
- Hip subluxation/dislocation
- Cervical spine instability
- Scoliosis
- Patellar instability

Children and Young People's Nursing at a Glance, First Edition. Edited by Alan Glasper, Jane Coad, and Jim Richardson.

Down's syndrome is a naturally occurring, congenital chromosomal disorder that has always been part of the human condition. It was first recognized as an entity in 1866, by Langdon Down (1828–1896), an English doctor working in Surrey, who first described the characteristics features of the syndrome. In most children with Down's syndrome, the condition is recognized at or shortly after birth. In most cases, the doctor will be quite certain of the diagnosis on the basis of the child's appearance alone.

Genetics

Down's syndrome, also known as trisomy 21, is a common chromosome disorder that results from changes on chromosome 21. Almost 95% of cases are triggered by non-disjunction, meaning the chromosome 21 pair fails to separate during cellular division (Nehring 2010). The second chromosomal defect is translocations – when a chromosomal segment moves to a new position (Tolmie 2002). The third chromosome defect is mosaicism, which arises when a mutation on chromosome 21 takes place later in cell division, subsequently in affected and normal cells. This mosaic arrangement of Down's syndrome is thought to affect individuals less severely than non-disjunction or translocation (Leshin 2000). Down's syndrome occurs in all racial and ethnic groups, and becomes more predominant with advanced parental age (Tolmie 2002). The incidence is approximately 1 in 800 live births (Aitken 2002).

Phenotype features

• **Face.** When looked at from the front the child with Down's syndrome typically has a rounded face. From the side, the face is apt to have a flat profile.
• **Head.** The occiput (back of the head) is slightly flattened in most children and adults with Down's syndrome. This is known as brachycephaly.
• **Eyes.** The eyes of nearly all children and adults with Down's syndrome slant upwards a little. In addition, they have a small fold of skin that runs vertically between the inner corner of the eye and the bridge of the nose. This is known as epicanthic fold or epicanthus. The eyes may have white or light yellow speckling around the rim of the iris (coloured part of eye). These specs are called Brushfield spots.
• **Hair.** The hair of children with Down's syndrome is often soft and straight.
• **Neck.** Newborn babies with Down's syndrome might have extra skin over the back of the neck, usually taken up as they grow. Older children and adults tend to have a short broad neck.
• **Mouth.** The mouth cavity is slightly smaller than average, and the tongue is slightly larger. This arrangement encourages the children to have the habit of putting their tongues out at all times.
• **Hands.** The hands of child with Down's syndrome tend to be broad, with short fingers. The little finger sometimes has two joints, and tends to be incurved towards the fourth finger, known

as 'clinodactyly'. The palm may have only one crease going across it, usually extending right across the hand.
• **Feet.** These incline to be stubby, and to have a wide space between the first and second toes known as 'sandal gap'. This may be associated with a short crease on the sole, which starts at this gap.
• **Muscle tone.** The limbs and necks of young children with Down's syndrome are often very floppy. This floppiness is called 'hypotonia', meaning low tone. As a result of this many children and adults with Down's syndrome become tired easily and find it hard to walk long distances.
• **Short stature.** Children with Down's syndrome tend to weigh less than average at birth. Their body length is similarly reduced. During childhood they grow slowly, and their ultimate height in adulthood is generally shorter than would be expected for their family and is usually near the bottom of the normal range (Selikowitz 2008).

Diagnosis

A number of tests can be undertaken to screen for Down's syndrome. These tests are offered to all pregnant women, regardless of their age, usually in combination to increase detection rates, while retaining a low false positive rate:

1 **Combined test:** ultrasound scan to measure nuchal translucency plus free beta-hCG and PAPP-A (pregnancy-associated plasma protein A)
2 **QUAD test:** this test measures maternal serum alpha-fetoprotein; unconjugated estriol, beta hCG, and inhibin-alpha
3 **Intergraded test:** uses measurements from first trimester combined test, and the second trimester Quad test to yield a more accurate result.

Specific medical problems in Down's syndrome

There are specific medical problems that occur more frequently in people with Down's syndrome, as a result of which all children with Down's syndrome should be offered regular medical review by a paediatric medical team throughout their childhood (Figure 128.2) (Marder and Dennis 2001).

Prognosis

Over the years there has been a profound change in people's outlook toward individuals with Down's syndrome. More and more parents have decided to rear children with Down's syndrome. The change in parental attitude has in turn resulted in the increased competence of individuals with Down's syndrome. Affected children should have regular child health surveillance checks so that any specific medical problems can be managed in a timely manner, increasing their quality of life.

129 Other genetic conditions

Figure 129.1 Main areas of muscle weakness affected Duchenne muscular dystrophy

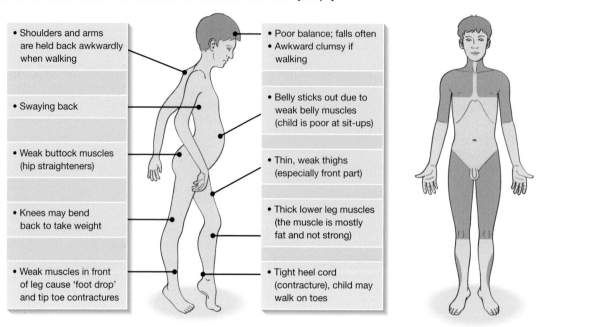

- Shoulders and arms are held back awkwardly when walking
- Swaying back
- Weak buttock muscles (hip straighteners)
- Knees may bend back to take weight
- Weak muscles in front of leg cause 'foot drop' and tip toe contractures

- Poor balance; falls often
- Awkward clumsy if walking
- Belly sticks out due to weak belly muscles (child is poor at sit-ups)
- Thin, weak thighs (especially front part)
- Thick lower leg muscles (the muscle is mostly fat and not strong)
- Tight heel cord (contracture), child may walk on toes

Figure 129.2 Phenylketonuria (PKU)

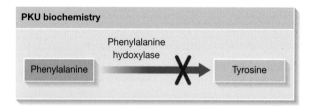

PKU biochemistry

Phenylalanine → ✗ → Tyrosine

Phenylalanine hydoxylase

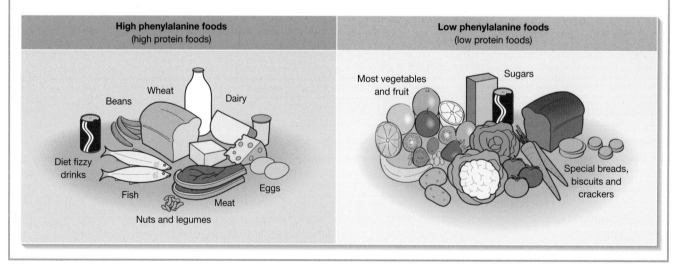

High phenylalanine foods (high protein foods)

Wheat, Beans, Dairy, Diet fizzy drinks, Fish, Nuts and legumes, Meat, Eggs

Low phenylalanine foods (low protein foods)

Most vegetables and fruit, Sugars, Special breads, biscuits and crackers

Children and Young People's Nursing at a Glance, First Edition. Edited by Alan Glasper, Jane Coad, and Jim Richardson.
© 2015 John Wiley & Sons, Ltd. Published 2015 by John Wiley & Sons, Ltd. Companion website: www.ataglanceseries.com/nursing/children

Phenylketonuria

Phenylketonuria (PKU) is an autosomal recessive human genetic disorder caused by a deficiency of hepatic phenylalanine hydroxylase enzyme activity, which prevents hydroxylation of phenylalanine into tyrosine.

PKU is a common inborn error of amino acid metabolism in Caucasian populations and approximately 1 in 50 are carriers of a PKU allele. The genetic disorder causes impairment of postnatal brain development, resulting in severe mental retardation in untreated children.

Phenylalanine is an essential amino acid provided by food that has a key role in the production of other amino acids. It is converted to tyrosine, used in the production of neurotransmitters.

How is PKU detected

- Every newborn baby is tested for PKU by taking a blood sample heel prick test measuring the level of phenylalanine.
- Normal range of phenylalanine average $<120\,\mu mol/L$ ($<2\,mg/dL$).
- In PKU, blood phenylalanine levels can range from normal level of <60–$7200\,\mu mol/L$ (1–$120\,mg/dL$), up to 80 times more than the normal level.
- If the babies' blood test results are outside the normal PKU range, they will be retested for confirmation and then immediately put on the standard treatment for PKU; a lifelong restricted diet.

Treatment

In PKU, encouraging adherence to diet includes continuing education, reinforcement and support from the family and professionals. All dietary proteins are roughly equally rich in phenylalanine, and a suitable diet can therefore be devised only by supplying the bulk of nitrogen as mixture of amino acids. While it would be possible to mix pure amino acids to obtain such a diet, the costs would render any long-term treatment of even a few cases impossible.

Prognosis

Researchers are studying whether the current standard therapy involving phenylalanine-restricted diet and meeting phenylalanine targets can still lead to changes in the brain. Some of the evidence gathered involves brain scans. So far, studies show that a large percentage of people with PKU may have some visible brain abnormalities and lifetime phenylalanine levels (the higher the phenylalanine levels, the more brain abnormalities).

Scientific evidence suggests that higher than normal blood phenylalanine levels can reduce the neurotransmitter dopamine in the brain of a person with PKU.

Duchenne muscular dystrophy

Duchenne muscular dystrophy (DMD) is the most common severe childhood form of muscular dystrophy resulting from gene mutation in the X-linked *DMD* gene. DMD is a recessive muscle disease that arises as a result of mutations caused in the gene responsible for dystrophin production, which is involved in mainiating the intergity of sarcolemma. DMD is severe progressive disease that affects 1 in 3600–6000 live male births. There is no cure, and management of DMD is limited to glucocorticoids that lengthen ambulation and drugs to treat cardiomyopathy.

Gene replacement

The molecular basis for DMD has been known for over 20 years. Several treatment strategies are under investigation and have shown promise for DMD. Procedures of molecular-based therapies that replace or correct the missing non-dysfunctional dystrophin protein have gained impetus. These approaches include gene replacement with adeno-associated virus, exon skipping with antisense oligo-nucleotides, and mutation suppression with compounds that 'read through' stop codon mutations. Other strategies include cell therapy and surrogate gene products to recompense for the loss of dystrophin. However, attempts to develop gene therapy for DMD have been problematic because of the massive size of the dystrophin gene.

When to suspect DMD

- Presence of Gower's sign in a male child, mainly if the child has a waddling gait. Gower's sign is a medical sign indicating weakness in the proximal muscles, explicitly those of the lower limbs.
- Delayed walking, frequent falls, or difficulty climbing stairs and running.
- Delays in attainment of childhood milestones, such as gross motor functions walking, running, climbing stairs and a positive family history of DMD.

Diagnosis

Diagnosis of DMD should be carried out by a neuromuscular specialist who can assess the child clinically and rapidly access and interpret appropriate investigations in the context of the clinical presentation. DMD is typically diagnosed at the age of 5 years, but may be suspected much earlier because of the delays in development milestones.

1 Observation of abnormal muscle function in a male child.
2 The detection of an increase in serum creatine kinase tested for unrelated conditions.
3 After the discovery of increased transaminases (aspartate aminotransferase and alanine aminotransferase, which are produced by muscle as well as liver cells). The diagnosis of DMD should therefore be considered in a child prior to a liver biopsy in any child with elevated transaminases.
4 Muscle biopsy demonstrates muscle degeneration, regeneration, isolated 'opaque' hypertrophic fibres, and significant replacement of fat and connective tissue.

Prognosis

Despite the current therapeutic methods under investigation, which are showing great potential for managing DMD, the challenge of finding a cure remains. Corticosteroids characterize the standard of care for treatment of this disease. These classes of drugs can make a change by extending ambulation and delaying or preventing scoliosis. Gene replacement approaches offer the potential for long-term correction.

References and further reading

2 SBAR framework

Institute for Healthcare Improvement. SBAR (situation, background, assessment, recommendation) tool. www.ihi.org (accessed 24 February 2014).

Morrow P. (2012) Interprofessional Assessment and Care Planning in Critical Care. In Corkin D, Clarke S, Liggett L (eds). *Care Planning in Children and Young People's Nursing*. Oxford: Wiley-Blackwell.

National Patient Safety Agency (NPSA). (2005) *How to confirm the correct position of nasogastric feeding tubes in infants, children and adults*. London: NPSA.

National Patient Safety Agency (NPSA). (2011) *Patient Safety Alert: Reducing the harm caused by misplaced nasogastric tubes in adults, children and infants*. London: NPSA.

3 The nursing process

Aggleton P, Chalmers H. (2000) *Nursing Models and nursing practice*. Mcmillan Basingstoke.

Casey A. (2007) Partnership model of nursing. In Glasper A, McEwing G and Richardson J. *Oxford Handbook of Children's and Young People's Nursing*. Oxford: Oxford University Press.

Chalmers H. (1990) Nursing models and their relationship to the Nursing process and Nursing theory. In Salvage J, Kershaw B (eds) *Models for nursing 2*. London: Scutari Press.

Colley S. (2003) Nursing theory: its importance to practice., *Nursing Standard* 17,46: 33–37.

De-Luc, K. (2000) Care Pathways: an evaluation of their effectiveness. *Journal of Advanced Nursing* 32 (2): 485–496.

Department of Health. (1997) *The New NHS: Modern, Dependable*. Leeds: Department of Health.

Department of Health. (1998) *A First Class Service Quality in the New NHS*. Leeds: Department of Health.

Department of Health. (2000) *The NHS Plan: A Plan for Investment – A Plan for reform*. London: The Stationary Office.

Department of Health. (2004) *Executive Summary, National Service Framework for Children, Young People and Maternity Services: Change for Children – Every Child Matters*. London: HMSO.

Glasper A. (1990) A planned approach to nursing children. In Salvage J, Kershaw B (eds). *Models for Nursing 2*. London: Scutari press.

Henderson V. (1960) Basic principles of nursing care. London: ICN.

Henderson V. (1978) The concept of nursing. *Journal of Advanced Nursing* 3: 113–130.

Herring L. (1999) Critical care pathways an efficient way to manage care. *Nursing Standard* 47: 11–17, 36–37.

Hurst. (1993) *Problem Solving in Nursing Practice*. London: Scutari Press.

McKenna H. (1997) *Nursing theories and models*. Routledge.

Nightingale F. (1859) *Notes on nursing: what it is and what it is not*. London: Duckworth and company (1970 reprint).

Norris AC, Briggs JS. (1999) Care pathways and the information for health strategy. *Health Informatics Journal* 1999; 5: 209–212.

Nursing and Midwifery Council (2004) *Professional Code of Conduct*. London: NMC.

Roper N, Logan W, Tierney A. (1983). A nursing model…why the nursing process is useful, when used in an explicit nursing framework. *Nursing Mirror* 156(21), 17–19.

Royal College of Nursing. (1992) *Paediatric Nursing; a Philososhy of Care*. London: Royal College of Nursing.

The United Nations Convention. (1991) London: HMSO.

Walsh M. (1997) 2002 Watson's clinical nursing and related sciences London: Balliere Tindall.

Walsh M. (2001) Models and Critical pathways in Clinical Nursing; Conceptual Frameworks for Care Planning. Edinburgh: Bailliere Tindall.

Wigfield A, Boon E. (1996) Critical care pathway development :the way forward. *BJN* 5 (12): 736–753.

Wimpenny P. (2002) The meaning of models of nursing to practicing nurses. *Journal of Advanced Nursing* 40(3): 346–354.

Wood CJ. (1888) The training of nurses for sick children. *The Nursing Recor*. Dec 6: 507–510.

4 Nursing models

Corkin D, Clarke S, Liggett L. (2012) *Care Planning in Children and Young People's Nursing*. Oxford: Wiley-Blackwell.

Cutliffe J, McKenna H, Hyrkas K. (2010) *Nursing Models: Application to Practice*. London: Quay Books.

Fitzpatrick L, Whall A. (2004) *Conceptual Models of Nursing: Analysis and Application*, 4th edition. USA: Prentice Hall.

McCrae N. (2012) Whither nursing models? The value of nursing theory in the context of evidence based practice and multidisciplinary health care. *Journal of Advanced Nursing* 68: 222–229.

5 The care plan

Alfaro-LeFevere R. (2009) *Applying Nursing Process: a tool for critical thinking*. Philadelphia: Lippincott Williams and Wilkins.

Barrett D, Wilson B, Woollands A. (2012) *Care Planning: A Guide for Nurses*. Pearson.

Corkin D, Clarke S, Liggett L. (2012) *Care Planning in Children and Young People*. Oxford: Wiley-Blackwell.

Lloyd M. (2010) *A Practical Guide to Care Planning in Health and Social Care*. Berkshire: Open University Press.

Nazarko L. (2007) *NVQs in Nursing and Residential Care Homes*, 3rd edition. Oxford: Blackwell Publishing.

7 Engagement and participation of children and young people

Department of Health (2011) You're Welcome Quality criteria for young people friendly health services. http://www.dh.gov.uk/en/Publicationsandstatistics/Publications/PublicationsPolicyAndGuidance/DH_126813 (accessed 29 January 2014).

Department of Health (2012) Report of the Children's and Young People's Health Outcomes Forum. http://www.dh.gov.uk/health/2012/07/cyp-report/ (accessed 29 January 2014).

National Children's Bureau (2012) Listening to children's views on health provision: a rapid review of the evidence. http://www.ncb

Children and Young People's Nursing at a Glance, First Edition. Edited by Alan Glasper, Jane Coad, and Jim Richardson.

© 2015 John Wiley & Sons, Ltd. Published 2015 by John Wiley & Sons, Ltd. Companion website: www.ataglanceseries.com/nursing/children

.org.uk/media/723497/listening_to_children_s_views_on
health-_final_report_july__12.pdf (accessed 24 February 2014).

NHS Institute for Innovation and Improvement (2010) Involving Children and Young People in Improving Local Healthcare services. http://www.institute.nhs.uk/images//documents/Quality _and_value/Focus_On/Microsoft%20Word%20-%20Involving% 20CYP%20Impact%20Evaluation%20Report%20April%20 2010%20FINAL.pdf (accessed 24 Febuary 2014).

NHS Institute for Innovation and Improvement (2013) Fifteen Steps Programme. http://www.institute.nhs.uk/productives/15stepschall enge/15stepschallenge.html (accessed 24 February 2014).

Royal College of Paediatrics and Child Health (RCPCH). (2010) Not Just a Phase: a guide to participation of children and young people in health services. http://www.rcpch.ac.uk/what-we-do/children -and-young-peoples-participation/publications/not-just-phase/ not-just-phase (accessed 24 Febuary 2014).

Unicef (2007) UN Convention on the Rights of the Child. http://www .unicef.org.uk/crc?gclid=CNDkjbT1zLQCFXHLtAodTVoA5w&si ssr=1 (accessed 24 Febuary 2014).

9 Observation of the sick child

Dougherty L. and Lister S. (eds) (2011) *The Royal Marsden Hospital Manual of Clinical nursing procedures*. (8th ed. Oxford: Wiley-Blackwell.

McCance, K. and Huether, S. (2010) Chapter 34 Alterations in Pulmonary function in children. In *Pathophysiology: The Biological Basis for Disease in Adults and Children. (6th ed.)*. Missouri: Mosby Elsevier.

National Institute for Health and Clinical Excellence. (NICE 2007) *Feverish Illness in children: Assessment and initial management in children younger than 5 years*. Guideline 47. London: NICE.

Royal College of Nursing (RCN). (2011) *Standards for assessing, measuring and monitoring vital signs in infants, children and young people*. London: RCN.

Spotting the Sick Child (2012) *Basic Child Assessment Transcript*. Accessed at: https://www.spottingthesickchild.com/basic-child -assessment/how-to/introduction/3 (accessed on 20.06.2014).

11 Advanced physical assessment

Advanced Life Support Group (ALSG). (2005) *Advanced Paediatric Life Support*, 4th edition. BMJ Books, Blackwell Publishing.

Cameron P, Jelinek G, Everitt I, et al. (eds) (2006) *Textbook of Paediatric Emergency Medicine*. Churchill Livingstone.

Glasper A, Aylott M, Battrick C. (eds) (2010) *Developing Practical Skills for Nursing Children and Young People*. Hodder Arnold.

Jarvis C. (2011) *Physical Examination and Health Assessment*, 6th edition. Saunders Elsevier.

Lissauer T, Clayden G. (2007) *Illustrated Textbook of Paediatrics*, 3rd edition. Mosby.

Royal College of Nursing (RCN). (2011) *Standards for Assessing, Measuring and Monitoring Vital Signs in Infants, Children and Young People*. London: RCN.

12 Developmental assessment

Bee H, Boyd D. (2012) *The Developing Child*, 13th edition. London: Pearson.

Glasper EA, McEwing G, Richardson J. (2007) *Oxford Handbook of Children's and Young People's Nursing*. Oxford: Oxford University Press.

17 Understanding blood chemistry

Metheny NM. (ed.) (2000) *Fluid and Electrolyte Balance, Nursing Considerations*, 4th edition. Philadelphia: Lippincott Williams and Wilkins.

21 Central venous devices

Great Ormond Street Hospital for Children (GOSH). (2013) Central venous access devices (long term) Clinical Practice Guideline. http://www.gosh.nhs.uk/health-professionals/clinical-guidelines/ central-venous-access-devices-long-term/ (accessed 24 February 2014).

Green J. (2008) Care and management of patients with skin-tunnelled catheters. *Nursing Standard* 22: 41–48.

Johnson KA. (2009) Power injectable portal systems. *Journal of Radiology Nursing* 28: 27–31.

Scales K. (2010a) Central venous access devices: Part 1. Devices for acute care. *British Journal of Nursing* 19: 88–92.

Scales K. (2010b) Central venous access devices: Part 2. For intermediate and long-term use. *British Journal of Nursing* 19(Suppl 1): 20–25.

26 Emergency care

Confidential Enquiry into Maternal and Child Health (CEMACH). (2006) Why Children Die: a pilot study. http://www.hqip.org.uk/ assets/NCAPOP-Library/CMACE-Reports/2.-May-2008-Why -Children-Die-A-Pilot-Study-2006-Children-and-Young-Peoples -Report.pdf (accessed 24 February 2014).

Grant K, Knight S. (2008) *Paediatric Emergency Nursing Competencies*. University Hospital Southampton NHS Foundation Trust.

Royal College of Paediatrics and Child Health (RCPCH). (2012) Standards for Children and Young People in Emergency Care settings. www.rcpch.ac.uk/emergencycare (accessed 24 February 2014).

27 Partnership

Casey A, Mobbs S. (1988) Partnership in practice. *Nursing Times* 84(44): 67–68.

Casey A. (1988) A partnership With Child and Family. *Senior Nurse Health Care Industry Journal* 8(4): 8–9.

Casey A. (1995) Partnership nursing: Influences on informal carers. *Journal of Advanced Nursing* 22: 1058–1062.

Coyne I, Cowley S. (2007) Challenging the philosophy of partnership with parents: A grounded theory study. *International Journal of Nursing Studies* 44(6): 893–904.

Coyne IT, O'Neill C, Murphy M, Costello T, O'Shea R (2011) What does family-centred care mean to nurses and how do they think it could be enhanced in practice. *Journal of Advanced Nursing* 67(12): 2561–2573.

Coyne IT. (1995) Partnership in care: parent's view of participation in their child's care. *Journal of Clinical Nursing* 4: 71–79.

Darbyshire P. (1994) *Living with a Sick Child in Hospital: The Experiences of Parents and Nurses*. Chapman & Hall, London.

Dearmun A. (1992) Perceptions of Parental Participation. *Paediatric Nursing* 4(7): 6–9.

Heimann K. (2000) Family needs: how do we know what they want? *Paediatric Nursing* 12: 31–35.

Hopwood B, Tallett A. (2011) Little voice: giving young patients a say. *Nursing Times* 107: 49/50, 18–20.

Hutchfield K. (1999) Family – centred care: a concept analysis. *Journal of Advanced Nursing* 29(5): 1178–1187.

Lee P. (2007) What does partnership in care mean for children's nurses? *Journal of Clinical Nursing* 16: 518–526.

Mountain G, Fallon S, Wood B. (2006) Preparing the family for stressful life events, child life and the role of therapeutic play. In E. A. Glasper and J. Richardson (eds). *A Textbook of Children's and Young People's Nursing*. Edinburgh: Churchill Livingstone Elsevier, pp. 197–210.

Mountain G. (2002) (2009) Parenting in society: A critical review. In L Smith and V Coleman (eds). *Child and Family Centred Healthcare: Concept, Theory and Practice*, 2nd Ed. Hampshire: Palgrave Macmillan.

Narramore NP. (2008) Meeting the emotional needs of parents who have a child with complex needs. *Journal of Children's and Young Peoples Nursing* 2(3): 103–110.

Noyes J. (2002) Barriers that delay children and young people who are dependent on mechanical ventilators from being discharged from hospital. *Journal of Clinical Nursing* 11(1): 2–11.

Shelton T, Smith Stepanek J. (1995) Excerpts from family centred care for children needing health and developmental services. *Pediatric Nursing* 21(4): 362–364.

Shields L. (2001) A review of the literature from developed and developing countries relating to the effects of hospitalization on children and parents. *International Nursing Review* 48: 29–37.

Shields L. (2010) Models of Care Questioning family-centred care. *Journal of Clinical Nursing* 19: 2629–2638.

Smith L, Coleman V, Bradshaw M. (2002) *Family Centred Care: Concept, Theory and Practice*. Hampshire: Palgrave Macmillan.

Smith L, Coleman V. (2010) *Child and family centred healthcare: Concept, theory and practice*, 2nd Ed. Hampshire: Palgrave Macmillan.

Towers C, Swift P. (2006) *Recognising fathers – Understanding the issues faced by fathers of children with a learning disability*. Mental Health Foundation. Available at: http://www.lul.se/Global/HOH/SUF_kunskapscentrum/Rapporter/FPLD_recognising_fathers_report.pdf (accessed 18.06.2014).

28 Family centred care

Casey A. (1988) A partnership with child and family. *Senior Nurse* 8: 8–9.

Smith F. (1995) *Children Nursing in Practice: The Nottingham Model*. Oxford: Blackwell Science.

29 Family health promotion

HM Government (2007) *PSA Delivery Agreement 22: Deliver a successful Olympic Games and Paralympic Games with a sustainable legacy and get more children and young people taking part in high quality PE and sport*. London: The Stationery Office.

HM Treasury (2002) *Spending Review: Public Service Agreements White Paper*. London: HM Treasury.

Morgan A. (2006) Needs assessment. In Macdowell W, Bonell C, Davies M. (eds) *Health Promotion Practice*. Maidenhead: McGraw-Hill Education, Open University Press, pp. 21–36.

Moyse K (Ed). (2009) *Promoting Health in Children and Young People*. Oxford: Wiley-Blackwell.

33 Collaboration with schools

Department of Health (2012) Report of the Children's Outcomes Forum. http://www.dh.gov.uk/health/2012/07/cyp-report/ (accessed 24 February 2014).

NHS Constitution (2012) http://www.dh.gov.uk/health/2012/03/nhs-constitution-updated/ (accessed 24 February 2014).

NHS Institute for Innovation and Improvement (2010a) Whole System Approach to Improving Emergency and Urgent Care for Children and Young People Guide. http://www.institute.nhs.uk/index.php?option=com_joomcart&Itemid=194&main_page=document_product_info&products_id=762&Joomcartid=4p6p553p1t895lv9ovh8v86e86 (accessed 24 February 2014).

NHS Institute for Innovation and Improvement (2010b) Involving Children and Young People in Improving Local Health Services: an impact evaluation of the engagement product and lesson plan. http://www.employment-studies.co.uk/pdflibrary/nhsi_0710.pdf (accessed 24 February 2014).

35 Safeguarding

Powell C. (2011) *Safeguarding and Child Protection for Nurses, Midwives and Health Visitors: a Practical Guide*. Open University Press.

36 Fabricated or induced illness

Department for Children, Schools and Families (DCSF). (2008) Incredibly caring. (Multidisciplinary training pack around issues of FII.)

Lazenbatt A, Taylor J. (2011) Fabricated or induced illness in children: a rare form of child abuse. Research Briefing NSPCC. https://www.nspcc.org.uk/Inform/research/briefings/fii_pdf_wdf83368.pdf (accessed 24 February 2014).

Royal College of Paediatrics and Child Health (RCPCH). (2009) *Fabricated or induced illness by carers (FII): a practical guide for paediatricians*. RCPCH.

37 Gaining consent or assent

Larcher V. (2005) Consent, competence, and confidentiality. *BMJ* 330: 353–356.

McAlinden O. (2012) Ethical and legal implications when planning care for children and young people. In Corkin D, Clarke S, Liggett L. *Care Planning in Children and Young People's Nursing*. Chichester: Wiley-Blackwell.

39 Breaking bad or significant news

Harrison ME, Walling A. (2010) What do we know about giving bad news? A review. *Clinical Pediatrics* 49: 619–626.

Price J, McNeilly P, Surgenor M. (2006) Breaking bad news to parents: the children's nurse's role. *International Journal of Palliative Nursing* 12: 115–120.

West Midlands Paediatric Macmillan Team (2005) *Palliative Care for the Child with Malignant Disease*. London: Quay Books.

48 Neonatal transport

Barry P, Leslie A. (2003) *Paediatric and Neonatal Critical Care Transport*. London: BMJ Publishing Group.

Byrne S, Fisher S, Fortune PM, Lawn C, Wieteska S. (2008) *Paediatric and Neonatal Safe Transfer and Retrieval: The Practical Approach*. Chichester: Wiley-Blackwell.

Jaimovich DG, Vidyasagar D. (1996) *Pediatric and Neonatal Transport Medicine*. St Louis: Mosby.

54 Nutrition in childhood

Change4Life.

Department of Health (2009) Healthy Child Programme: pregnancy and the first five years of life.

Department of Health (2009) Healthy Child Programme from 5 to 19 years old.

NICE Public Health Programme Guidance (2008) Maternal and child nutrition: guidance for midwives, health visitors, pharmacists and other primary care services to improve the nutrition of pregnant and breastfeeding mothers and children in low income households.

56 Bottle feeding

Food Safety Authority of Ireland (2011) *Best practice for infant feeding in Ireland: From preconception through the first year of an infant's life*. Dublin: Food Safety Authority of Ireland.

58 Percentile charts

Further information can be found on the Royal College of Paediatrics and Child Health website or on the growth charts themselves. http://www.rcpch.ac.uk/growthcharts (accessed 24 February 2014).

Glasper E, McEwing G, Richardson J. (Eds) (2009) *Oxford Handbook of Children's and Young People's Nursing*. Oxford: Oxford University Press.

Lindley AA, Benson JE, Grimes C. (1999) The relationship in neonates between clinically measured head circumference and brain volume estimated from head CT scans. *Early Human Development* 56: 17–29.

Macqueen S, Bruce EA, Gibson F. (Eds) (2012) *The Great Ormond Street Hospital Manual of Children's Nursing Practices*. Oxford: Wiley-Blackwell.

NHS Choices (2011) Your baby's screening programme. http://www.nhs.uk/conditions/pregnancy-and-baby/pages/baby-screening.aspx#close (accessed 24 February 2014).

Royal College of Nursing (RCN). (2010) *Standards for the weighing of infants, children and young people in the acute healthcare setting*. London: RCN.

Royal College of Paediatrics and Child Health (RCPCH). (2013) UK-WHO growth charts. http://www.rcpch.ac.uk/growthcharts (accessed 24 February 2014).

Sutter K, Engstrom JL, Johnson TS, Kavanaugh K, Ifft DL. (1997) Reliability of head circumference measurements in preterm infants. *Pediatric Nursing* 23: 485–490.

Weller B. (ed.) (2002) *Nurses' Dictionary, 23rd edition.* London: Bailliere Tindall.

59 Child development: 0–5 years
Devitt P, Thain J. (2011) *Children and Young People's Nursing Made Incredibly Easy.* London: Lippincott Williams.
Miall L, Rudolf M, Smith D. (2012) *Paediatrics at a Glance: Evaluation of the Child, Development and Developmental Assessment,* 3rd edition. Wiley & Sons.
Sidwell RU, Thomson MA. (2011) *Easy Paediatrics.* London: Hodder Arnold.

60 Child development: 5–16 years
Gogtay N, Giedd JN, Lusk L, et al. (2004) Dynamic mapping of human cortical development during childhood through early adulthood. *Proceedings of the National Academy of Sciences* 101: 8174–8179.

63 Adolescent development
Bronfenbrenner U. (1979) *The Ecology of Human Development.* Cambridge, MA: Harvard University Press.
Erikson EH. (1950) *Childhood and Society.* New York: Norton.
Piaget J. (1951) *The Child's Conception of the World.* London: Routledge and Kegan Paul.

64 Child health promotion
Department of Health (2012) Making every contact count. http://cno.dh.gov.uk/2012/04/20/stepping-up-to-the-challenge-how-nurses-can-improve-public-health/ (accessed 24 February 2014).
Ewles L, Simnett I. (2003) *Promoting Health: A Practical Guide to Health Education,* 5th edition. Edinburgh: Bailliere Tindall.
Nursing and Midwifery Council (NMC). (2010) *Standards for Pre-registration Nursing Education.* London: NMC.
Prout A, Hallett C. (2003) Introduction. In Hallett C, Prout A. (eds). *Hearing the Voices of Children: Social Policy for a New Century.* London: Routledge Falmer.
World Health Organization (WHO). (1984) *Health Promotion: A Discussion Document on the Concept and Principles.* Copenhagen: WHO.
World Health Organization (WHO). (2005) *The European Health Report 2005. Public health action for healthier children and populations: Executive Summary.* Copenhagen: WHO.

65 Immunity and immunization
Department of Health (2006) *Immunisation Against Infectious Disease.* TSO.
Wakefield AJ, Murch SH, Anthony A, et al. (1998) Ileal-lymphoid-nodular hyperplasia, non-specific colitis, and pervasive developmental disorder in children. *Lancet* 351: 37–641.

69 The NHS change model
Department of Health (2003) Getting the right start: National Service Framework for Children, Young People and Maternity Services: Standard for hospital services. http://webarchive.nationalarchives.gov.uk/20130107105354/http://www.dh.gov.uk/en/Publicationsandstatistics/Publications/PublicationsPolicyAndGuidance/DH_4006182 (accessed 3 March 2014).
Department of Health (2012) Report of the Children and Young People's Health Outcomes Forum. http://www.dh.gov.uk/health/2012/07/cyp-report/ (accessed 24 February 2014).
NHS Change Model (2013) www.changemodel.nhs.uk (accessed 24 February 2014).
Office for National Statistics (2010) http://www.ons.gov.uk/ons/publications/all-releases.html?definition=tcm:77-22371 (accessed 24 February 2014).
Pearson GA, Ward-Platt M, Harnden A, Kelly D. (2011) Why children die: avoidable factors associated with child deaths. *Archives of Disease in Childhood* 96: 927–931.
Wolfe I, Cass H, Thompson MJ, et al. (2011) Improving child health services in the UK: insights from Europe and their implications for the NHS reforms. *BMJ* 342: d1277.

74 Preoperative preparation
Royal College of Nursing (RCN). (2005) *Peri-operative Fasting in Adults and Children.* London: RCN.

World Health Organization (WHO). (2009) Patient safety: tools and resources. www.who.int/patientsafety/safesurgery/tools_resources/ (accessed 24 February 2014).

75 Postoperative care
Moules T, Ramsay J. (2008) *The Textbook of Children's and Young People's Nursing,* 2nd edition. Oxford: Blackwell Publishing.
Royal College of Nursing (RCN). (2011) *Standards for Assessing, Measuring and Monitoring Vital Signs in Infants, Children and Young People: RCN guidance for children's nurses and nurses working with children and young people.* London: RCN.

76 Pressure area care
European Pressure Ulcer Advisory Panel and National Pressure Ulcer Advisory Panel (2009) *Prevention and Treatment of Pressure Ulcers: Quick Reference Guide.* Washington DC: National Pressure Ulcer Advisory Panel. http://www.npuap.org/wp-content/uploads/2012/02/Final_Quick_Prevention_for_web_2010.pdf (accessed 11 July 2014).
NICE (2014) *Pressure ulcers: prevention and management of pressure ulcers. NICE guideline CG179. London National Institute for Health and Care Excellence.* https://www.nice.org.uk/guidance/CG179 (accessed 11 July 2014).
Wounds UK (2013) *Best Practice Statement: Eliminating Pressure Ulcers.* London: Wounds UK http://www.wounds-uk.com/best-practice-statements/best-practice-statement-eliminating-pressure-ulcers (accessed 11 July 2014).

78 Administering medication
British National Formulary for Children. http://www.bnf.org/bnf/org_450055.htm (accessed 24 February 2014).
Chang YK, Mark B. (2011) Effects of learning climate and registered nurse staffing on medication errors. *Nursing Research* 60: 32–39.
Crawford D. (2012) Maintaining good practice in the administration of medicines to children. *Nursing Children and Young People* 24: 29–35.
Department of Health (2012) Report of the Children and Young People's Health Outcomes Forum. http://www.dh.gov.uk/health/2012/07/cyp-report/ (accessed 24 February 2014).
Medicines for Children. www.medicinesforchildren.org.uk (accessed 24 February 2014).
National Institute for Health and Clinical Excellence (NICE). (2009) Medicines adherence: involving patients in decisions about prescribed medicines and supporting adherence. http://www.nice.org.uk/CG76 (accessed 27 February 2014).
National Patient Safety Agency (NPSA). (2009) Review of patient safety for children and young people. http://www.nrls.npsa.nhs.uk/resources/?entryid45=59864 (accessed 27 February 2014).
Nursing and Midwifery Council (NMC). (2010) Standards for medicines management. http://www.nmc-uk.org/Documents/NMC-Publications/NMC-Standards-for-medicines-management.pdf (accessed 27 February 2014).

79 Drug calculations
Blair K. (2011) *Medicines Management in Children's Nursing.* Exeter: Learning Matters.
Fry MM, Dacey C. (2007) Factors contributing to incidents in medicines administration. *British Journal of Nursing* 16: 676–681.
Hutton M. (2009) Numeracy and drug calculations in practice. *Primary Health Care* 19: 40–45.
Nursing and Midwifery Council (NMC). (2010a) *Essential Skills Clusters (2010) and Guidance for Their Use (guidance G7-1.5b). Annexe 3 Standards for Pre-registration Nursing Education: Final.* London: NMC.
Nursing and Midwifery Council (NMC). (2010b) *Standards for Medicines Management.* London: NMC.
National Patient Safety Agency (NPSA). (2009) *Safety in Doses: Improving the Use of Medicines in the NHS.* London: NPSA.
Nursing Times (2012) How to ensure patient safety in drug dose calculations. *Nursing Times* 108: 12–13.

Warburton P. (2010) Numeracy and patient safety: the need for regular staff assessment. *Nursing Standard* 24: 42–44.

Wright K. (2009) Resources to help solve drug calculation problems. *British Journal of Nursing* 18: 878–883.

81 The feverish child

Glasper A, Aylott M, Battrick C. (2010) *Developing Practical Skills for Nursing Children and Young People*. Hodder Arnold.

McCance K, Heuter S. (2010) *Pathophysiology: The Biological Basis for Disease in Adults and Children*, 6th edition. Elsevier.

National Institute for Health and Clinical Excellence (NICE). (2007) *Feverish Illness in Children*. NICE Guideline 47.

Pocock G, Richards CD. (2004) *Human Physiology: The Basis of Medicine*, 2nd edition. Oxford University Press.

82 Infectious childhood diseases

National Institute for Health and Clinical Excellence (NICE). (2013) Feverish Illness in children: assessment and initial management in children younger than 5 years. http://www.nice.org.uk/nicemedia/live/14171/63908/63908.pdf (accessed 24 February 2014).

84 Prevention of infection

Department of Health (DoH). (2010) *The Health and Social Care Act 2008. Code of practice on the prevention and control of infections.* London: DoH.

Foster CB, Sabella C. (2011) Health care-associated infections in children. *Journal of the American Medical Association* 305: 1480–1481.

National Institute for Health and Clinical Excellence (NICE). (2011) *Prevention and Control of Healthcare-Associated Infections: Quality Improvement Guide*. London: NICE.

Thousand Lives Plus (2012) Reducing healthcare associated infections. www.1000livesplus.wales.nhs.uk (accessed 27 February 2014).

85 Hyponatraemia and its prevention

Playfor S. (2013) Reducing the risk of hyponatraemia when administering intravenous fluids to children. www.bmj.com (accessed 24 February 2014).

86 Thermal injuries

Betts M, Pomeroy S. (2010) Caring for children suffering from burn injuries. In Glasper A, Aylott M, Battrick C. (eds). *Developing Practical Skills for Nursing Children and Young People*. London: Hodder Arnold.

Devitt P, Thain J. (2011) *Children and Young People's Nursing Made Incredibly Easy*. London: Wolters Kluwer/Lippincott Williams & Wilkins: pp. 544–551.

www.clicknow.org.uk

www.rospa.com

87 Childhood fractures

Dandy D, Edwards D. (2009) *Essential Orthopaedics and Trauma*. Edinburgh: Churchill Livingstone.

Hamblen D, Simpson A. (2007) *Adams's Outline of Fractures*, 12th edition. Edinburgh: Churchill Livingstone.

Royal College of Nursing (RCN). (2010) *Guidance on Pin Site Care*. London: RCN.

88 Plaster care

Miles S, Burden J, Prior M, Johnson C. (2000) *A Practical Guide to Casting*, 2nd edition. Hull: BSN Medical Ltd.

90 Neurovascular observations

Dykes PC. (1993) Minding the five P's of neurovascular assessment. *American Journal of Nursing* 6: 38–39.

Ferlic PW, Singer G, Kraus T, Eberl R. (2012) The acute compartment syndrome following fractures of the lower leg in children. *Injury* 43: 1743–1746.

Great Ormond Street Hospital (GOSH). (2011) Neurovascular observations: methods. http://www.gosh.nhs.uk/health-professionals/clinical-guidelines/neurovascular-observations-method/ (accessed 01 July 2014).

Nursing and Midwifery Council (NMC) (2008) *The NMC Code: standards for performance, conduct and ethic of professional conduct.* London, NMC.

Royal College of Nursing (RCN). (2009). The recognition and assessment of acute pain in children. www.rcn.org.uk/development/learning/learningzone/clinical_skills/pain_in_children (accessed 01 July 2014).

Wright E. (2009) Neurovascular impairment and compartment syndrome. *Paediatric Nursing* 21: 26–29.

91 Neurological problems

Forsyth R, Newton R. (2007) *Paediatric Neurology: Oxford Specialist Handbooks in Paediatrics*. Oxford, New York: Oxford University Press: p. 274.

Fullerton H, Chetkovich D, Wu Y, Smith W, Johnston S. (2002) Deaths from stroke in US children, 1979 to 1998. *Neurology* 59: 34–39.

Ganesan V, Prengler M, McShane M, Wade A, Kirkham F. (2003) Investigation of risk factors in children with arterial ischemic stroke. *Annals of Neurology* 53: 167–173.

World Health Organization (WHO). (2001) International Classification of Functioning, Disability and Health (ICF). Geneva: WHO.

92 Brain injury and coma

National Institute for Health and Clinical Excellence (NICE). (2007) Triage, assessment, investigation and early management of head injury in infants, children and adults. http://www.nice.org.uk/cg56 (accessed 24 February 2014).

Ragheb J. (2008). Accidental head injuries. In Albright A, Pollack I, Adelson P (eds). *Principles and Practices of Pediatric Neurosurgery*, 2nd edition. New York; Stuttgart: Thieme, pp: 803–808.

Sharples PM. (1998) Head injury in children. In Ward Platt MP, Little RA. (eds). *Injury in the Young*. Cambridge: Cambridge University Press, pp. 151–175.

93 Seizures

Epilepsy Action (2013) Advice and information. https://www.epilepsy.org.uk/info/children/childreith-epilepsy (accessed 27 February 2014).

Great Ormond Street Hospital. (2014) Neurology information for health professionals. http://www.gosh.nhs.uk/health-professionals/clinical-specialties/neurology-information-for-health-professionals/ (accessed 24 February 2014).

National Institute for Health and Clinical Excellence (NICE). (2012) The epilepsies: the diagnosis and management of epilepsies in adults and children in primary and secondary care. Clinical guideline CG137. http://guidance.nice.org.uk/CG137/NICEGuidance/pdf/English (accessed 25 February 2014).

94 Meningitis

National Institute for Health and Clinical Excellence (NICE). (2010) Bacterial meningitis and meningococcal septicaemia: Management of bacterial meningitis and meningococcal septicaemia in children and young people younger than 16 years in primary and secondary care. http://publications.nice.org.uk/bacterial-meningitis-and-meningococcal-septicaemia-cg102/guidance (accessed 3 March 2014).

95 Septicaemia

Brierly J, Carcillo JA, Choong K, et al. (2009) Clinical practice parameters for hemodynamic support of pediatric and neonatal septic shock: 2007 update from American College of Critical Care Medicine. *Critical Care Medicine* 37: 666–688.

97 Asthma

British Thoracic Society Guidelines (2008) revised (2012) & Scottish Intercollegiate Guidelines (2008) revised (2012) Guidelines Network. British Guideline on the Management of Asthma: A National Clinical Guidelines. http://www.sign.ac.uk/pdf/sign101.pdf (accessed 01 July 2014).

Asthma UK. http://www.asthma.org.uk/ (accessed 01 July 2014).

100 Inflammatory bowel disease

Beattie RM. (2010) Symposium 6: Young people, artificial nutrition and transitional care. Nutrition, growth and puberty In children and adolescents with Crohn's Disease. *Proceedings of the Nutrition Society* 69: 174–177.

Crohn's and Colitis UK (2011) *lBD in Children: a Parents' Guide*. Hertfordshire: Crohn's and Colitis UK.

IBD Working Group of British Society of Paediatric Gastroenterology and Nutrition (BSPGHAN). (2008) *Guidelines for the Management of IBD in Children in the United Kingdom*. London: BSPGHAN.

Mamula P, Markowitz J, Baldassano R. (2003) Inflammatory bowel disease in early childhood and adolescence: spectal considerations. *Gastroenterology Clinics of North America* 32: 967–995.

101 Gastro-oesophageal reflux

Martin J, Pratt N, Kennedy JD, et al. (2002) Natural history and familial relationships of infant spilling to 9 years of age. *Pediatrics* 109: 1061–1067.

National Institute for Health and Clinical Excellence (NICE). (2014) GORD in children. NICE Clinical Knowledge Summaries. http://cks.nice.org.uk/gord-in-children (accessed 24 February 2014).

Vandenplas Y, Rudolph CD, Di Lorenzo C, et al. (2009) Pediatric Gastroesophageal Reflux Clinical Practice Guidelines: Joint Recommendations of the North American Society for Pediatric Gastroenterology, Hepatology, and Nutrition (NASPGHAN) and the European Society for Pediatric Gastroenterology, Hepatology, and Nutrition (ESPGHAN). *Journal of Pediatric Gastroenterology and Nutrition* 49: 498–547.

102 Coeliac disease

Husby S, Koletzko S, Korponay-Szabo IR, et al., for the ESPGHAN Working Group on Coeliac Disease Diagnosis, on behalf of the ESPGHAN Gastroenterology Committee. (2012) European Society for Pediatric Gastroenterology, Hepatology, and Nutrition (ESPGHAN) Guidelines for the Diagnosis of Coeliac Disease. *Journal of Pediatric Gastroenterology and Nutrition* 54: 136–159.

National Institute for Health and Clinical Excellence (NICE). (2009) Coeliac disease: Recognition and assessment of celiac disease. Nice Clinical Guideline 86. http://www.nice.org.uk/cg86 (accessed 24 February 2014).

What is coeliac disease? http://www.coeliac.org.uk/ (accessed 24 February 2014).

103 Appendicitis

Royal College of Nursing (RCN). (2005) *Perioperative Fasting in Adults and Children*. London: RCN.

104 Constipation

Beattie RM, Dhawan A, Puntis JWL. (2009) *Paediatric Gastroenterology, Hepatology, and Nutrition*. Oxford: Oxford University Press.

Benninga MA, Voskuijl WP, Taminiau JA. (2004) Childhood constipation: is there new light in the tunnel? *Journal of Pediatric Gastroenterology and Nutrition* 39: 448–464.

Borowitz SM, Cox DJ, Tam A, et al. (2003) Precipitants of constipation during early childhood. *Journal of the American Board of Family Practice* 16: 213–218.

British Medical Association and Royal Pharmaceutical Society of Great Britain (2009) *British National Formulary for Children*. London: BMJ Group, RPS Publishing, RCPCH Publications.

Di Lorenzo C. (2000) Childhood constipation: finally some hard data about hard stools! *Journal of Pediatrics* 136: 4–7.

Leung AK, Chan PY, Cho HY. (1996) Constipation in children. *American Family Physician* 54: 611–618, 627.

Loening-Baucke V. (1994) Management of chronic constipation in infants and toddlers. *American Family Physician* 49: 397–400, 403–6, 411–3.

Loening-Baucke V. (1996) Encopresis and soiling. *Pediatric Clinics of North America* 43: 279–298.

Murphy SM, Clayden GS. (1996) Constipation. In Walker WA (ed). *Pediatric Gastrointestinal Disease: Pathophysiology, Diagnosis, Management*. St Louis: Mosby, pp. 293–321.

National Institute for Health and Clinical Excellence (NICE). (2010) *Constipation in children and young people*. NICE clinical guideline 99.

Partin JC, Hamill SK, Fischel JE, Partin JS. (1992) Painful defecation and faecal soiling in children. *Pediatrics* 89: 1007–1009.

Squires RH, Doerck M. (1993) Constipation. In Eichenwald HF, Buchanan W, Stroder J (eds). *Pediatric Therapy*. St Louis: Mosby Year Book, pp. 127–131.

105 Renal problems

Glasper A, Richardson J. (2011) *A Textbook of Children's and Young People's Nursing*, 2nd edition. Edinburgh: Elsevier.

Glasper A, McEwing G, Richardson J. (2012) *Emergencies in Children's and Young People's Nursing*. Oxford: Oxford University Press.

Kelsey J, McEwing G. (2008) *Clinical Skills in Child Health Practice*. Edinburgh: Elsevier.

National Institute for Health and Clinical Excellence (NICE). (2007) *Urinary Tract Infection in Children*. Clinical Guideline 54. London: NICE.

107 Musculoskeletal problems

Bessette A, Rousseau C. (eds). (2012) *Scoliosis: Causes, Symptoms and Treatment*. New York: Nova Science.

Clarke S, Dowling M. (2003) Spica cast guidelines for parents and health professionals. *Journal of Orthopaedic Nursing* 7: 184–191.

Linehan K, O'Sullivan M. (2011) The non-surgical management of congenital talipes equino varus (CTEV) in the first year of life: an Irish perspective. *International Journal of Orthopaedic and Trauma Nursing* 15: 71–75.

109 Skin conditions

British Dermatological Nursing Group. http://www.bdng.org.uk (accessed 24 February 2014).

NZ DermNet. www.dermnetnz.org (accessed 24 February 2014).

Office for National Statistics (2001) KS02 Age structure: Census 2001, Key Statistics for Local Authorities. http://www.ons.gov.uk/ons/publications/re-reference-tables.html?edition=tcm%3A77-211026 (accessed 3 March 2014).

Schofield, J, Grindlay, D, Williams, H (2009). Skin Conditions in the UK. A Health Care Needs Assessment. Centre of Evidence Based Dermatology, University of Nottingham. http://www.nottingham.ac.uk/research/groups/cebd/documents/hcnaskinconditionsuk2009.pdf

111 Living with chronic illness

Eiser C. (1997) Effects of chronic illness on children and their families. *Advances in Psychiatric Treatment* 3: 204–210.

Lazarus RS, Folkman S. (1984) *Stress, Appraisal and Coping*. New York, Springer.

113 Juvenile idiopathic arthritis

Arthritis Research UK. (2014) http://www.arthritisresearchuk.org/arthritis-information.aspx (accessed 6 March 2014).

Great Ormond Street Hospital for Sick Children (GOSH). (2014) Medical conditions. http://www.gosh.nhs.uk/medical-conditions (accessed 24 February 2014).

Royal College of Nursing (RCN). (2009) *Assessing, Managing and Monitoring Biologic Therapies for Inflammatory Arthritis: Guidance for Rheumatology Practitioners*. London: RCN.

114 Epilepsy

National Epilepsy Society (2011). www.epilepsysociety.org.uk (accessed 24 February 2014).

122 Self-harm in childhood

Cooper J, Kapur N, Webb R, et al. (2005) Suicide after deliberate self-harm: a 4 year cohort study. *American Journal of Psychiatry* 162: 297–303.

Evans J, Evans M, Morgan HG, Hayward A, Gunnell D. (2005) Crisis card following self-harm: 12 month follow-up of a randomised controlled trial. *British Journal of Psychiatry* 187: 186–187.

Favazza A. (1998) The coming of age of self mutilation. *Journal of Nervous and Mental Disease* 186: 259–268.

Madge N, Hewitt A, Hawton K, et al. (2008) Deliberate self harm within an international community sample of young people: comparative findings from the Child and Adolescent Self Harm in Europe (CASE) Study. *Journal of Child Psychology and Psychiatry* 49: 667–677.

Mangnall J, Yurkovich E. (2008) A literature review of deliberate self-harm. *Perspectives in Psychiatric Care* 44: 175–184.

National Institute for Clinical Excellence (NICE). (2004) Clinical Guideline 16. *Self-harm: The Short-term Physical and Psychological Management and Secondary Prevention of Self-harm in Primary and Secondary Care.* London: NICE.

National Suicide Research Foundation (NSRF). (2011) *National Registry for Deliberate Self Harm. Annual Report.* Cork: NSRF.

NHS Centre for Reviews and Dissemination (2000) *Deliberate Self Harm.* University of York: NHS Centre for Reviews and Dissemination.

Platt S, Bille-Brahe U, Kerkhoff J, et al. (1992) Parasuicide in Europe: the WHO/EURO multicentre study on parasuicide: 1. Introduction and preliminary analysis for 1989. *Acta Psychiatrica Scandinavia* 85: 97–104.

126 Positive behavioural support

Emerson E, Barrett S, Bell S, et al. (1987) *Developing Services for People with Severe Learning Disabilities and Challenging Behaviours.* Kent: Canterbury Institute Of Social and Applied Psychology.

127 Atrioventricular septal defect in children with learning disability

Down's Heart Group (DHG). (2014) http://www.dhg.org.uk/resources .aspx (accessed 24 February 2014).

128 Genetic conditions: Down's syndrome

Aiten DC. (2002) Prenatal screening for neural tube defects and aneuploidy. In Rimoin DL, Connor JM, Pyeritz RE, Korf BR (Eds). *Emery and Rimoin's Principles and Practices of Medical Genetics*, 4th edition. New York: Churchill Livingstone, pp. 763–801.

Leshin L. (2000) Mosaic Down syndrome. http://www.ds-health.com/ mosaic.htm (accessed 24 February 2014).

Marder E, Dennis A. (2001) Medical management of children with Down's syndrome. *Current Paediatrics* 11: 57–58.

Nehring W. (2010) Down syndrome child with a chronic condition. In Allen PV (ed.) *Down Syndrome Child with a Chronic Condition*, 5th edition. St Louis: Mosby, pp. 447–469.

Selikowitz M. (ed.) (2008) *Down Syndrome*, 3rd edition. Sydney, Australia: Oxford University Press, pp. 25–33.

Tolmie JL. (2002) Down syndrome and other autosomal trisomies. In *Emery and Rimion's Principles and Practices of Medical Genetics*, 4th edition. New York: Churchill Livingstone, pp. 1129–1183.

Index

NOTE: The sorting ignores spaces so that, for example, 'headache' comes before 'head boxes'.
Page numbers in *italic* refer to figures.